D0764539

Good for You!

Books Published by the American Cancer Society

A Breast Cancer Journey: Your Personal Guidebook

American Cancer Society's Complementary and Alternative Cancer Methods Handbook

American Cancer Society's Guide to Complementary and Alternative Cancer Methods

American Cancer Society's Guide to Pain Control

Cancer in the Family: Helping Children Cope with a Parent's Illness, Heiney et al.

Caregiving: A Step-By-Step Resource for Caring for the Person with Cancer at Home, Houts and Bucher

Colorectal Cancer: A Thorough and Compassionate Resource for Patients and Their Families, Levin

Coming to Terms with Cancer: A Glossary of Cancer-Related Terms, Laughlin

Consumers Guide to Cancer Drugs, Wilkes et al.

Crossing Divides: A Couple's Story of Cancer, Hope, and Hiking Montana's Continental Divide, Bischke

Informed Decisions, The Complete Book of Cancer Diagnosis, Treatment, and Recovery, 2nd Edition, Eyre et al.

Our Mom Has Cancer, Ackermann and Ackermann

Prostate Cancer: What Every Man—and His Family—Needs to Know, Revised Edition, Bostwick et al.

Women and Cancer: A Thorough and Compassionate Resource for Patients and Their Families, Runowicz et al.

Also by the American Cancer Society

American Cancer Society's Healthy Eating Cookbook: A Celebration of Food, Friends, and Healthy Living, 2nd Edition

Celebrate! Healthy Entertaining for Any Occasion

Kids' First Cookbook: Delicious-Nutritious Treats to Make Yourself

Good for You!

Reducing Your Risk of Developing Cancer

Published by
American Cancer Society
Health Content Products
1599 Clifton Road NE
Atlanta, Georgia 30329, USA

Printed in the United States of America
Designed by Jill Dible
Cover designed by Jill Dible

5 4 3 2 1   02 03 04 05 06

Library of Congress Cataloging-in-Publication Data

Good for you! : reducing your risk of developing cancer.
        p. cm.
Includes index.
   ISBN 0-944235-38-7 (pbk. : alk. paper)
   1. Cancer--Prevention. I. American Cancer Society.
   RC268 .G663 2002
   616.99'4052--dc21

                              2001008075

A NOTE TO THE READER
The information contained in this book is not intended as medical advice and should not be relied upon as a substitute for consulting with your physician. This information may not address all possible actions, precautions, side effects, or interactions. All matters regarding your health require the supervision of a physician who is familiar with your medical needs. For more information, contact your American Cancer Society at 1-800-ACS-2345 (www.cancer.org).

Good for You!

Reducing Your Risk of Developing Cancer

Managing Editor
Katherine Bruss, Psy.D.

Editor
Anneke Smith

Production Editors
Lisa Dunlap
Beverly Greene
Thomas J. Gryczan, M.S.

Contributor
Sandra J. Wendel, Consumer Health Writer

Editorial Review
Terri Ades, R.N., M.S., A.O.C.N.
Rick Alteri, M.D.
Colleen Doyle, M.S., R.D.
Ted Gansler, M.D., M.B.A.
Marji McCullough, Sc.D., R.D.
Mary O'Connell
Robert Smith, Ph.D.
Michael Thun, M.D.
Ron Todd, M.S., Ed.D.

Editorial and New Media Director
Chuck Westbrook

Director, Publishing Strategy
Diane Scott-Lichter

Book Publishing Manager
Candace Magee

CONTENTS

Foreword

Cancer is one of the most feared words among the American population. The impression most people have, despite advances in treatment, is pain, suffering, and an untimely death. What this book demonstrates is that you can take charge of your lifestyle and your health. You are clearly in the driver's seat when it comes to your own health. You're in charge, and you can definitely decrease your risk for cancer.

I have had more than 50,000 patient encounters over the course of my career as a cancer doctor. If I could have talked with my patients years before they came into my exam room at the Mayo Clinic, this is what I would have shared with them: well over half of all cancers are related to lifestyle issues—smoking, alcohol, lack of exercise, too much sun exposure, and an unhealthy diet. If detected early, many cancers can be effectively treated. So we can be proactive and shift the odds in our favor to minimize our risks for cancer. How? By being attentive to how we live and making some changes in our lifestyle and finding cancer early.

Cancer is not a genetically "done deal." In other words, if you have a strong family history of cancer, you are not destined to develop cancer and succumb to this disease. Nor is cancer a case of roulette, a random selection of cards, or a roll of the dice. By ignoring our choices, we can put ourselves behind the 8-ball, deal ourselves a lousy hand, or give ourselves an unplayable lie; however, with smart choices, we can position ourselves so that our lives can be productive, creative, and meaningful. We each can indeed make the world a little better than it is right now. But we have to be here to do that.

The choice is always yours. The information is available, right here, to help guide you in appropriate directions. I urge you to use this book as a practical, user-friendly, and "hands on" guide, compass, and lighthouse to help you navigate through the stormy waters of understanding your cancer risk.

I cannot emphasize enough the importance of early detection and screening. For the vast majority of cancer types, the earlier they are detected, the greater the probability of cure.

With the bewildering variety of information available through print and the Internet, it is very difficult for the informed consumer to know where to turn. This book presents some easy-to-understand recommendations so that you can clearly position yourself to make responsible and credible choices. Please join us on this journey. The road to good health starts with your first step. Simply turn the page (literally and symbolically).

I am humbled and honored to have been asked by the American Cancer Society to write the foreword for this must-read book.

EDWARD T. CREAGAN, M.D.
Professor, Mayo Clinic Medical School
American Cancer Society Professor of Clinical Oncology
John and Roma Rouse Professor of Humanism in Medicine
Associate Medical Editor, MayoClinic.com

Introduction

Be aware of wonder. Live a balanced life — learn some and think some and draw and paint and sing and dance and play and work every day some.
— ROBERT FULGHUM

How would you answer this question?

Thinking of all types of health problems, what do you feel is the single most important health problem that you could personally face in the future?

If you were like most Americans polled by the American Cancer Society (ACS), you would likely respond, "Cancer." Heart disease was the second response and only serious contender. Other than cancer and heart disease, what health issues should we worry about? Just a handful of people named diabetes, high blood pressure, AIDS, or obesity as their health problems of greatest concern.

Clearly, as the survey showed, Americans are concerned about cancer. Yet, in reality, more people die of heart disease.

The Disease Americans Fear Most . . .
and Why You Don't Need to Be Afraid

Cancer is the number one day-to-day health concern in America, even though heart disease is the number one killer. According to a nationwide poll, conducted by the ACS and the Discovery Health Channel, most Americans really don't understand cancer—its causes and risk factors. And most of us are woefully unaware of what we can do to lower our risks for developing cancer.

So buckle up your safety belt. We're going to set the record straight! The reality about cancer might come as a surprise to you. In the poll, most people surveyed did not know these cancer facts.

- Age is the single most important risk factor for developing cancer—not family history, as most people surveyed incorrectly believed. Inherited risk factors account for less than 15 percent of all cancers.

- More than two-thirds of cancer deaths are related to lifestyle and other controllable risk factors—one third of them are related to diet alone.

- Lung cancer, for example, is a common and deadly form of cancer, but many people surveyed thought that pollution is as much a cause for lung cancer as smoking. It is not.

- Men are at a higher lifetime risk of developing cancer in general than women.

- African Americans are more likely to develop cancer than people from any other racial or ethnic group.

- Alcohol use increases risk of developing several forms of cancer.

- Cervical cancer is most often caused by sexually transmitted viruses, which are largely preventable and certainly treatable when detected early.

- Nearly half of all women believe the breast self-exam is the best method to detect cancer of the breast, when, in fact, the ACS recommends a combination of mammography, breast exam by a professional, plus the self-exam as the best way to detect it early.

- Women underestimate the importance of age in the development of breast cancer. Many think that if they have no family history and reach their mid-forties or older, they're relatively home free, when, in fact, their risk increases.

- Younger men are at the greatest risk of developing testicular cancer, while men over age forty are at much lower risk, although most think the opposite is true.

- Men also underestimate the importance of age over family history in assessing cancer risk, and they do not know that more than two-thirds of all fatal cancers are related to lifestyle choices.

The take-home message is that cancer risk is controllable and you can do a lot of things every day to reduce your risk. The other startling news from the poll is that many of us know *what* to do to reduce our risk of cancer but are not taking action to lower our risks.

If the pollsters called you today, what steps would you say you are taking to reduce your risk of getting cancer? Here are some steps that people surveyed were asked to report on.

- Do you work with your doctor to make sure you have early detection tests and cancer screenings?

- Do you watch your weight and try to maintain a healthy weight?

- If you smoke or use other tobacco products, what steps have you taken to reduce your use or quit smoking entirely?

- Are you eating more fruits and vegetables (at least five servings a day)?

- What are you doing to protect your skin from the sun?

- Have you reduced the fat in your diet (such as limiting high-fat foods, eating leaner meat, adding several servings of grain each day)?

- Do you watch how much you drink?

- Are you living a more active lifestyle (and reducing stress in your life)?

Of those surveyed, 14 percent said they have taken no action at all to reduce their cancer risk. More than one-fourth of the people surveyed had not undertaken early detection or screening tests for cancer. That's perhaps because we don't know how often we need to be screened. The ACS recommends a cancer-related checkup every three years for anyone between twenty and thirty-nine years of age and then every year after that, as well as additional early detection tests at intervals that vary according to your age (see Chapter 9).

Take the First Step

Take the first step in faith.
You don't have to see the whole staircase,
just take the first step.
—MARTIN LUTHER KING, JR.

Happily, you have the answers to all these questions in your hands right now. The information in this book can help you understand your risks. Knowledge is powerful medicine when it comes to understanding lifestyle choices, reducing your cancer risk, and finding cancer early, when it can be treated most successfully.

Lifestyle change begins with you. Your first action step to live a healthful, cancer-free life is to allow yourself to take charge of your health. Form a partnership with your doctor because, believe it or not, your doctor can become your teacher, not just someone to see when you have a sore throat. Your doctor can teach you about how early detection and screening are important for you, as well as how your lifestyle choices affect your health. Chapter 1 will help you choose the right doctor and explain how to talk so your doctor will listen. An ounce of prevention really is worth a pound of cure. You can identify and control your risk factors, with the help of your health care team.

What you put on your plate is your decision. What you eat or don't eat can make a difference in your cancer risk. The foods you choose can lower your cancer risk—or make it greater. In Chapter 2 we discuss why calories do count, why not all fats are bad fats, the good foods that may play a protective role against cancer, and how you can develop your game plan for successful eating.

Together, diet and exercise are a powerful one-two punch to reduce excess weight (a cancer risk factor) and keep it off. If you really want to guarantee success with healthful eating, you must get yourself moving. And we're not talking about sweat-busting, heavy breathing, heart-pounding exercise. We're talking about the type of moderate physical activity the Office of the Surgeon General recommends that you do for at least thirty minutes nearly every day. You really can fit fitness into your busy day—no excuses. Take our Fit Test and determine which activity is right for you. In Chapter 3, we'll show you what physical activity can do for you and how being active can reduce your risk of cancer. After all, adults need recess too.

It's no secret—cover up. While you're outside enjoying the great outdoors on your new walking program, you'll need to protect yourself from the sun's harmful rays. A little ultraviolet light goes a long way—into your skin to cause the most common type of cancer: skin cancer. It's largely preventable with the right clothing, sunscreen, and the intelligence to use them. Chapter 4 describes how sun sense makes sense. Compare your skin type and find out if you're among the groups most at risk for various types of skin cancer and how you can recognize whether that wayward mole or funny-looking freckle might be a skin cancer.

If you don't smoke, that's great. But you may not want to skip Chapter 5. You may want to know how much you are at risk for illness (such as headaches, nausea, or lung cancer) even if you are not a smoker. The truth about tobacco and secondhand smoke may surprise you. If you are a smoker, you'll learn why it is so hard to quit. We'll explain the strategies for quitting and discuss ways to quit for good.

Viruses can cause more than the common cold. Not only do infections cause colds, but certain viruses and bacteria can also trigger some types of cancer. Some infections that can lead to cancer, such as HIV (the virus that causes AIDS), are transmitted through sexual contact. But other infections, such as *Helicobacter pylori* (the bacterium thought to be a risk factor for stomach cancer), are not transmitted through sexual contact. Chapter 6 explains the relationship between infections and cancer and what you can do to protect yourself.

Stress less so you can make better lifestyle choices. These days, everyone is stressed to some degree. When stressed, we make unhealthy lifestyle choices, such as drinking more alcohol, exercising less, smoking more, or eating poorly. This is where learning how to manage stress comes into play. You can learn how to recognize stress early and deal with it in healthy ways so you can make better lifestyle choices. Chapter 7 helps you learn how to manage your stress.

The world within you—and around you—can make or break your cancer risk. As we've discussed, lifestyle choices determine some cancer risks. But other aspects of your environment have a role to play as well. Chapter 8 looks at the world around you and where those hazards to your health may be. We can't live our lives in a bubble, so it's best to know where the risks are (or aren't) in our food and drinking water, in our homes, in our workplace, in our gardens, and even at the doctor's office. Once we know which exposures increase our risk of cancer, we can learn to take steps to avoid them.

What's your action plan? Screening and early detection of cancer (and any disease) are the most important life-saving gifts you can give yourself and your family. But knowing when to have which tests is still not routine for most people. The worksheets in Chapter 9 can help. Talk with your doctor to decide when *you* should have certain screening tests.

Risk, Reason, and Reality

The signs and symptoms of some forms of cancer were described as far back in history as 3000 B.C. The physicians of Ancient Egypt treated their patients for several forms of cancer by prescribing pills and pigs' ears. Some early writings describe surgery for cancer.

With the abundance of information that is reported about new cancer studies, one of challenges to the public is to sort through and understand what cancer really is and what it is not. This book explains the many faces of cancer, the reality behind what causes it, and what you can do to prevent it.

Cancer is not inevitable based on your family history. If your mother developed lung cancer or your father has skin cancer, you are not destined to follow that pattern. When it comes to cancer risk, Americans severely underestimate other, more powerful, risk factors. They overlook the critical importance of age, ethnicity, lifestyle, alcohol use, and diet in determining cancer risk. Our environment plays a role, but a smaller one than most people think.

The genes you inherit are certainly important in setting the stage for cancer, but how important? What you eat and drink, how physically active you are, where you live and work, how much time you spend in the sun, your age, and your gender are all things that determine if you develop cancer, which type, or whether you develop cancer at all.

The ACS recognizes that cancer is a group of complex diseases and no *one* cause is responsible. We also recognize that many factors influence whether a person has cancer or not. Some of these factors cannot be changed. For example, we cannot change our age and we know that cancer is more common as we get older. But, there are things that we do, that is, our lifestyle, which can influence whether we develop cancer.

Although we recognize that no lifestyle change can guarantee full protection against any disease, we believe that taking the steps outlined earlier (pages 4–7) offer the best information currently available to help Americans reduce their risk of cancer. The sooner you start, the longer you will benefit. You'll immediately begin to be healthier and reduce your cancer risk.

To help you understand the task at hand, it is essential to understand what we're up against. Let's look at what cancer is and how it develops to gain a better understanding of what we're actually preventing.

What Is Cancer?

Normal cells grow, divide, and die in an orderly fashion. During the early years of life, normal cells divide more rapidly until a person becomes an adult. After that, cells in most parts of the body divide only to replace worn-out or dying cells and to repair injuries.

Cancer occurs when cells in some part of the body begin to grow out of control. Although there are many kinds of cancer, they all come about because of uncontrolled growth of abnormal cells. Cancer cells develop because of damage to DNA, the substance in every cell that directs all its activities. We inherit our DNA from our parents and, unfortunately for some, we can inherit mistakes in our DNA that can make us more likely to develop cancer. More often, though, a cell's DNA becomes damaged from exposure to something in the environment, like cigarette smoke.

In many cases, scientists and doctors still do not understand *why* a cell's DNA becomes damaged. Most of the time when DNA is altered, the body is able to repair it. In cancer cells, such damaged DNA has not been repaired.

Cancer cells differ from normal cells in that they continuously grow and divide, even when they shouldn't. They outlive normal cells and continue to produce new cancer cells. This disruptive cell growth can affect the organ where it is taking place, preventing it from performing its vital functions. This can lead to serious disability, or even death.

Most types of cancer form a lump, called a tumor. Some cancers, such as leukemia, do not form tumors. Instead, these cancer cells involve the blood and blood-forming organs (these include bone marrow, the lymphatic system, and the spleen) and circulate through other tissues where they accumulate.

Often, cancer cells travel to other parts of the body where they begin to grow and replace normal tissue. This process, called metastasis, occurs as the cancer cells accumulate and get into the bloodstream or lymph channels of the body. It is important to remember that when cells from a cancer, such as breast cancer, spread to another organ such as the liver, the cancer cells in the liver are still "breast cancer" cells, not liver cancer.

Not all tumors are cancerous (or malignant). Benign (noncancerous) tumors do not metastasize, but they can be life-threatening if they grow in a vital area.

Different types of cancer can behave differently. Lung cancer and breast cancer, for example, are very different diseases. They grow at different rates, respond to different drugs, and often spread to different parts of the body. That is why people with different types of cancer need treatment that is aimed at their particular type of cancer.

Cancer is not like the flu or a cold. You cannot "catch" the disease from someone else. Nor will you get cancer by being around or by touching someone with cancer (see Chapter 6.)

How Do We Know?

This book offers a lot of advice about reducing your risk of developing cancer and finding cancer early, when it is most likely to be curable. Some of this advice may contradict information from other sources. Some may seem contrary to what you would expect. It's natural for you to wonder how scientists and doctors decide what causes cancer, how to best prevent cancer, and how to find the disease as early as possible.

The answer to these questions is "science." There are scientific methods for answering these questions. By looking at evidence from a number of different types of scientific studies, researchers are able to put together pieces of this very complex puzzle.

But even within the realm of science, sometimes there are differences between what we know and what we think we know. Scientists develop theories, logically based on the available facts, to explain how or why something happens. For example, based on the ability of antioxidants (such as vitamins A, C, and E) to protect our DNA from damage, it makes sense that they may play some role in reducing one's risk of cancer. So should we all start taking antioxidant supplements?

Just because a theory makes sense doesn't mean that it's necessarily true. Scientific studies must be done to prove a theory is correct before we start drawing conclusions and making recommendations. In the case of antioxidant supplements, we still don't have any solid proof that they reduce cancer risk. In some cases, they might even increase your risk of cancer or other health problems (see Chapter 2).

There is an important difference between scientific studies and personal testimonials, also known as anecdotal reports. Just because someone ate a pickle every day for forty years and didn't develop cancer does not mean that pickles prevent cancer; or just because someone who used an antiperspirant later developed breast cancer doesn't mean the two are related. Testimonials can sound very convincing, even moving. But scientifically they are meaningless, unless combined with solid evidence.

Scientific studies are designed to try to weed out all the other possible factors that could come into play, so that we are left with a clearer understanding of the relationship between the particular factor we are studying and cancer.

Results from individual studies can, and sometimes do, contradict previous results. When conflicting results are reported in the media, it may seem as though little or no progress is being made at times. But the fact is that science is always moving forward, even if slowly.

Scientific methods are not perfect, and we're not claiming that we have all the answers. A few may turn out to be wrong after more research is done. In many cases, the honest answer is that we're still not certain, but we can suggest some ideas based on the available evidence. In still other cases, we have no clue and need to be honest when that is the case. But in all cases, our answers should be based on science.

Kinds of Scientific Studies

There are many kinds of scientific studies and many ways to classify them. For example, in the area of cancer prevention (or treatment, for that matter), it's often useful to distinguish laboratory studies from human studies and to distinguish observational studies from interventional studies.

Laboratory Studies

Test Tube Studies. These are the *in vitro* (Latin for "in glass") studies that use bacteria, animal, or human cells grown in laboratory dishes or test tubes. For example, researchers add suspected carcinogens and then examine the DNA of the cells for mutations. Or, they might add vitamins or other nutrients they suspect might protect DNA against cancer-causing mutations. These studies are often the first ones done after a potential cancer-causing (or cancer-preventive) agent is identified because they are easy to do, are relatively inexpensive, and take a short amount of time to complete. But they provide only a limited amount of information because they don't look at whole organisms.

Animal Studies. These are often an important next step after test tube studies. Animals are more complex than cells, and, unlike humans, laboratory animals can be studied in a well-controlled environment. It's much easier to make sure that they eat the same diet, get the same amount of exercise, or even have the same genetic makeup, and then vary the level of exposure to a potential carcinogen. The cause of any differences in cancer rates is then clear-cut. These studies often provide good information, but they are not the last word on the subject. A substance that causes cancer in mice, for example, may or may not cause cancer in humans, and the level of exposure needed to cause cancer may be far above any dose a person would be exposed to.

Human Studies

Epidemiologic studies are scientific investigations of the factors that influence occurrence of diseases in human populations. There are two general categories of epidemiologic studies—observational studies and interventional studies.

Observational Studies. These studies are done in real life, looking at real people. They often provide the first indication that something might cause (or prevent) cancer and are really the only way to determine if an agent causes cancer in humans. Therefore they are the first and last steps in proving an association. They often follow a logical progression.

Ecological studies compare the risk of a disease such as cancer in different populations (groups of people) These studies might tell researchers that the risk of developing lung cancer is higher among Americans studied during the 1980s than among those studied during the 1950s, or that lung cancer is more common in the United States and

Western Europe than in most African countries. But there are so many differences to be looked at (genetics, diet, environmental exposures, and so on) that these studies are generally only useful in creating theories, which can then be tested in other types of studies.

Case-control studies often provide the first indication that a particular substance may be associated with an increased (or decreased) risk of a disease such as cancer. These studies look at people (the "cases") with a certain type of cancer and then compare their histories to those of other people (the "controls") in similar situations who did not develop cancer. If exposure to a particular agent is different between the two groups, an association between the agent and cancer is possible. For example, case-control studies showing that smoking was more common among people hospitalized for lung cancer than among patients in the same hospital for noncancerous problems were among the earliest evidence that eventually led to the conclusion that smoking causes lung cancer.

Cohort studies follow a group of people over a period of time. In most cohort studies, participants answer questions about exposures at the start of the study, before the researchers know who will eventually be diagnosed with diseases such as cancer. As with case-control studies, the cancer risk among people with an exposure (smokers, for example) is compared to the risk of people who are not exposed.

One of the strengths of cohort studies is that information about exposures is more accurate. For example, some cohort studies ask participants to fill out a detailed record of what they eat over a certain period of time. This approach is more accurate than asking people with a particular disease to recall what they usually ate many years ago. The disadvantage of cohort studies is that they take much longer to complete than case-control studies do.

These three types of studies are all *observational*, because they involve analyzing people but not actively changing their risk factors or other exposures. One weakness of any observational study is the possibility that exposures to other agents might be confusing the results. For example, several case-control and cohort studies have found that people who eat a high-fiber diet are less likely to develop colon cancer. But these studies don't tell us whether this statistical link occurs as a direct result of the fiber. In fact, most researchers now believe the reason is that a high-fiber diet usually includes plenty of fruits and vegetables, which contain vitamins and countless other substances, one or more of which are probably responsible for the protective effect of this diet. Researchers can use statistical methods to address these issues, but this is sometimes difficult. This is one reason they often undertake interventional studies.

Interventional Studies. With interventional studies, the researchers intentionally change at least one exposure they believe to be related to risk of a disease.

Randomized controlled clinical trials are intervention trials where people are randomly assigned (like flipping a coin) to one group or another, and some factor is intentionally kept different between the two. They are most often used to study new treatments but can also be used in prevention (studying vitamin supplement use, for example).

Randomized controlled clinical trials are the "gold standard" for proof, but they are often difficult to do because of ethical concerns or cost. For example, it's virtually impossible to do a clinical trial to study the value of breast self-exams to detect breast cancer, because it would be very difficult to find women who would be willing not to do them if they were randomly assigned to that group.

We mentioned that it could be difficult for observational studies to be sure that a particular exposure is truly responsible for a difference in cancer risk, because of its complex relationships to other risk factors. Randomized controlled clinical trials are intended to solve this problem. If a large enough group of people is randomly assigned to the intervention (such as a vitamin supplement, an exercise program, or smoking cessation program) or the control group, all other exposures should "average out" between the two groups. However, even this approach is not perfect or simple. If the intervention is exercise, for example, people in the intervention group may start feeling healthier and become motivated to quit smoking and eat a healthier diet. This makes it more difficult to say which change is responsible for any observed differences in cancer risk.

Studying people in their day-to-day lives (as opposed to a controlled laboratory setting) is complicated, especially when it comes to cancer prevention. There is often a long period of time between exposure and the development of cancer—sometimes decades. By the time a study is finished and a conclusion is reached, many more people may have been exposed to the agent in question. Especially when an association between an agent and a type of cancer is small, it may take huge numbers (tens or even hundreds of thousands) of people to find a link. Needless to say, these studies are often difficult to do and can be very expensive, but these epidemiologic studies are still the best way to guide decisions about your health.

What Do the Headlines Really Mean?

As we mentioned earlier, scientific studies have not convincingly proven that antioxidant supplements can reduce the risk of cancer. But that may not be so obvious if you pay attention to health headlines in news stories or on the Internet.

With the amount of information we have at our fingertips today, it's difficult—if not downright frustrating—to try to sort through it all. We would all love to wake up one morning and hear that someone has finally discovered a magic pill (or food) that prevents cancer.

Unfortunately, media stories can be overenthusiastic at times. Experimental breakthroughs are just that—experimental—and some that receive media attention are still theoretical, or in very preliminary stages, and completely unproven in humans. While they may indeed hold promise, often they are years away from providing benefits to patients. This is because of the amount of testing that is needed—in test tubes, animals, and humans—to ensure that they are what we think they are.

Rarely does a month go by without a new dietary supplement being touted as a prevention or cure for cancer or other serious diseases. Often this is based on a study or studies that found people eating certain foods that contain this substance have lower rates of disease. The fact is that there are

How to Sort Through the Facts and Stats

Of course, there are also people who are simply out to make a profit, without regard for whether or not something might help you. Consider the following the next time you hear or read about something that reduces (or increases) the risk of cancer:

- Realize that no one study is the last word on any subject. Every study has strengths and limitations, and each study should be considered in light of other studies. Health recommendations from organizations such as the ACS are not based solely on one study because each one contributes only a piece to a larger puzzle.

- Use common sense. It is never wise to change your diet, for example, based on a single study or news report, particularly if the data are considered "preliminary."

- Be skeptical about claims of miracle cures, breakthroughs, and healing medicines you read or hear about and any advertised "cures" for cancer on the Internet. Advertising is done for a reason—to get you to buy a product. Unfortunately at the present time there is very thousands of chemicals that make up the foods we eat, and knowing which ones in which combinations are important is very difficult to tease out.

Because each type of scientific study discussed above has its limitations, the results of different kinds of studies need to be looked at in a larger context if we are to get anything truly meaningful out of them. Remember, each one is only a small part of a much larger picture. When we put them all together and the laboratory studies support the human

little regulation concerning what people can and can't claim on a web site, and many people are taking advantage of this (and you).

- Read (or listen to) more than just the headlines. Interpreting scientific studies can be very tricky, and writers who try to condense results into a few catchy words sometimes miss the actual point of the study. While it's not always easy, try to get at what a new study actually does prove. Don't rely on the writer's interpretation.

- Risk factors for cancer are just that—factors that may increase or decrease your risk. It is extremely unlikely that exposure to any one factor will absolutely guarantee that you will (or will not) get cancer.

- Risk factors affect your *relative risk*. But you need to know what your *absolute risk* is before you can decide if it's something you need to worry about. As an example, if you are a man, you might be alarmed to learn that a certain substance increases your risk of breast cancer (yes, men get breast cancer!) by 300 percent, while you might be less worried about something that increases your risk of prostate cancer by only 50 percent. But a man's risk of developing breast cancer in the first place— your *absolute risk*—is so low that tripling it isn't really changing it much at all. On the other hand, your absolute risk of developing prostate cancer is rather high to begin with (about one in six). Increasing this risk is more likely to affect you, even though the number appears smaller.

studies (and vice versa), we can be much more confident about the conclusions we reach, and therefore about the recommendations we make.

Can We Live Forever?

Americans on average are living longer than ever before, and much of this is due to the progress we've made in fighting diseases that account for a majority of deaths in the country. But we can do even more by eating right, exercising regularly, and taking other simple steps to promote good health and prevent serious illness and disease.
—TOMMY G. THOMPSON, Secretary of Health and Human Services

Life expectancy continues to increase as death rates for leading causes of death, including cancer, go down. In 2000, life expectancy was boosted to a record high of 76.9 years old, according to the Centers for Disease Control and Prevention. Death rates are now lower for heart disease and cancer, in particular—the two diseases that account for more than half of all deaths in the United States. Death from cancer has been on the decline since 1990.

While cancer remains the second leading cause of death in the U.S. (behind heart disease), half of all men and a third of all women in the U.S. will develop cancer during their lifetimes. Today, almost 9 million people are living with cancer or have been cured of the disease. Prevention and early detection efforts have contributed significantly to this number. The risk of developing most types of cancer can be reduced if you make changes in your lifestyle, such as quitting smoking or eating a healthier diet. And the sooner cancer is found and treatment begins, the better your chances are for cure.

You *can* take control of your health. No one else will do it for you. Start slowly. Don't try to do everything all at once. Small steps in the right direction add up to big changes in your path to healthy living. And your first step is turning the page.

CHAPTER 1

Take Charge of Your Health

If you're not ready, it's like trying to make a garden
without preparing the soil.
—JAMES O. PROCHASKA, PH.D.

Let's face it: there are some things in life over which you have no control. There's not much you can do about your height, age, or color of your eyes. But sometimes you do indeed have control over what happens to you—probably more often than you think. You can make better lifestyle choices that can help reduce your risk of serious illness. You can choose to be different. You already are, judging by the fact that you've picked up this book.

It's *never* too late to make life-saving changes. In fact, those who've already survived serious illness often say they are in better health now than they were before they became ill. They're getting regular preventive care, eating a healthy diet, and getting information about specific diseases. More are exercising regularly, drinking or smoking less, and controlling their weight.

Disease is not inevitable. If you are like the majority of people, you are not destined to develop breast cancer just because your mother did, or prostate cancer for the simple reason that your Uncle Joe had it. In fact, up to 70 percent of serious diseases can be prevented or delayed if we make healthful lifestyle choices. Most people would bet on those odds.

You don't have to wait for a life-threatening illness to change your life course. You can start on a healthier path right now.

Why? Because only you can take control of your health. No one else has a greater stake in your health than you do. This book will help you make smart lifestyle choices to help you live well and stay well. Consider it your guidebook to helping reduce your risk of cancer and other potentially serious diseases as well. While there is no guarantee that you will never get sick if you follow these guidelines, they can help you stay on track for healthy living.

Change Begins with You

Habits are at first cobwebs then cables.
—Spanish proverb

Have you ever tried to quit smoking, only to pick up a pack six months later during a particularly stressful event? You probably made a bargain with yourself, "I promise I'll quit for good the next time." And what about dieting? How many times have you been down that road? You made drastic changes, lost weight, but felt miserable, deprived, and disappointed. You decided you couldn't eat like that forever, so you ended up putting the pounds back on. Remember the health club membership? A year's worth of dues, paid up front, was supposed to guarantee that you'd drag yourself in there on a regular basis. A week's worth of sore muscles later, and those workout clothes were back in the closet where they continue to collect dust.

Why is change so difficult?

Our intentions are good, but we often try to do too much, too soon. We are used to having things happen quickly, and we think we can make huge changes in our lives in short periods of time. We tend to concentrate on the short term. When we try to do things that require major behavioral changes, such as eating well or becoming (and staying) physically active, we often fall short. In the end, we get very little accomplished and end up more discouraged than we were before we started.

James O. Prochaska, Ph.D., a behavioral scientist and Director of the Cancer Prevention Research Center at the University of Rhode Island, and his colleagues have identified five stages of behavior change, and it all boils down to this: If you're not ready, you can't change your behavior. Simple as that.

The goal is to move yourself forward through the stages of change to a point where you're ready to make a behavior change—for good. Are you ready?

What lifestyle changes are you thinking about making? At which stage are you in your decision making?

For the researcher or behavioral scientist who figures out how to move people from one stage to the next, the Nobel Prize awaits. Just what is it that motivates someone to make a lasting behavior change? No one knows for sure. But if you think about what helped you make a change in the past, you just might hone in on the reason so that you will be able to make more changes in the future.

Listen to your body. Listen to yourself. And when it comes to making changes in your health, seek out the best information available to make the smartest choices you can. Understand that the changes you make could have consequences far beyond simply reducing your risk of cancer. You're reading this book because you seek more information. We don't plan to disappoint you.

Moving Through the Stages of Change

STAGE 1 – Precontemplation: If you're in this stage, you are not even thinking about making a lifestyle change. Your mantra is "no way." You may feel your situation is hopeless ("I can't quit smoking"), or you might deny you need to make a change ("I'm not gaining weight"). To move yourself forward from this stage, a doctor's advice may be just what you need to start thinking about making a change. Or a major life event might jumpstart your thinking, and this could even be a life-threatening illness.

STAGE 2 – Contemplation: You begin to consider making a change when you reach this stage. Maybe you've been thinking, "It's about time I started…" But when? You weigh the pros and cons, and the scales start tipping toward doing something different. You can even imagine yourself making a change—walking or lifting weights, choosing fruit for dessert, managing stress. But be careful. Some people get stuck here waiting for the "magic moment" to smoke that last cigarette or switch to skim milk. And some never move from here. Keep tipping those scales for the better.

You Can Make a Difference

An ounce of prevention is worth a pound of cure.
—HENRY DE BRACTON

A risk factor is anything that increases your chance of developing a disease such as cancer. Different cancers have different risk factors. Smoking, for example, is a risk factor for lung cancer and for cancers of

STAGE 3 – Preparation: OK, you're starting to gear up for the change. You say, "Let's do it." You are planning to take action within a month, and you feel a real commitment to your new behavior change. At this point, you are making your action plan and taking small steps: smoking fewer cigarettes, eating smaller portions, buying comfortable walking shoes, joining a fitness center, reading about healthful food choices.

STAGE 4 – Action: You're there. "Hey, look at me!" You are practicing the behavior change you envisioned. Keep rewarding yourself. Hang in there. It's hard work.

STAGE 5 – Maintenance: Success is yours. "I did it!" you say. Keep up your guard so you're not lured back into old habits during times of stress. Sure, you might crave a cigarette once in a while, but you don't give in. You might stay in bed instead of heading to the gym one morning, but you stick to your overall plan for physical activity. You have incorporated your behavior change into your life, and you wonder why you didn't do this sooner. And you feel great.

the mouth, throat, larynx, bladder, kidney, and several other organs. Smoking increases your risk but does not always cause the disease. In fact, many people who smoke never develop cancer, and others who have never smoked may develop cancer.

Some risk factors, including lifestyle choices such as smoking, being overweight, or getting too much sun, can be modified. Other risk factors such as your age and the genes you inherited from your parents cannot be changed. Risk does not equal "cause."

So what about those risk factors you can change? Some things are in your control. What you eat, what you do and don't do (exercise, smoke), whether you protect yourself from the sun—these risk factors are all within your control. Certain environmental choices are also within your control to a certain extent: where you live, what you do for a living, the water you drink.

And for the things that are not in your control, you can minimize your risk by monitoring yourself closely, with the help of a doctor who is your partner in good health, to prevent, detect, and treat any problems that may come along.

Your best protection is doing what you can to help reduce your risk of cancer.

Prevention and early detection are two of the most important and effective strategies for saving lives from cancer, diminishing suffering due to cancer, and eliminating cancer as a major health problem.

Prevention (sometimes called *primary prevention* by public health professionals) is the reduction of cancer risk by eliminating or reducing contact with factors that cause cancer. For example, a change in lifestyle, such as quitting smoking, reduces the risk of lung and other cancers. Prevention also includes active measures that can help reduce the risk of developing cancer, such as engaging in regular physical activity and eating a healthful diet. This book looks at these vital areas of cancer prevention.

- How what you eat may help to reduce your risk of developing cancer (see Chapter 2).

- How starting with just thirty minutes of moderate physical activity (let's not even call it exercise if that word makes you sweat!) on most days of the week can keep you healthy (see Chapter 3).

- What you can do to protect your skin from damaging sun rays—the cause of over a million cases of skin cancer each year (see Chapter 4).

- How to be successful at quitting smoking, or reduce your risk from others who do (see Chapter 5).

- Surprising information about infections, including some sexually transmitted diseases that can increase your risk for cancer (see Chapter 6).

- How you can control stress before it controls you (see Chapter 7).

- How you can understand the risks in the world around you, and reduce your risk of cancer due to factors you may not even know exist (see Chapter 8).

Early detection (sometimes called *secondary prevention* or *screening*) includes examinations and tests intended to find cancer as early as possible (ideally, before it has spread), when it can be treated most effectively and with the fewest possible side effects. Secondary prevention may also refer to the removal of precancerous growths. This book concludes with detailed worksheets to help you develop your action plan for preventing and detecting cancer (see Chapter 9).

Regular health screening can detect cancers of the breast, colon, rectum, cervix, prostate, testis, mouth and throat, and skin at earlier stages when treatment is more likely to be successful. If all Americans participated in regular cancer screenings, the five-year survival rate for these cancers would increase from 80 percent to 95 percent.

You and Your Doctor: A Partnership for Life — Your Life

There's one more person to listen to as you ponder a healthful future, and that's your doctor. We use that term to mean any number of health care professionals. Like the American Express card, don't leave on your healthful journey without a doctor as your partner in health. Here's why you need a medical partner and how to find the one you like.

You rely on your doctor to provide you with an accurate assessment of your health or a diagnosis of your condition. You depend on your doctor to provide trustworthy information about your health and to maintain an intimate knowledge of your medical history. Similarly, your doctor depends on your description of any medical conditions you may be experiencing. He or she requires feedback from you about how certain medications affect you, how you feel in a given situation, and whether or not your condition changes. That's how this partnership works.

A Little Advice Goes a Long Way

More and more, doctors are becoming involved in prevention. They're not just somebody with a cold stethoscope and a handy prescription pad. They have come to realize their importance as key players in the prevention game—not just treating illnesses but also stopping them before they start. Health insurance providers, too, have realized it's usually less expensive for them to pay for preventive care than it is to foot the bill once someone has developed a serious problem. In the long run, you'll be the one likely to benefit from all of this.

Many people like to have their doctors offer suggestions about staying healthy. For example, when it comes to physical activity, a little doctorly advice goes a long way.

Recent research conducted at eleven medical centers across the country showed that a little help can make a big difference in getting inactive adults off the couch and into activity. Overall, researchers found that doctor's advice and health education in various forms, including behavioral counseling, phone calls, a monthly newsletter, a step counter (pedometer), and a calendar, resulted in gains in physical activity and cardiovascular fitness. At the start of the study, only about 1 to 2 percent of the volunteers were moderately active thirty minutes on five or more days. After the study, about 10 to 30 percent met the Surgeon General's guidelines for activity levels.

In regular daily practice, this means that an important part of good health care is a solid relationship between you and your doctor—in sickness and in health. You must be able to communicate well with each other so your needs are met.

Types of Health Care Professionals

Your relationship with your health care professional is the foundation for maintaining wellness and reducing your risk of developing disease. And by developing this relationship *before* you get sick, you will have already established a baseline of trust and communication to build upon if you do become ill.

Knowing who's who among the medical specialists, nurses, and other health care professionals involved in your care empowers you to take an active role in your health, as well as to work together with your health care team in making informed decisions.

Medical Doctors

What is a doctor? And what makes him or her qualified to give you medical advice? Certainly you've heard of professionals outside of medicine, such as dentists, veterinarians, and other people with advanced degrees (such as Ph.D.s) who are referred to as "Doctor." Each of these people has earned this title through years of training and hard work. But obviously you don't want that rash on your arm examined by someone whose advanced degree is in economics or history.

There are also some professions slightly outside of the medical mainstream whose practitioners refer to themselves as doctors. And, believe it or not, some people confer this title upon themselves.

But how do you tell all of these people apart? And how do you know where to turn for the most credible, accepted standards when it comes to keeping yourself in good health? You can usually get a good idea about someone's qualifications by looking at the alphabet soup of capital letters after his or her name.

Medical doctors generally have to complete four years of college plus four years of medical school. The majority of doctors in the United States attend a traditional allopathic (Western) medical school, leading to an M.D. (Medical Doctor) degree upon graduation. Some doctors attend an osteopathic medical school and receive a D.O. (Doctor of Osteopathy) degree after graduating. Osteopathic medicine focuses on a more holistic (whole person) approach to medicine that includes osteopathic manipulative treatment (OMT). Doctor using OMT use their hands to treat structural abnormalities and apply corrective forces to relieve joint restrictions and misalignments. Much of the difference between the two types of schools is in the way the material is taught (and learned), not in the subject matter itself.

Doctors with either degree may then go on to complete an additional year of internship, which is required (along with passing a series of exams) by most states before they can become licensed to practice medicine. Doctors with this basic level of training are often referred to as generalists or general practitioners (GPs). Of course, doctors can (and often do) go on to specialize in a particular area of medicine.

Many doctors undergo two to six years of additional training (a residency) to become specialists in one of about two dozen specialties recognized by the American Board of Medical Specialties (ABMS) (see page 33). In recent years, family medicine has developed into a specialty of its own; those who complete the additional training are usually called family practitioners.

Collectively, GPs, family practitioners, and doctors who specialize in pediatrics, obstetrics/gynecology, geriatrics, and internal medicine (known as internists) are considered to be primary care doctors. The term *primary care* reflects the fact that these doctors are usually consulted first when a medical need arises, or they are the ones you turn to for your annual physical exam (sometimes referred to as a "well visit"). These visits are often the best time for you and your doctor to discuss what you can do to stay healthy.

If something unexpected is found or more complex tests are needed, your primary care doctor may refer you to a specialist for further care or testing.

Doctors who specialize in a particular field of medicine, such as dermatologists (skin doctors), cardiologists (heart doctors), and oncologists (cancer doctors), generally do not provide primary care. In other words, you wouldn't see them normally without being referred by your primary care doctor. And even though gynecologists are considered to be primary caregivers, some may not be able to give you the best advice on prevention of cancers outside of their specialty, such as colorectal or skin cancer. In the end, your primary care doctor is your most valuable partner in helping you to reduce your risk of cancer and many other diseases.

Nurses and Physician Assistants

You may see other health care professionals as well during your doctor visits. Physician assistants (PAs), nurse practitioners (NPs), and advanced practice registered nurses (APRNs) can assess your condition and, depending on the state in which they are licensed, may write orders for tests or prescriptions. These caregivers usually work in collaboration with a doctor.

To earn a nursing degree and a license to practice nursing, registered nurses (RNs) earn an associate degree (two years) or a bachelor's degree (four years) in nursing from a school accredited by the National League for Nursing and pass a state licensing exam. Nurses use the scientific knowledge of diagnosis and treatment and provide a caring relationship that promotes healing. They can provide you with the most up-to-date information about cancer prevention and detection and may have more time to answer your specific questions.

Advanced practice registered nurses are registered professional nurses with a master's or doctoral degree and are recognized as such by their State Board of Nursing. Working independently and collaboratively with doctors and other health care professionals, APRNs exercise specialized judgment, experience, and skill. Their scope of practice is to provide expert, quality, and comprehensive nursing care. The APRNs that can help take care of you are clinical nurse specialists (CNSs) and NPs.

Clinical nurse specialists are registered nurses with a master's or other advanced degree who specialize in the direct care of patients in specific areas, such as oncology or mental health nursing (Psych CNS). They usually work in institutions such as hospitals or long-term care facilities.

Nurse practitioners have additional training in primary care and other specialties, like oncology (cancer care) and acute care, and share many tasks with doctors, such as taking patient histories, conducting physical exams, and prescribing medications within their scope of practice.

Physician assistants generally have to complete at least two years of college (although most have a bachelor's or master's degree) along with work experience in the health care field. Many have backgrounds in nursing or emergency medicine. They must complete a two-year training program and pass an examination before becoming a certified physician assistant (PA-C). While they can go on to specialize, PAs generally see patients under the supervision of a doctor.

Other Health Care Professionals

Through a variety of wellness programs (offered in your community or workplace), you can learn safe and effective techniques that lead to positive, permanent changes in health behaviors, such as weight management, smoking cessation, and stress management. The following professionals offer services to promote your physical, emotional, and social well-being.

Dietitians and nutritionists plan food and nutrition programs and supervise the preparation and serving of meals. They help prevent and treat illnesses by promoting healthy eating habits, scientifically evaluating people's diets, and suggesting ways to improve them. A registered dietitian (R.D.) has at least a bachelor's degree and has passed a national competency exam; the term nutritionist is also used, but there are no educational requirements associated with this title.

Psychiatrists, who hold M.D. degrees, and psychologists, who hold a Ph.D., Psy.D., or Ed.D. degree (those with a master's degree also may provide some services), may suggest behavioral or cognitive approaches that can relieve stress. Some also offer psychosocial workshops (such as stress management), which can be useful in maintaining healthy relationships or reducing anxiety. Psychiatrists can prescribe medications to treat symptoms that may be hindering your mental health, such as depression, anxiety, and fatigue. (See Chapter 7 for tips on managing stress.)

Social workers have a degree in social work (B.S.W, M.S.W, or D.S.W) and in most cases must be licensed or certified by the state in which they work. They are trained to help people deal with a range of emotional and practical issues, such as childcare, finances, emotional issues, family concerns and relationships, transportation, and problems with the health care system. Some are also trained as health educators to provide education related to wellness and healthy lifestyles.

Choosing the Right Doctor for You

Skill, compassion, education, and a pleasant bedside manner—all of these qualities and many more go into making a great doctor or health care professional. But how do you find one? A bit of investigation can help you find someone who can provide not only the best care but also the kind of care you want.

Many people already have a relationship with at least one primary care doctor. Members of Health Maintenance Organizations or similar health plans may be assigned to a primary care doctor or may be asked to select one from a list. Usually, the members of these plans need written referrals from their primary caregiver before they can see a specialist.

But what if you don't have a primary care doctor, or you don't think you have the right one for you? Or perhaps you just want to learn more about the one you have.

Places to Start

Before making phone calls or stopping by a physician's busy office, you may want to find out what you can about a specific doctor on the Internet or at your local library.

A good starting point may be the American Medical Association's web site (www.ama-assn.org), which provides a service called Doctor Finder. This database provides the name, phone number, office address, medical school and residency program attended, and board certification status of nearly all licensed physicians in the U.S. One catch is that you need to know in what state your doctor is licensed—not always as obvious as you might think.

Many libraries carry *The Official American Board of Medical Specialties (ABMS) Directory of Board Certified Medical Specialists*, which lists those doctors who have had additional training and who have passed special qualifying tests. The National Cancer Institute also maintains a computer database called PDQ, or Physician Data Query, that can provide information for callers through the Cancer Information Service toll-free line (see Resources for more specific information). Among other things, the database contains a directory of doctors whose practices center on cancer treatment.

State, county, and local health departments can provide further information about doctors, as can the web site of the Association of State Medical Board Executive Directors (www.docboard.org) through DocFinder, which provides links to some state medical licensure boards that list background information on doctors. For further information, each state's medical board has current disciplinary information.

Board Certification

Board certification indicates that a doctor has studied an area of medicine intensely and devotes much of his or her practice to it. Doctors can become certified specialists by completing training and passing a test given by an accreditation board. To maintain their certification, doctors must undergo continuing education after passing the exam. Most certification boards require doctors to continue their education and retest every seven to ten years. Specialists who have reached a higher plateau of achievement are rewarded with the title of Fellow.

Doctors need not be board certified to become specialists and to achieve a high level of accomplishment in their careers. Indeed, many good doctors, particularly those in certain primary care fields, may not be board certified. Increasingly, however, even primary care doctors seek these additional qualifications.

The ABMS maintains a list of all board-certified physicians (at www.abms.org, click on "Who's Certified"), information about a doctor's certification status, and a list of certified specialists by geographic area, if the doctor subscribes to the ABMS service. The ABMS cannot provide doctor referrals. They can only provide verification of ABMS board certification.

Experience and Expertise

The years teach much which the days never knew.
—Ralph Waldo Emerson

Experience is an important consideration. Years in practice are one measure, but the number of patients that your doctor has seen is also significant. You may want to ask about the doctor's patient load and the types of conditions he or she is experienced in treating.

Perhaps more importantly, find out about his or her philosophy when it comes to keeping you in the pink. Some doctors are better than others about

Doctor, Tell Me About Yourself

A simple but effective strategy for learning more about your doctor's (or prospective doctor's) qualifications is to ask about his or her qualifications directly. The following questions may be helpful. The answers you may expect are explained further on.

- Where did you attend medical school, internship, and residency?

- How long have you been practicing?

- What types of conditions are you experienced in treating?

- Are you board certified?

- What is your specialty? Do you do research in your specialty? Do you have a subspecialty?

- Are you or others in your practice involved in experimental or new treatments?

- What hospitals are you affiliated with? What hospitals do you have privileges with?

- What are your office hours?

- Can you be contacted outside those hours? How?

- Do you accept my insurance plan?

- Who supervises your patients when you are on vacation?

Doing the research can be time consuming—but worth it. Putting in the effort upfront means finding a doctor who is best for you and may save time and hassle in the long run.

guiding you down the right path, even when you may be perfectly healthy.

Many doctors are involved in research to some extent at some point during their careers. Whether or not a doctor continues to be active in research while practicing may or may not influence your decision to see him or her. Some doctors at respected hospitals, particularly specialists, may only see patients in the context of clinical trials. Many primary care doctors, on the other hand, choose to focus on patient care. Others fall somewhere in between these two extremes.

Doctors don't have to do research to be good at what they do, but if yours does, it might provide some insight into the doctor's philosophy and approach. Because doctors involved in research usually publish their findings in medical journals, you might ask for copies of articles. If you have the time and know-how, you may want to research online medical databases, such as PubMed, which is available through the National Library of Medicine's web site (www.ncbi.nlm.nih.gov/PubMed).

Practice Environment and Hospital Affiliations

What is the nature of the doctor's practice? Different types of practices have their own advantages and disadvantages. Continuity and consistency can be provided in the environment of a solo practice where all patients see the same doctor for each appointment. A group practice may offer more expertise and resources, as well as increased flexibility with scheduling. A practice group that has multiple specialties in one facility may be able to offer increased experience in many areas, whereas a single-specialty group is able to concentrate on one area of medical care.

Because doctors can send patients only to those facilities (such as hospitals and clinics) where they have admitting privileges, you should know where you would go if needed for surgery or other care. You may want to check with your health insurance company to see which doctors and treatment facilities your particular plan includes.

Teaching Affiliation

A teaching affiliation, especially with a prestigious medical school, may indicate that a doctor is a respected leader in the field. Academic physicians who maintain practices are often in close touch with experts around the country and may be well versed in the latest therapies. You can ask if your doctor is affiliated with a medical school or teaching hospital.

Many educators are leaders in their fields and are knowledgeable about research and treatments, but doctors affiliated with smaller hospitals are also highly skilled and knowledgeable.

If you have a complex health problem, you will want to know if the doctor is involved in research and teaching. On the other hand, if you are looking for someone who can take care of your general needs, who will listen and respond to your questions, and with whom you feel comfortable, these issues may not be as important to you.

Doctor's Reputation

A doctor's reputation is less easily evaluated, but no less important in choosing the one that is right for you. Sometimes asking others can tell you a lot about the way a doctor practices. Friends, family members, and coworkers can provide important referral information about their own doctors. You may want to inquire about the rapport the person has with the doctor, and whether or not they felt comfortable asking questions and discussing care options with their doctor.

Other Considerations

A good head and a good heart are always a formidable combination.
—NELSON MANDELA

Other factors may also affect your choice of a doctor. If a doctor's office is difficult to reach or the drive is too long, the chances that you will make regular appointments may decrease. Inconvenience may add an unnecessary complication to your health care.

Style of practice and personality are two imprecise attributes that can factor into your decision for choosing a doctor. A doctor who has good communication skills is critical. His or her personality may be difficult to quantify, but genuine concern, understanding, and support from your doctor are relevant to superior health care. In other words, is the chemistry right? Do you have a good feeling about this doctor? Is this person going to help coach you in lifestyle issues?

One question that people frequently ask is, "Do I have to like my doctor?" The answer is "No"—to a point. While it can be helpful to have someone you can relate to or easily converse with about topics other than your health, trust is the most important thing you should feel toward your doctor.

At the very least you need to be able to talk openly and honestly with each other, and should respect each other's point of view. If your doctor is hard to talk to and abrupt when talking to you, yet still very capable of providing you the best care possible, consider asking more questions and informing him or her of your desire for more information. Sometimes the problem is simply a lack of communication, which can be easily resolved.

If, on the other hand, you feel that an uncomfortable relationship with your doctor is affecting your care, you might need to consider changing doctors.

Talking with Your Doctor

Like all successful relationships, your bond with your doctor is a two-way street. It is your responsibility to ask questions and become educated about your health and how to reduce your risk for developing certain diseases. Doctors differ in how much information they give to patients. Likewise, people differ in the amount of information they need or want. It is up to you to tell your doctor if he or she is giving you too much or too little information. Doctors often do not know what information you need unless you tell them. They will take their cues from you, so it is important to work on communicating with your doctor.

Assessing Practice Style and Philosophies

Ask yourself these questions once you've had an appointment with a doctor, or ask these questions of others who are recommending a particular doctor.

- Are appointments easy to make, and is the interval between your call and your appointment short?

- Can you speak to your doctor personally before or after your scheduled appointment?

- Are phone calls returned promptly?

- Are the waiting room and office area clean and comfortable?

- Is the doctor's staff courteous and professional?

- Is the doctor punctual, or are you kept waiting for an indeterminate amount of time? Does the doctor apologize for being late?

- Do you get to see your doctor at each visit, or are you shuffled between a series of partners or other health professionals?

You should feel at ease with your doctor. A good relationship with your doctor is worth the effort needed to create it. If you and your doctor have similar viewpoints about sharing facts, making choices, or joining self-help groups, you are likely to have a good relationship.

- Does your doctor make recommendations regarding ways you can stay healthy?

- Does your doctor listen to you?

- Is your doctor open to answering your questions, or do you feel rushed through your examination and discussion? Do they take place in private?

- Is it acceptable to bring a family member, friend, or child with you to your appointment?

- Does your doctor appear open to assistance from other health care professionals such as social workers, nurses, therapists, and other specialists?

- Is your doctor willing to provide referrals or recommendations for second opinions?

- Is the office staff prepared to answer your questions and provide information as needed? Do they appear well trained?

- Is the office staff helpful with insurance matters? Is your doctor's office agreeable to negotiating terms of payment?

- How would you rate the follow-up to your appointment? Are you informed of test results promptly?

For you, what is the first step in creating good communication with your doctor?

Ask Yourself, "How Much Do I Want to Know?"

You may want a lot of details. Some people feel much better when they know all the facts about what they should be doing to stay healthy. If you are like this, you should ask the doctor for exact details and information.

Or you may want only the overview. You may want simple directions—what early detection tests will be needed and when they should be done. Don't be afraid to tell your doctor how much, or how little, information you want.

Sharing Information

We each have our own way to communicate. That's why the perfect doctor for one person may not be a good match for another. You may want your doctor to be business-like. Some people prefer doctors who are direct and to the point. They don't need a warm relationship—just a sharing of needed facts. Or you might prefer a doctor with a more friendly style.

After you know what you want as a patient, the next step is looking at how you talk with your doctor.

Understanding the Words

There may be times when you are anxious or feeling overwhelmed with information, and it's hard to listen well and understand. Even if the doctor is very thorough, you may not hear or remember what is being said. Bring a list of questions and take notes to help recall what your doctor says. Or ask if you can tape-record your talk for later review. Better yet, bring a family member or friend with you to take notes and act as your eyes and ears. They can remind you of questions you want to ask and help you remember what the doctor said.

Some doctors try to share information but use terms you may not know. If you don't understand something, ask your doctor to explain it to you.

Asking Questions

He who asks a question is a fool for five minutes;
he who does not ask a question remains a fool forever.
—Chinese proverb

Here are some questions your doctor can usually answer for you about reducing your risk of cancer and finding it early.

- What should someone of my age and gender be concerned about?

- What are my risk factors for specific diseases? Which of these can I do something about?

- What else can I do to decrease my risk of developing these diseases?

- What wellness programs do you suggest for me?

- What early detection tests should I consider? How often should I have them done?

- How good are these tests? What do they involve? Are they painful?

- What do I need to do to prepare for the tests?

- Will my insurance pay for the tests?

- What is the best time to call if I have a question? (Some doctors have a special time for callbacks. Expect your doctor to return your calls, but remember that a quick response may not be possible if another patient is having a crisis.)

When you get instructions from your doctor, write them down. Make sure you understand them before you leave the office. Then follow them. Keep written notes and bring them with you, if needed.

Above all, your doctor should take your questions seriously. He or she should be interested in your concerns and not make you feel rushed. If your doctor does not respond this way, bring it up at your next visit. If you don't, communication may be blocked and your relationship may suffer.

Problems Talking with Your Doctor

People choose to change doctors for different reasons. You may feel your doctor is not listening to you, or you're just having trouble communicating. Maybe you do not have confidence in the way your doctor treats you. Don't stay with a doctor only to protect his or her feelings. You have the right to find the best doctor for you.

Some people find that they can get their questions answered from a nurse or another medical professional. If this isn't an option, it may be time to find a new doctor.

Building a relationship with your doctor doesn't just happen. It takes care and effort on both sides. Chances are, you'll both benefit.

The Doctor-Patient Relationship

Here's how to improve communication with your doctor, as well as how to maintain a good doctor-patient relationship.

- Make and bring a list of things you would like to discuss with your doctor. Include a list of all your questions. Take it with you to your doctor visits. Don't be ashamed or shy about asking these questions. *There is no such thing as a dumb question.*

- Bring a list of the medications you are taking currently, including vitamins, supplements, and herbals. Include how much and how often you take them. Or, even better, bring the medications with you so your doctor can see them. Make a separate list of those medications to which you are allergic.

- Begin your appointment with the most important item on your list.

- Tell your doctor if you don't understand certain medical tests or terms. Ask him or her to review complicated information or procedures.

- Realize that if you bring in information you've found at the library or on the Internet, your doctor may not have time to go over it with you. Instead, consider asking your doctor about the sources he or she uses or relies on for reliable health information. Or leave the information for your doctor to review and get back with you later.

- Talk over your concerns with your doctor. Mention lifestyle habits, even if it's something you're not proud of, such as smoking. Never hold back information—something you think is minor could affect your health, or something you think is serious might be easily relieved. Remember, your doctor is there to help, and he or she may not be able to do it to the best of his or her ability without all the facts.

CHAPTER 2

What's Your Food Attitude?

Why the Foods You Choose May Lower Your Cancer Risk

If we could give every individual the right amount of nourishment and exercise, not too little and not too much, we would have found the safest way to health.
— HIPPOCRATES

Hippocrates had it right — even then. We've known for a long time that eating right and being active are important for achieving and maintaining good health *and* for reducing your risk of cancer. Even if you have a family history of the disease, your food choices and physical activity habits can influence your own risk of developing cancer. In fact, if you do not smoke, the most important ways for you to influence your cancer risk are to eat a healthy diet, be physically active on a regular basis, and maintain a healthy body weight.

That's the good news. And these are relatively easy things you can do to improve your health and reduce your risk of developing cancer, as well as heart disease, diabetes, and obesity. The challenge is that many aspects of modern life make healthy eating more difficult. The places where we live, work, and play do not always encourage us make healthy food choices.

Food is everywhere—in vending machines at gas stations, bus stations, hospitals, and schools; in fast food outlets in shopping malls; and on almost every street corner. Billions of dollars in advertising encourage all of us—and especially children—to eat too much food, as well as many foods that are not nutritional. We're eating out more frequently, where portion sizes are often larger than what we eat at home. Even the average plate size has increased over the years! Add this to our fast-paced lifestyles, where we're lucky to grab a quick lunch during the week or get a balanced meal on the table at home for dinner, and you can begin to see the impact these issues are having on our health. Now over 55 percent of American adults are overweight, and obesity rates in our youth have more than doubled in the last two decades.

This chapter will highlight the best of what is known about reducing your risk of cancer through healthy eating and weight control, provide you some practical tips for making changes in your own eating habits and those of your family, and give you some food for thought on how you can make a difference in your community, your worksite, and your school so that the *healthiest* choices become the *easiest* choices.

Getting Started

Since you're reading this chapter, it's likely that you've been thinking about making some changes to your diet—maybe you want to lose weight and feel better, or maybe you're concerned about your risk of cancer or heart disease. Whatever your reason for wanting to eat more healthfully, you're in the right place! Before you make any changes to your diet, it's a good idea to take a look at your current habits—what things you are currently doing that you should keep doing and where some opportunities are to make some healthy changes. Take the following quiz to get some insight on times, places, and ways you can start eating your way to good health.

Take the Food Attitude Quiz

This quiz is designed to reveal why, when, where, and how you eat. Mark *true* or *false* next to each statement. Be as honest as you can. Your responses should give you an idea about your eating style and your perceptions about food, and give you some ideas on where to start making healthy changes in your eating patterns.

_____ **1.** I usually eat breakfast.

_____ **2.** I never skip a meal.

_____ **3.** I don't often eat out or buy meals away from home. (often = twice per week for any meal)

_____ **4.** I usually eat dinner no later than 7 P.M.

_____ **5.** When I eat a snack, I try to eat something nutritious.

_____ **6.** I don't have a tendency to overeat on special occasions or when I'm out with friends.

_____ **7.** I like eating a variety of foods and trying something new.

_____ **8.** I avoid eating when I'm bored, stressed, or lonely.

_____ **9.** I don't eat when I'm watching TV or socializing with other people.

_____ **10.** I rarely eat meals and/or snacks in the car.

_____ **11.** I never eat in my bedroom.

_____ **12.** I don't usually have uncontrollable cravings for certain foods.

_____ **13.** I like nutritious food—I think it tastes good.

_____ **14.** I'm pretty clear on what foods I should be eating. I think I eat healthfully.

_____ **15.** I stay away from sweets and salty snacks.

_____ **16.** I make time to eat right. I'm never too busy.

(continued on page 48)

(continued from page 47)

_____**17.** I keep healthy foods readily available at home and at work.

_____**18.** I drink plenty of water and juice.

_____**19.** I only drink alcohol occasionally (or not at all).

_____**20.** I limit my servings to small portions at meals.

Count and tally your answers: _____ **True** _____ **False**

What Your Answers Mean

If you answered *true* to 15–20 statements: You're on your way! Keep up the good work! You practice good eating habits and you like healthy foods. If you answered *false* to any of the questions, keep reading for some ideas on how you might answer *true* the next time! Continue doing what you're doing and look for even more ways to improve your eating habits.

If you answered *true* to 8–14 statements: You've got great opportunity to make some changes! You're on your way, and can probably now identify some easy things to do to keep heading in the right direction. Your true statements reveal that the healthy eating habits you already have are actions you do without thought. That's great—you've got some good habits! Keep reading to learn how the statements you answered *false* to can help jumpstart your thinking on some other habits you can work on.

If you answered *true* to 7 or fewer of the statements: All is not lost! You do have some things going for you, although you could very much benefit from taking a serious look at your eating patterns (see later section on "Your Food Diary"). Take heart, though, it's not as difficult as you might think. Look at the statements you marked *false* and read the following comments to learn more.

NOTE: This quiz is intended to be used for informational purposes only. Scoring and results are not based on scientific research.

Simple Steps to Healthy Eating

Take a look at those statements you answered *false*. These statements provide you with insight on how you can start to take simple steps to improve your eating habits—today!

1. **If you don't usually eat breakfast:** Breakfast eaters are less likely to be overweight than people who do not eat breakfast. That's because people who eat breakfast tend to eat less fat and calories throughout the day. Don't have time for breakfast? That morning meal doesn't have to take a long time. Some good options include cereal and milk, toast with jelly, or grab-and-go items such as fresh fruit, a bagel with low-fat cream cheese, or yogurt.

2. **If you sometimes skip meals:** Skipping any meal during the day can lead to inconsistent nutrient intake, poor food choices later in the day, and overeating. You can avoid this habit by planning ahead. For example, if you have a meeting at 11 A.M. and another at noon, eat a "mini-meal" at 10:30 A.M. and another at 2 P.M.

3. **If you often eat out or buy meals away from home:** Keep in mind that meals eaten away from home tend to be higher in fat and calories than home-cooked meals. Portion sizes also tend to be larger, so enjoy half your meal and pack up the rest for tomorrow's lunch.

4. **If you usually eat dinner after 7 P.M.:** The later you eat at night, the less likely you are to burn off those calories. Try eating more of your calories earlier in the day. Get in the habit of making lunch your biggest meal of the day.

5. **If it's hard to find a nutritious snack:** Many fruits, such as bananas, apples, and citrus fruits, are completely portable. Other good choices include sliced or chopped veggies, baby carrots, pretzels, plain popcorn, yogurt, and low-fat cheese and crackers. All fit nicely in pockets, purses, book bags, glove compartments, and desk drawers.

(continued on page 50)

(continued from page 49)

6. If you tend to overeat on special occasions or when you're out with friends: We all splurge from time to time. They key is to plan ahead for those occasional indulgences! If you know you're going to be eating out at a special restaurant or enjoying your favorite dessert, watch what you eat throughout the day. Better yet, add more physical activity to your day to balance those extra calories.

7. **If you don't like eating a variety of foods or trying something new:** Tempt your taste buds with a variety of different fruits, vegetables, and grain-based products. Who knows, you may even find some new favorites! Commit to trying something new each week. Go for it!

8. **If you sometimes eat when bored, stressed, or lonely:** Many of us eat for emotional reasons, and often this leads to overeating or making poor nutritional choices. Keeping a food diary can help you identify those situations that cause you to overeat, or to eat when you're not really hungry (see "Tips for Keeping a Food Diary" on page 86).

9. **I eat when I'm watching TV or socializing with other people:** These habits can be distracting and often lead to overeating because it's easy to overeat when you're doing more than "just eating." Try turning off the TV when you eat. To help focus on what's on your plate, save mealtime for the dinner table. If you are planning on going to a party, you can bring healthy choices to the gathering yourself. Don't go to the party hungry. Make only one trip to the buffet table.

10. **I sometimes eat meals and snacks in the car:** For many Americans, cars and public transportation have become a dining room away from home. Certainly, eating while driving can be as distracting and dangerous as talking on a cell phone. Drive-up and dine-through has created a fast way to eat on the run. If you're traveling, pack foods that transport well such as dried fruits, individually packaged raisins, carrots, or apricots. Vacuum-packed juices and bottled juices or water are also good choices.

11. If you eat in the bedroom…or the family room…or the den: Eating in multiple rooms in your house isn't necessarily a dietary no-no, but it can lead to food associations and snack cravings when you're in that room. Commit to eating in just one room in the house —like the kitchen or dining room.

12. **If you sometimes get uncontrollable cravings for certain foods:** Control your cravings by moderating your portions and choosing a variety of foods, including *some* of those high in fat and calories. If you can identify the foods that you crave the most and the times when you feel vulnerable, you may be able to prevent future overeating or poor dietary choices.

13. **If you don't like nutritious food—or don't think it tastes good:** Americans (44 percent) don't want to give up foods they like, especially when those foods are not the best choices, according to a survey by the American Dietetic Association (ADA). This reinforces the fact that food habits are hard to change. But the real facts of the matter are that nutrition and flavor can go hand in hand—you don't have to sacrifice one for the other. There are plenty of tasty foods that are nutritious. And if you put some thought into it, you should be able to replace the unhealthy items currently on your favorite food list.

14. **If you're not really clear on what foods you should be eating:** The same ADA survey found that nearly 30 percent of Americans who had not changed their eating habits in the past few years say they have not done so because they didn't "know or understand nutrition guidelines." Despite the fact that food labeling has become more specific and easier to read, more information about general nutrition guidelines and diet needs to be clearly spelled out. This chapter hopes to fill some of those gaps.

15. **If you have trouble staying away from sweets and salty snacks:** Chocolate and other sweets usually contain fat and sugar, while salty snacks, especially fried ones, are often high in fat and calories. You

(continued on page 52)

(continued from page 51)

don't have to totally give up your favorite snack foods to eat healthy—the key is watching how often you consume these foods and watching your portion sizes. Buy snacks that are packed in individual packages, like small bags of chips. Instead of the package of full-size candy bars, buy the smaller snack sizes. Moderation is the key.

16. **If you don't have the time to eat right:** Among those Americans who have not changed their eating habits in recent years, nearly 40 percent feel that "it takes too much time to keep track" of their diet. With some helpful hints in this chapter, you can make your dietary goals become habits, and then you won't need to "keep track" of your portions and food choices.

17. **If you don't buy healthy food because it costs more:** You may run into increased expense for healthy food if you buy prepackaged low-fat, reduced-fat, or fat-free food or if you eat out. Otherwise, healthy food doesn't cost anymore than any other kind of food. You can buy fresh fruits and veggies from the farmers market or roadside stands in season when they are least expensive. Think about how you can freeze or preserve them. Depending on the season, canned and frozen fruits and vegetables may be less expensive than buying fresh, and they can be just as nutritious.

18. **If you have trouble drinking plenty of water and juice:** Staying hydrated is essential to good health. Drink at least eight glasses of water, juice, or skim milk per day and more during summer months and while performing physically strenuous activities. Caffeinated drinks, such as tea, colas, and coffee, and alcoholic beverages can actually dehydrate you. They don't count toward your eight glasses of water a day.

19. **If you drink alcohol:** If you choose to drink, try to limit your consumption of alcohol to one drink per day for women and two drinks per day for men, and accompany these drinks with water.

20. **If you overeat during meals:** Smaller portion sizes are an easy way to limit the amount you eat. Instead of loading your plate with large portions, use ½-cup servings.

Eating Your Way to Good Health

Nutritious food and healthy choices are your best protection in preventing and controlling not only cancer but a number of other lifestyle-related illnesses, including heart disease and diabetes. And the good news is that eating a healthy diet does not have to feel agonizing or depriving.

Want even better news? You don't have to give up all your favorite foods to eat a healthful diet! The key is balancing out healthier choices with not-so-healthier choices. Evidence suggests that one-third of the 500,000 cancer deaths that occur each year are related to what people eat—or don't eat.

Go for the Green and Other Colors

You've heard it many times before, and your mother was right! Eating more vegetables and fruits is an easy—and delicious—way to reduce your risk of cancer. Strive to eat at least five servings of vegetables and fruits each day. Serving sizes are small, so eating five or more doesn't have to be a challenge. Adding fruits and vegetables to your diet may help you reduce your risk of developing certain cancers. Research has shown significant benefit and protective effects of eating fruits and vegetables. They do, in fact, contain compounds that appear to block or inhibit carcinogens (cancer-causing agents).

What is it about vegetables and fruit that make them so beneficial to our health? It could be the variety of cancer-protective antioxidants that vegetables and fruit contain. These are the compounds that provide the beautiful array of colors in vegetables and fruit, and they help protect our cell membranes and DNA from damage. Vegetables and fruits are also low in fat and high in fiber.

The American Cancer Society Guidelines on Nutrition and Physical Activity for Cancer Prevention

Below are the ACS Guidelines on Nutrition and Physical Activity for Cancer Prevention—the best of what we currently know that can help you reduce your risk of cancer, starting today! (See the next chapter to learn more about how physical activity can help reduce your risk of cancer.)

1. Eat a variety of healthful foods, with an emphasis on plant sources.

- Eat five or more servings of a variety of vegetables and fruits each day.

- Choose whole grains in preference to processed (refined) grains and sugars.

- Limit consumption of red meats, especially those high in fat and processed.

- Choose foods that help maintain a healthful weight.

2. Adopt a physically active lifestyle.

- Adults: engage in at least moderate activity for thirty minutes or more on five or more days of the week; forty-five minutes or more of moderate to vigorous activity on five or more days per week may further reduce the risk of breast and colon cancer.

- Children and adolescents: engage in at least sixty minutes per day of moderate-to-vigorous physical activity at least five days per week.

3. Maintain a healthful weight throughout life.

- Balance caloric intake with physical activity.

- Lose weight if currently overweight or obese.

4. If you drink alcoholic beverages, limit consumption.

While no diet can guarantee full protection against any disease, following these Guidelines is your best bet for reducing the risk of cancer.

It's Your Serve

Eating at least five servings of fruits and vegetables each day is pretty simple when you consider the size of an actual serving. Look below to see how small one serving really is:

1 medium piece of fruit (banana, apple, orange)
¼ cup of dried fruit
½ cup of frozen, cooked, or canned fruit or vegetable
1 cup of leafy greens
6 ounces of 100% fruit or vegetable juice

Suggestions:

Eat five or more servings of fruits and vegetables each day.

- Include fruits or vegetables in every meal and for snacks. In general, those with the most color—green, red, yellow, and orange—tend to have the most nutrients.

- Eat a variety of vegetables and fruits. In addition to eating different types, also use different ways to prepare them so you won't get bored eating the same things over and over. Also, keep in mind that canned and frozen fruits and vegetables can be just as nutritious as fresh ones and, depending on the season, may be less expensive than buying fresh.

- Limit French fries, snack chips, and other fried vegetable products. Although they are technically from plants, they can be loaded with fat and extra calories because of the way they are cooked.

- Choose 100% vegetable and fruit juices, rather than "juice drinks." Look for "100% juice" on the label. If it doesn't say that, it's likely made with sugar and flavoring, with just a little bit of juice.

- Add vegetables and fruits to the foods you're already eating: sliced bananas on your cereal, lettuce and tomato on your sandwich, black beans in your burritos.

- Try a new vegetable or fruit each week.

- Keep vegetables and fruit handy and ready-to-eat for snacks: baby carrots and celery sticks in your refrigerator, a bowl of apples and oranges on your counter, mini-boxes of raisins in your desk. And don't forget dried fruits—they are excellent as an alternate choice.

Choose whole grains in preference to processed (refined) grains and sugars.
- Include whole grain products such as breads, cereals, rice, or pasta in every meal. Whole grains have more fiber and are generally more nutritious.

- Limit your consumption of "refined carbohydrates," such as pastries, sweetened cereals, soft drinks, and sugars.

In the majority of scientific studies on this subject, greater consumption of vegetables, fruits, or both together has been associated with a lower risk of lung, esophagus, oral, stomach, and colon cancers. Evidence is less strong for those types of cancers considered to be hormonally related, such as breast and prostate.

Because it's not known which components—or combination of components—are most beneficial to reduce the risk of cancer, the best advice is to eat at least five servings of vegetables and fruit each day, eat a variety of vegetables and fruits in their various forms (fresh, frozen, canned, dried, and juiced), and focus especially on those that have the most color.

Antioxidants and Cancer

The idea that foods may play a role in reducing the risk of cancer first emerged from findings that linked fruit and vegetable consumption with lower cancer risk. Researchers are learning that certain nutrients in fruits and vegetables appear to protect the body against the damage to tissues that constantly occurs as a result of normal metabolism.

Because such damage is associated with increased cancer risk, antioxidant nutrients are thought to protect against cancer. Antioxidants include

The Scoop About Bioengineered Foods and Food Additives

Bioengineered foods are made by the combination or breeding of genes from different plants or other organisms to increase resistance to pests, to retard spoilage, or to improve transportability, flavor, nutrient composition, or other desired qualities. In theory, these foods might create substances that could cause adverse reactions among sensitized or allergic individuals. However, there is currently no evidence that the substances found in bioengineered foods now on the market are harmful or that they would either increase or decrease cancer risk because of bioengineering (the added genes).

Bioengineered foods are different from food additives, which are substances added to foods to preserve them and to enhance color, flavor, texture, or nutritional value. Additives are usually present in very small quantities in food. No convincing evidence exists that any additives at these levels cause cancer in humans.

In fact, some additives actually promote better health. Certain foods are "fortified" with nutrients that we sometimes don't get enough of in our regular diets. For example, milk is fortified with vitamin D, while grain products, such as breads, cereals, and pasta, are fortified with folic acid. Foods containing added nutrients must be labeled as such.

vitamin C, vitamin E, selenium, carotenoids (relatives of vitamin A), and some other phytochemicals that occur naturally in plant foods. Studies suggest that people who eat more fruits and vegetables containing these antioxidants have a lower risk for some types of cancer. But there seems to be something important about getting the nutrients from foods themselves, because studies of antioxidant supplements have not shown a reduction in cancer risk. In fact, for beta-carotene, supplements have been associated with a higher risk of lung cancer in cigarette smokers.

Cut the Meat and the Calories Will Follow

The major source of saturated fat and cholesterol in the American diet comes from foods derived from animal sources, especially red meat. Even though meat is an excellent source of protein and certain vitamins and minerals, it's not necessary to eat meat every day because these nutrients can be obtained from other foods.

The way meat is prepared may also play a role in promoting cancer. For example, some research suggests that frying, broiling, or grilling meats at very high temperatures creates chemicals that might increase cancer risk. Although these chemicals cause cancer in animal experiments, it is uncertain whether they actually cause cancer in people.

Rather than drastically changing your diet or deciding to become a vegetarian, the following suggestions are designed to help you change your habits gradually and easily.

Suggestions:
Limit consumption of red meats, especially those high in fat and processed.

- Choose fish, poultry, or beans as an alternative to beef, pork, and lamb. Beans are a great source of vitamins, minerals, and fiber. Select beans, either canned or dried, as a low-fat, high-protein alternative to meat.

- When you eat meat, select lean cuts and smaller portions. (Lean cuts have the words *loin* and *round* in them, such as tenderloin and top round.)

Phytochemicals At-A-Glance

The term *phytochemicals* refers to a wide variety of compounds produced by plants. Some have either antioxidant or hormone-like actions both in plants and in people who eat them.

Because consumption of fruits and vegetables reduces cancer risk, researchers are searching for specific compounds in these foods that might account for the beneficial effects.

- Lycopene, a red-orange carotenoid (a type of pigment) antioxidant found in tomatoes and tomato products, is thought to protect cells from damage.

- Soy contains several phytochemicals, some of which appear to protect against hormone-dependent cancers in animal studies. Soy supplements, on the other hand, may increase the risk of estrogen-responsive cancers, such as breast or endometrial cancer.

- Sulphoraphane, commonly found in broccoli, can encourage the body to produce protective enzymes that may prevent cell damage that can lead to cancer.

- Ellagic acid, found in raspberries, strawberries, cranberries, walnuts, pecans, and pomegranates, has been shown to slow the growth of tumors in animal studies. Further research is needed to determine if the results apply to humans.

There are thousands of phytochemicals, but we don't know which are most effective for disease prevention. There is no evidence that phytochemicals taken as supplements are as beneficial as the vegetables, fruits, beans, and grains from which they are extracted. Your best bet right now is to eat a mostly plant-based diet, which includes at least five servings of a variety of fruits and vegetables each day.

- Prepare meat by baking, broiling, or poaching, rather than by frying or charbroiling. Meat should be cooked thoroughly to destroy harmful bacteria and parasites but should not be charred.

Choose foods that help maintain a healthful weight.

- When you eat away from home, choose food low in fat, calories, and sugar and avoid large portion sizes. Check food labels and use them as a guide in making healthier choices. You may be surprised. What you think is low in fat may actually be quite high in fat and/or calories, such as a breakfast muffin. (See page 81 for a guide to healthy weight.)

How to Eat Healthy When Dining Out

- Choose restaurants that offer healthy entrees (such as baked chicken or fish).

- Don't be afraid to ask how a dish is prepared, or ask for a lower-fat version of your meal in a restaurant. Many will prepare your meal to order or offer a healthier choice.

- Consider a salad instead of an appetizer. But be careful—dressings are often loaded with calories, and other salad bar items such as potato salad and macaroni salad are high in fat. Ask for oil and vinegar dressing.

- Split an entree with a friend.

- Choose an entree other than red meat, especially if it is high-fat or processed.

- Ask for a to-go box before you begin your meal. Keep a portion for another meal.

- Eat smaller portions of high calorie foods. Be aware that "low-fat" or "non-fat" does not mean "low-calorie" and that low-fat cakes, cookies, and similar foods are often high in calories. If you do choose high-fat foods, choose those that contain polyunsaturated or monounsaturated fats, such as those in certain salad dressings, cooking oils, fish, and nuts.

- Substitute vegetables, fruits, and other low-calorie foods for calorie-dense foods such as French fries, cheeseburgers, pizza, ice cream, doughnuts, and other sweets.

- For special meals, allow yourself to indulge in something you enjoy. Just remember to be moderate and return to foods that are healthier the next day.

- Try an ethnic restaurant, and ask about dishes that are cooked in healthy ways.

- Eat a healthy snack or drink some juice before you arrive at a special event. Then you're not completely starved and don't find yourself standing at the appetizer table stuffing yourself with bacon-wrapped sausages.

- If you order dessert, choose healthier dishes, such as angel food cake, sherbet, or fresh berries or fruit.

- If possible, bring your toothbrush and toothpaste with you wherever you go. If you brush, you may be less likely to continue nibbling.

- If there appears to be no healthy choice at your event, just eat a smaller portion. You don't always have to "clean your plate!"

As a Matter of Fat

The word *fat* is scary to many people on a diet or who are conscious about maintaining their weight. Fat is also a necessary nutrient. Among the many essential functions it serves, fat helps the body absorb certain vitamins, stores energy, helps maintain hair and skin, and protects vital organs.

The problem that Americans run into is that fat is also the ingredient that makes food smell and taste good and gives us a satisfied feeling after we eat it. Our bodies have evolved to recognize that fat gives us more energy (in the form of calories) than other types of foods. While at one time in the distant past this was important for our survival, it's now the cause of many of our health problems.

People who eat high-fat diets tend to be heavier, eat more meat, and eat fewer fruits and vegetables, so their risk of cancer is increased for other reasons. High-fat diets have been associated with an increase in the risk of cancers of the colon, rectum, prostate, and endometrium. The association between dietary fat and breast cancer risk is not as strong. Whether these associations are due to the total amount of fat, the particular type of fat, the calories contributed by fat, or some other factor in the food has not yet been determined. These relationships to cancer and cancer risk are actively being studied.

Although overall fat consumption is down to about 34 percent of calories in the average American diet, compared to 40 percent a few years ago, Americans continue to eat far too many calories despite (or because of) the increased availability of fat-free and reduced-fat foods.

Because a gram of fat contains more than twice the calories of a gram of protein or carbohydrate (9 versus 4 kilocalories per gram), it's difficult to tell if the negative effects of fat are from the fat itself or from the calories it contains. "Low-fat" or "non-fat" on the label just tells you about the fat content. The other important number to know is the number of calories.

Have you ever thought, "This is a fat-free food, so I can eat more"? Colleen Doyle, M.S., R.D., Director of Nutrition and Physical Activity at the ACS, counters, "These may be fat-free foods, but if you eat too many calories, your body turns those extra calories into fat." Maintaining a healthy weight and lifestyle has more to do with eating fewer calories, choosing healthful foods, and being physically active, rather than simply eating low-fat foods.

All Fats Are Not Created Equal

Triglycerides, good cholesterol, bad cholesterol, omega-3 fatty acids, monounsaturated fats—these terms are confusing enough. Add to the confusion the fact that there are several kinds of fat we eat in our diet and that they are all very different, especially in their effects on cholesterol levels. You might think you need a college degree in nutrition to understand the differences. Well, you don't need a degree; you just need to read the food label.

Current evidence indicates that saturated fat may increase your risk for cancer as well as for heart disease. Many foods contain a combination of different types of fats (see chart), and it's usually difficult to tell which is the predominant fat. While modifying your fat intake to include more unsaturated and less saturated fats is important, it's even more important to lower the total amount of fat in your diet because fat is still high in calories.

A Toast: To Your Health?

Whether you drink hard liquor, wine, or beer, studies clearly show that cancer risk increases with the amount of alcohol consumed. This means that your choice of alcoholic beverage may be less important than how much you drink.

For men, the recommendation is to limit alcohol to two drinks a day. For women, one drink a day. A drink is defined as twelve ounces of regular beer, five ounces of wine, or one and a half ounces of eighty-proof distilled spirits. For comparison, a bottle of beer, a glass of wine, a shot of liquor, or a mixed drink all have about the same amount of alcohol in them.

	Saturated Fats	Monounsaturated Fats
Other Names	Saturated fatty acids	Monounsaturated fatty acids
Examples	Butter/shortening, egg yolks, chocolate, dairy products, meats and poultry with skin, palm and coconut oil	Olive, canola, and peanut oils; avocados; plant foods; some seafood
Effect	Raises blood cholesterol May increase risk of heart disease	May lower blood cholesterol May lessen the risk of heart disease
What You Should Do	Cut back on foods from this list	Choose more of your fat-containing foods from this list

Risk increases substantially with even moderate drinking, defined as more than two drinks per day. Alcohol consumption increases the risk for cancers of the mouth, throat, esophagus, liver, and, for women, cancer of the breast. It may also be related to the risk of colorectal cancer. Cancer risk is directly related to the amount, not the type (beer, wine, or hard liquor), of alcohol consumed.

Why alcohol increases risk is still unknown, but researchers think alcohol may bring about changes in hormones in the blood or that alcohol and the substances produced in its breakdown might have a cancer-causing effect on breast tissues, for example. This risk may be especially strong for women who drink every day and whose mother, sisters, or daughters have breast cancer, according to a Mayo Clinic study. Another possibility is that people who drink have lower levels of folic acid, a B vitamin that plays a key role in maintaining healthy DNA.

Polyunsaturated Fats	Trans Fats
Polyunsaturated fatty acids	Trans fatty acids
Corn, soybean, sesame, and safflower oils; plant foods; some seafood	Partially hydrogenated vegetable oils, beef, pork, lamb, dairy products, many fast foods and baked goods, including most commercially produced white breads
May lower blood cholesterol May lessen the risk of heart disease	Raises blood cholesterol May increase risk of heart disease
Choose more of your fat-containing foods from this list	Limit intake of foods from this list

Drinking and smoking together greatly increase the risk of mouth, throat, and esophagus cancers compared to drinking or smoking alone. Certainly other hazards are associated with drinking as well, including alcoholism, binge drinking, violence, liver damage, and social problems.

There's a big difference between someone who enjoys an occasional glass of wine with dinner and the person who must drink daily. A good

Alcohol As a Direct Cause or Increased Risk for These Types of Cancer	Liver cancer, Oral cavity (mouth, tongue, and throat) cancers, Esophagus cancer, Breast cancer
Alcohol Suspected As a Likely Contributing Cause for These Types of Cancer	Colorectal cancer

frame of reference is two drinks for men and one drink for women per day.

Heavy drinking is also related to poor nutrition. People who drink large amounts of alcohol are susceptible to malnourishment. Alcohol provides "empty calories" in the form of carbohydrates that make the drinker feel full. Poor nutrition can lead to a weakened immune system, which may contribute not only to cancer but to other health problems as well.

Beyond increasing the risk for cancer, most people are aware that drinking can lead to other health problems. It is well known that alcohol can have serious effects on the liver, pancreas, and even the nervous system. It can increase blood pressure and can cause gastrointestinal bleeding. Excessive drinking can also have serious social and psychological consequences.

Some people should not drink alcohol at all. This includes children and adolescents, pregnant women, people taking certain prescription medications affected by alcohol (such as antidepressants), and those who are driving, operating machinery, or unable to limit themselves to moderate drinking.

For some people, especially men over fifty and women over sixty, the heart-protective benefits of *moderate* drinking may outweigh the risk of cancer. But there is no compelling reason for those who do not drink alcohol to start drinking. Discuss your risk factors for both heart disease and cancer with your health care team and make an informed decision about your own use of alcohol.

Water: The Essential Drink

Fluid loss throughout the day is normally about ten cups—from sweat, urine, air exchange (in the lungs), and bowel movements. This water must be replaced to maintain fluid balance. Food provides some water, but it's usually difficult to estimate how much. Thirst is your

Stay in Control: Some Tips to Avoid Drinking Too Much

- Quench your thirst before you drink an alcoholic beverage. Knocking back alcoholic drinks when you're thirsty can be dangerous because of the dramatic increase in alcohol levels in the bloodstream.

- Order water or other nonalcoholic drinks at the same time as your alcoholic beverage. (Staying hydrated also prevents hangover effects the next day.)

- Sip your drink slowly.

- Try a nonalcoholic beer or wine. Soft drinks, as well as club soda or sparkling water with lemon or lime, are always an acceptable choice at any social function.

- If you drink heavier in the company of certain people, try to avoid or limit social situations where you know they will be.

- Order a diluted drink, such as a mixed drink with less alcohol or a wine spritzer.

body's way of telling you that you are dehydrated (although older individuals are less aware of thirst). A lack of concentration and energy is a common side effect of even slight dehydration.

Drinking plenty of liquids is very important to good health, and your body must have water to live and carry out its normal functions. The cells in our body are about 70 percent water. Drinking enough water helps us maintain muscle tone, keeps skin soft, lubricates joints and organs (providing protection), regulates body temperature, and discards wastes. And these are just a few of the many ways that water is essential to life.

Dieters sometimes think they can drink away their food cravings with water. Or they think drinking a glass of water before a meal staves off hunger. While that's actually not true (water does not take up a lot of volume in the stomach), foods high in water content are good for increasing volume — leading to a fuller sensation in the stomach. Juicy fruits such as grapefruits and oranges contain larger amounts of water.

Eating water-rich foods can lower the number of calories you take in during a meal. Such foods are water-based soups, for example. Start your meal with a hearty tomato soup made with water, and you'll feel full and satisfied on fewer calories. Water-based soups usually contain less fat than cream-based ones. Other ways to put water into your meals are by eating pasta salad or chili bulked up with vegetables and beans or adding lettuce and tomato to a sandwich. A bowl of grapes will be much more satisfying than a handful of raisins and will make you feel much more full, in addition to supplying water to your diet.

Drinking water during the day may also have other health benefits, such as decreasing the chances of developing kidney stones or urinary tract infections. Recent studies have suggested that drinking more liquids might lower the risk of bladder and colon cancer, although these effects will need to be confirmed with further research.

Eight glasses of water a day is a good rule of thumb, but your body has its own needs, and the amount varies depending on your weight and level of activity. People who live in high altitudes or in hot, humid conditions certainly need to drink more fluid. For a good estimate of how much water you need each day, divide your body weight (in pounds) in half. The result is the approximate number of ounces of water you should drink daily. You can include fluids other than water, but do *not* count alcoholic beverages and caffeinated drinks. They can actually cause fluid loss through urination.

What's Your Alternative?

Many complementary and alternative therapies claiming to prevent cancer involve specific foods or nutritional supplements. However, increasing scientific evidence suggests that a diet high in fruits, vegetables, and whole grain products can help protect the human body against cancer. These foods contain enough vitamins and minerals necessary for normal growth and development, health, and well-being, without the need for additional supplemental products.

It is strongly recommended that you check with your doctor before taking any herbs, botanical teas, vitamin supplements containing doses above the daily value (formerly known as the recommended daily allowance or RDA), or other dietary supplements, particularly if you are being treated for a medical condition. If you are taking medication, serious interactions may occur. Contact the ACS for more information about complementary and alternative cancer methods.

Definition of Terms

Although complementary and alternative methods have been around for a long time, they have grown in popularity in recent years. The words *complementary* and *alternative* are often used interchangeably; however, there are very important distinctions between the two terms.

- *Complementary therapies* are those that patients use *along with* conventional medicine and practices. *Complementary* refers to supportive methods that are used to complement, or add to, mainstream treatments. Examples might include dietary supplements, massage therapy, or meditation. *Integrative therapy* is a term that refers to the combining of evidence-based mainstream and complementary therapies.

- *Alternative therapies* are unproven treatments that people use *instead of* conventional therapy in an attempt to prevent, lessen, or cure disease.

They are considered unproven because they have not been scientifically tested; or they were tested and found to be ineffective or less effective than conventional treatment; or the test results were inconclusive. Alternative therapies may be harmful in and of themselves or because they are used instead of conventional means.

Supporters may claim that different complementary or alternative methods have a direct effect on different types of cancer. For example, based on results from an animal study, ginseng is sometimes promoted as an herbal remedy for preventing lung cancer. Garlic is sometimes said to reduce the risk of stomach and colon cancers. Some claim that drinking green tea can help prevent prostate, stomach, and esophageal cancers. In many cases, these claims are based on animal or laboratory studies or comparisons of populations in different regions of the world, but they have not been confirmed to be effective in humans through controlled clinical trials.

The establishment of the Office of Alternative Medicine within the National Institutes of Health (NIH) was a major step by the U.S. Government toward objective evaluation of complementary and alternative therapies. Today, this Office has been elevated to a National Center within the NIH and renamed the National Center for Complementary and Alternative Medicine. The Center is responsible for providing oversight to government-sponsored research into specific therapies.

Dietary Supplements

This category of foods has received a tremendous amount of attention over the past decade. What exactly is a dietary supplement? If you take a vitamin regularly, you are taking a dietary supplement. That is, you are adding something to your diet of foods, most likely in an attempt to make up for a less-than-perfect diet, to promote good health, or to help speed healing when illness strikes.

The term *dietary supplement* includes vitamins, minerals, herbs, amino acids, and other products that, according to current regulations, are not considered to be "drugs." Dietary supplements are sold in grocery stores, health food shops, drug stores, and national discount chain stores and through mail-order catalogs, television programs, the Internet, and direct sales. Vitamins are the supplements most often purchased in this country.

The category of dietary supplements also includes botanical products such as herbal remedies, skin care products, and oils, teas, or capsules, which are derived from a part or multiple parts of a plant. It is estimated that nearly 80 percent of the world's population currently uses herbals as medicine for some aspect of health care.

In many countries other than the United States, botanicals are sold as drugs and undergo certain regulatory requirements. In the U.S., botanicals are sold as dietary supplements and regulated in much the same way as food products. They are self-prescribed and can be purchased in the same locations as vitamins and minerals.

Only a few special groups of people need dietary supplements in addition to a balanced diet. These include pregnant and breast-feeding women, young children, vegans (people who eliminate all meat and dairy from their diets), alcoholics, and people who are frail or ill and unable to eat normally. Women may also benefit from taking calcium supplements to help prevent osteoporosis. However, it is dangerous to take a single supplement (whether it is an herb, vitamin, or mineral) in excess beyond the recommended dosage. If you have a serious problem or illness related to the use of a supplement, you should call your doctor immediately. You or your doctor can report the adverse reaction to the Food and Drug Administration (FDA) at 800-FDA-1088 or http://www.fda.gov/medwatch.

Buyer Beware

Unlike prescription and over-the-counter products with standard labeling and regulation, dietary supplements are not regulated as drugs by the FDA, nor are they required to live up to high standards set for these items. Dietary supplements are defined as a separate category of foods in the 1994 Dietary Supplement Health and Education Act. Manufacturers do not need to show proof of safety or proof that the product provides a health benefit, and they are not even required to list the amount of ingredients on labels. In other words, manufacturers of a dietary supplement (such as a vitamin or herbal product) can make certain types of health claims on the label without having to prove them.

What's Safe: Nine Common-Sense Guidelines When Using Dietary Supplements

Rule One: Investigate before you buy or use. There are many resources in libraries and on the Internet. However, promoters produce much of this information, so it may contain biased or incorrect information. Rely on materials from a trained expert or government agency.

Rule Two: Check with your doctor before you try a dietary supplement. He or she may or may not be thoroughly versed in all of the product areas, but your doctor may be able to prevent you from making a dangerous mistake.

Rule Three: Do not take any self-prescribed remedy instead of the medicine prescribed by your doctor without discussing it first.

Rule Four: Try one new product at a time. Be alert to any negative effects you experience while taking the product. Any product that produces a rash or a feeling of sleeplessness, restlessness, anxiety, gastrointestinal disturbance (nausea, vomiting, diarrhea, or constipation), or severe headache should immediately be stopped, and the reaction should be reported to your doctor.

There is a great need for public protection and consumer awareness in the area of dietary supplements. A "buyer beware" caution is needed when it comes to nutritional supplements and herbal medicines. Prescription medication can interact with supplements. Potential drug-supplement dangers include affecting the way drugs exert their activity on the body, either by increasing the drug's activity or by blocking it. Furthermore, many dietary supplements contain ingredients that can cause adverse side effects or allergic reactions by themselves. Taking

Rule Five: Avoid any dietary supplements not prescribed by a licensed doctor or nurse during pregnancy or if you are breast-feeding. Few, if any, of these products have been studied for safety, and their effects on the growing fetus are largely unknown.

Rule Six: Do not depend on any nonprescription product to cure cancer or any other serious disease. Regardless of the claims you might hear, "if it sounds too good to be true, it probably is." Some signs of possible fraudulent products include claims of a "miracle cure," that the product can be used for multiple conditions, or that it is based on a "secret" ingredient or method.

Rule Seven: Never give a product to a baby or child under eighteen years of age without consulting a doctor first. Their bodies metabolize nutrients and drugs differently than an adult's body, and the effects of many products, including supplements, in children are not known.

Rule Eight: Always read the label on the bottle first. Are you buying what you think you are? Are there any added ingredients? How do you know what dose to take? Overdoses could be deadly. Do not take a dietary supplement any longer than experts recommend.

Rule Nine: Try to avoid mixtures or combinations. The more ingredients, the greater the possibility for harmful effects.

combinations of dietary supplements could be even more dangerous. Pharmaceutical companies do not usually conduct research on drug-supplement interactions, and dietary supplement manufacturers generally do not have the resources to perform that kind of research. The burden of responsibility is left to you—the consumer.

The challenge to consumers is to determine which products are safe and which are not. You should read the product label to be sure you are purchasing what you are intending. If a label on a dietary supplement makes a claim that the product can diagnose, treat, cure, or prevent disease, the product is being sold illegally as a drug.

Cancer Risk and the Foods You Choose

When you go to the grocery store, what determines which foods you buy? According to the Shopping for Health 2000 survey by the Food Marketing Institute, more than 70 percent of consumers fill their grocery carts with foods they think will reduce their risk of specific illnesses. And more than nine out of ten people surveyed think, and correctly so, that fruits, vegetables, and grains contain natural substances that can help reduce the risk of diseases such as cancer.

Overall, about one-third of all cancers deaths are diet related—what you eat, how much you eat, what you don't eat. In fact, nutrition has been implicated as an important factor in several types of cancer (see pages 76–77, "Can Diet and Activity Reduce Your Risk of Cancer?"). There are many dietary factors that may affect cancer risk: the types of foods eaten, the way the food is prepared and stored, the amount eaten, the variety of foods, and the overall balance of calories.

A smart plan would be to fill your plate with foods that can reduce your risk and avoid foods that increase your risk for cancer and other diseases.

Your Weight and Your Health

*We've adopted a fast-food, high-fat diet
to complement our fast-paced, high-stress lifestyles.*
—COLLEEN DOYLE, M.S., R.D., Director of Nutrition and
Physical Activity for the American Cancer Society

Food, in its basic sense, is fuel. Our bodies are like machines. They need food for energy and normal body functions—it is a necessity. Yet over time, food has taken on a totally different meaning. For example, delicacies such as chocolate and ice cream were at one time reserved for royalty or special occasions. Today, those foods are accessible and, in fact, are staples in some households. "Ritual feasts" such as Thanksgiving give us a reason to stuff ourselves. Advertisements equate burgers, fries, and beer to having a good time.

Because we live in a time of plenty, people use food for comfort or reasons other than need. Increasingly, Americans "live to eat" and not "eat to live." This is due to greater availability of food and drink, foods with higher calorie and fat content, and the growth of the fast-food and snack-food industries. Admittedly, eating fast food and prepackaged or processed foods is easy, convenient, and timesaving, but eating healthfully can be the same way if you form and adopt good habits.

The problem with eating too much, eating an unhealthy diet, and getting little or no exercise is that excess calories are stored as body fat. The combination of too many calories and a low activity level can lead to being overweight. Complex interactions among diet, metabolism, physical activity, hormones, and growth factors become altered when a person becomes more than overweight and becomes obese. And being overweight or obese is associated with serious health problems such as cancer, heart disease, stroke, respiratory problems, sleep apnea, and type II diabetes, as well as other conditions.

Can Diet and Activity Reduce Your Risk of Cancer?

Type of Cancer	Convincing Evidence of Reducing Cancer Risk
Colorectal cancer	Physical activity Avoiding being overweight
Breast cancer	Physical activity Avoiding being overweight
Prostate cancer	
Lung cancer	
Stomach cancer	
Oral and esophageal cancer	Limiting alcohol intake
Bladder cancer	
Pancreatic cancer	
Endometrial cancer	Avoiding being overweight

As early as the 1940s, researchers found that laboratory animals that were placed on calorie-restricted diets appeared to be less likely to develop cancer. More recently, an ACS study published in the *New England Journal of Medicine* reported that heavier men and women in all age groups had an increased risk of death and that the heaviest individuals had a 40 to 80 percent increased risk of dying from cancer.

Probable Evidence of Reducing Cancer Risk	Possible Evidence of Reducing Cancer Risk
Eating lots of fruits and vegetables Limiting intake of red meats	Limiting alcohol intake
Limiting alcohol intake	Eating lots of fruits and vegetables
	Eating lots of fruits and vegetables Limiting intake of red meats
Eating lots of fruits and vegetables	
Eating lots of fruits and vegetables	
Avoiding being overweight Eating lots of fruits and vegetables	
	Eating lots of fruits and vegetables
	Eating lots of fruits and vegetables Limiting intake of red meats Limiting alcohol intake Avoiding being overweight
Physical activity	Eating lots of fruits and vegetables

Being Overweight Versus Obese — What's the Difference?

Except for smoking, obesity is now the number one preventable cause of death in this country.
— DR. C. EVERETT KOOP, former U.S. Surgeon General

Because Americans eat more now than ever, the average body weight has increased over the past twenty years. In fact, more than 55 percent of American adults are now overweight, and nearly 25 percent are obese. Overweight refers to an excess of body weight compared to set standards (see body mass index on page 80). The excess weight may come from muscle, bone, fat, and/or body water. Obesity is determined by excess body fat, not just excess weight. It specifically refers to having an abnormally high proportion of body fat.

Obesity among Americans is an epidemic. Even though the prevalence of obesity for both men and women has increased in recent years regardless of age, race, marital status, education level, or leisure time activity, women are more likely to be overweight or obese than men. Similarly, obesity in American children and teens has also increased throughout the 1990s.

Poor habits in childhood, such as reliance on soft drinks, are often difficult to change as children grow into adulthood. So children who are overweight may be at an even greater risk for adult obesity.

Obesity and the Risk of Cancer

Several types of cancer are associated with being obese. For obese women, their risk increases for breast cancer (particularly among postmenopausal women) and for cancer of the endometrium. Cancers more common in all obese people include colon, esophagus, gallbladder, pancreas, and kidney cancer. Evidence is accumulating that being overweight or obese may increase the risk of other cancers as well.

Where Do You Fit In?

Weight is a very individual thing. Many factors influence your weight, including genes (which play a direct role in determining your height, body frame, and shape), activity level, age, and the amount and type of foods you eat. Because these factors vary from person to person, your weight by itself may not be a good indicator of your risk for disease. You can use a number of different methods, other than simply looking in the mirror, to determine if you are overweight or obese and therefore at increased risk of disease and disability.

Body Shape and Weight Distribution

Apple and *pear* are the descriptions of body shape often used by health care professionals to determine your risk for future disease. Apple refers to a top-heavy body shape, in which a larger distribution of fat exists above your hips. Fat in this area appears to increase a person's risk of diabetes, high cholesterol, and cardiovascular disease. Men are more likely to have apple-shaped body types. Pear-shaped people, mostly women, have extra weight on their hips and thighs. This type of body shape or weight gain poses less of a concern for risks of certain diseases. Although you cannot control how fat is stored in your body, if you have an apple-shaped physique, you will need to make sure you stay fit by getting plenty of exercise and eating a healthy diet.

Waist Circumference

The amount of fat around your abdomen can be an important aspect in determining your risk of disease. The waist-to-hip ratio classifies fat deposition into two patterns, as do the apple or pear descriptions, but the ratio uses a formula to identify people with higher risk of disease. To find your waist-to-hip ratio, use a measuring tape and measure the distance around your waist and then around your hips. Divide the number of inches around your waist by the number of inches around your hips, using the following formula:

$$\textbf{Waist-to-Hip Ratio} = \frac{\text{Waist size (inches)}}{\text{Hip size (inches)}}$$

Lower ratios are better for health. Ratios higher than 0.8 for women and 1.0 for men are associated with increased health risks (such as heart disease).

Skinfold Thickness

Using calipers (an instrument that measures thickness), a health care professional can measure your skin-to-skin thickness and the amount of fat in select areas, such as the back of the arm, front of the leg, shoulder blades, and waist. Some health clubs and fitness centers offer this type of body fat measurement as part of an overall fitness assessment. Make sure whoever performs this measurement is well trained in the technique and explains what your results mean.

Body Mass Index (BMI)

Body mass index or BMI is probably the single best indicator of the amount of body fat. It is a formula that uses weight and height to determine levels of body fat for adults aged twenty and older.

Body mass index is really a ratio of your weight to your height. You can't change your height, so the only number you can really modify is your weight (especially if the ratio is not within the healthy range of 18.5 to 25 kg/m²). Technically, BMI is your weight in kilograms divided by your height in meters squared. Put away your slide rules and use the chart on page 81.

Your Game Plan for Success

Today is the day that you keep putting off.
—Unknown

For many of us, changing what we eat comes about by learning more about good foods and then making a conscious decision to eat differently. The combination—increasing food knowledge followed by actively adopting new habits—will only happen if you are motivated.

If you don't smoke cigarettes, then the most important lifestyle choices in lowering your cancer risk come from what you choose to eat and whether you get enough physical activity. These behavioral factors do

Are You at a Healthy Body Weight?

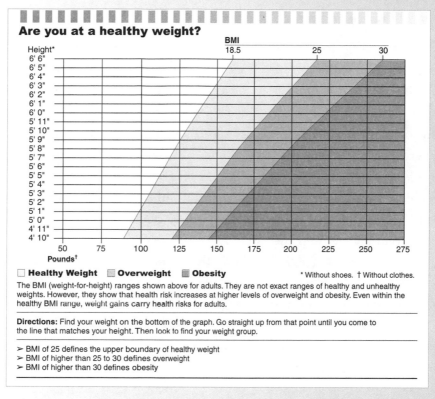

Are you at a healthy weight?

Healthy Weight ☐ Overweight ☐ Obesity ■

* Without shoes. † Without clothes.

The BMI (weight-for-height) ranges shown above for adults. They are not exact ranges of healthy and unhealthy weights. However, they show that health risk increases at higher levels of overweight and obesity. Even within the healthy BMI range, weight gains carry health risks for adults.

Directions: Find your weight on the bottom of the graph. Go straight up from that point until you come to the line that matches your height. Then look to find your weight group.

➤ BMI of 25 defines the upper boundary of healthy weight
➤ BMI of higher than 25 to 30 defines overweight
➤ BMI of higher than 30 defines obesity

Table reprinted from *The Report of the Dietary Guidelines Advisory Committee on the Dietary Guidelines for Americans, 2000,* United States Department of Agriculture.

Keep in mind that people who are over the normal weight limits for their group but are very muscular are not necessarily overweight. Likewise, those at or below the weight standard for their height may have excessive body fat and little muscle. Ideally, it's best to maintain a healthy weight throughout life, with a BMI below 25, but studies show that significant health benefits can be had by losing as few as ten to twenty pounds.

indeed make a difference in your cancer risk, and the ACS guidelines concerning nutrition and physical activity discussed in this book can be used as your roadmap to healthy living.

Take It One Bite at a Time

You don't have to submit yourself to a drastic name-brand diet to change your eating habits. If you set realistic goals, you are more likely to be successful. Many people think they have to give up everything—chocolate, French fries, and fast food. But moderation is the key word; cut down and attempt to make those changes slowly over time and not overnight. Don't quit "cold turkey." Instead of eating a piece of chocolate every day at 3 P.M., eat a half piece, and on some days eat a piece of fruit in its place. An occasional fast food is okay but not every day. Eating healthy is often viewed negatively because people feel they have to give up everything they like. And this just isn't so.

Making the choice to buy—and then prepare and eat—healthful foods is the next step. If you set short-term goals for changing your diet and tackle them one at a time, you might very well be successful. Here's why.

Researcher Tracy Sbrocco, Ph.D., Co-Director of the Uniformed Services University Weight Management Program, suggests that you don't have to worry so much about weight. Just make very small, permanent changes in your behavior. For example, if you usually eat two donuts with your morning coffee, try eating just one donut for a week. Okay, you can do that. No scales, no special shopping lists, no food deprivation. Get used to this little change and keep it up. The next week, switch from 2% milk to 1%. Eventually, you'll make another switch to skim milk. Simple. Another small step in a healthy direction. How about a piece of fruit with every lunch? One scoop of ice cream instead of two? Splitting a ten-ounce steak with a friend? Make it a regular practice to order your salad dressing on the side and use just half.

These small changes build slowly over time to become natural, normal behavior. All are designed to lower your caloric intake and will eventually help you lose—and keep off—weight. Use the food diary described below to decide which behavior changes you can make and maintain—one at a time.

Your Food Diary

There are no junk foods, only junk diets.
—ANN GRANDJEAN, PH.D., Executive Director,
Center for Human Nutrition, University of Nebraska Medical Center

A stick of gum after lunch, a handful of potato chips while making dinner, a soft drink during a mid-afternoon work break, a late-night refrigerator raid—these are the items we forgot we ate because they weren't part of a planned meal or eaten during a regular meal time. Most of us would be amazed to learn what we actually put into our mouths in the course of a day.

The best way to get an accurate picture of what (and how much) you eat and drink is to write it down. A food diary is a record of everything you eat and drink for a day (or longer). The idea is to write down not only everything you eat and drink but when and how much, as well as a description of the circumstances surrounding your food and drink intake. Try to be as detailed as possible and include how the food was prepared, quantity in terms of estimated cups and tablespoons, condiments you added, nutritional supplements such as vitamins or calcium, candy or gum, and anything else. You may find that keeping track of what you eat makes you more conscious of your eating habits and food choices on your plate.

If you are motivated, you can calculate the number of calories and fat grams you consumed. Without any complicated calculations, you can look at your diary and see where you can cut back or improve your choices, such as eating more foods from plant sources.

Time	Food/Drink	Amt/Portion	Extras	Amt	Preparation
7:30 AM	coffee	1 cup (8 oz.)	sugar; half & half	2 Tbsp. each	
8:20 AM	yogurt	6 oz.			
	cinnamon-blueberry bread	1 slice			homemade
10:25 AM	banana water	1 2 cups			
12 noon	bread water refill	½ slice 2 cups			homemade
1:00 PM	soup crackers lentil soup cup	2 servings 10 fl oz.			add hot water
1:30 PM	orange	1			
2:00 PM	sugar cookies	1½			
	water refill	2 cups			
3:00 PM	chocolate	2 pieces			
6:00 PM	crackers	½ cup			
8:30 PM	rice chicken breast dijon sauce	1 cup 1 breast ½ cup			browned in olive oil ½ cup of water, dijon mustard, onions—peeled & raw
	cucumbers	1 cup	sauce: mayo, sour cream, dill, salt & pepper	2 Tbsp.	
	juice	2 cups			

* *This is a sample of a diary for an average size woman.*

Total Servings: Bread/Cereal = approx. 6, Fruits/Vegetables = 5, Meat/Poultry = 2.5, Dairy = 1, Fat/Oil = approx. 1, Liquids = 9 cups (not including coffee)

Emotions/Setting	Additional Comments	Food Group	Serving	Liquids
drank while commuting	routine one cup of coffee to get me going in the AM	Fat/Oil Sugar; Dairy	½	1 cup
ate yogurt because it was getting warm ate at desk		Dairy	1	
		Bread/Cereal	1	
	hungry! keep cup at desk	Fruit/ Veg	1	2 cups
ate at desk	hungry!	Bread/Cereal	½	2 cups
ate at desk ate at desk	1 serv = 60 cal; 1.5 g fat 250 cal; 2 g fat	Bread/Cereal Meat?	2 ½	1 cup
ate at desk still hungry		Fruit/ Veg	1	?
crave sweets after lunch	110 cal; 5 g fat	Bread/Cereal	¾	2 cups
craving sweets	chocolates	Fat/Oil	½	
munchies after work	1 serv = 150 cal	Bread/Cereal	1	
ate in front of TV		Bread/Cereal Meat/Poultry Fat/Oil	1 2 ½	
		Fruit/Veg	1	
				2 cups

How can I improve my diet today? <u>Eat more fruits and vegetables; eat better quality bread/ cereal products; reduce sugar intake.</u>

Tips for Keeping a Food Diary

- Write down *anything* that goes in your mouth. Don't forget candy, lozenges, gum, breath mints, vitamins, and other supplements— ANYTHING.

- Try to keep your diary with you at all times and fill it out immediately after each meal, drink, or snack.

- Note the time the item was consumed.

- Indicate how the food was prepared: raw, broiled, fried, steamed, and so on. Be as detailed as possible. Write down things such as the type of bread (wheat, rye, white) or type of dairy product (2%, skim, fat-free).

- Note the amount of your portions in cups, tablespoons, or serving size as listed on a food label.

- Include items you add to your food and drinks, such as sugar, sauce, dressing, butter, cheese, ketchup, mayonnaise, toppings, gravy, and so on.

- Consider allowing space to write additional comments, such as these:

  Specific ingredients added to fat content: vegetables sautéed in butter, skin on chicken, or casserole made with cheese, for example

  Information from product packaging, such as fat, cholesterol, or sodium

  Your emotions surrounding the consumption of the food, whether or not you felt full before or after you ate it, enjoyment or dislike, the setting, and so on

  Cravings you encounter throughout the day

- You may want to place the foods you eat into food groups and keep track of the number of servings you eat from each.

- Keep a running tab of how much water, juice, or milk you drink. Caffeinated soft drinks, tea, and coffee should also be recorded, but remember that these items actually dehydrate the body and don't count toward your recommended eight glasses of water per day.

Are You Ready?

It's never too late to change your dietary habits. Results from your efforts will be felt, if not seen, almost immediately. Eating a healthy diet—low in animal fat, high in whole grains, and rich in fruits and vegetables—can give you a real sense of satisfaction. People who change their eating habits for the better often report having more energy, increased concentration, improved mood, and an overall better feeling about their health and themselves. Your outlook and attitude can also affect the people around you—your family, coworkers, and friends. Encourage them to join your healthy lifestyle.

Please note that we did not discuss any particular diet or diet plan in this entire chapter. Tens of millions of Americans are dieting at any given time and spending millions on weight-reduction products such as diet foods and drinks. The key is to focus less on "dieting" and more on healthy eating. Popular diets and diet books are quick fixes; they all work in the short term, but they're not healthy and can do major damage to your body. Truly the best solution is smart eating and making wise food choices taken in small steps.

Let's be realistic. No diet or lifestyle change can guarantee protection against disease. But it is safe to say that a combination of a variety of healthy foods, maintaining a healthy weight, and regular physical activity lowers cancer risk and contributes to overall good health.

Eating Right Can Start with Small Steps — Right Now

- Identify where you need improvement, and note your strengths as well. Use your food diary to help in this assessment.

- Start making changes in the most comfortable way possible. Give yourself plenty of time to make small steps toward small goals.

- You may want to pick an eating habit in which you can be successful and conquer it first, and then move on to the bigger challenges. As you achieve each goal, make more changes.

- Think "variety, balance, and moderation" for your overall diet.

- Include snacks and treats in your diet. But remember that moderation is the key.

- Make food choices that match your lifestyle and balance the food groups within your diet.

- Ask for help from a professional if you need it. Registered dietitians, certified nutritional experts, and your health care team can provide additional guidance.

CHAPTER 3

How to Get Yourself Moving One Step at a Time

Everyone should walk their dog thirty minutes a day,
whether you have one or not.
—KENNETH COOPER, M.D., M.P.H.

If a Fountain of Youth truly exists, then you can find it at your local gym, neighborhood park, shopping center, walking and bike paths, or anywhere people go for activity. Even your own garden or home treadmill will do. Whatever you call it—exercise, movement, activity, or physical fitness—all are names for exerting your body in the name of health.

Defining the "E" Word

Our view of exercise is changing. It's no longer limited to gyms, Spandex, or exercise machines. The Office of the Surgeon General promotes a kinder, gentler exercise in the form of physical activity and movement. Regular physical activity is fundamental to healthy living. This is not a secret.

One thing we do know is that a lack of physical activity directly contributes to the development of chronic illness and to being overweight. We've become a nation of "watchers" rather than "doers." Indeed, Yankee Stadium replaced its seats with bigger seats, and it wasn't because they wanted to give their diehard fans more "elbow" room. Nature's own Fountain of Youth—physical activity—is part of the solution along with diet.

So the big question is, "What's holding us back from physical activity?" and more importantly, "What's holding *you* back from putting more movement into your day?" In this chapter, you'll learn what might motivate you for long-term success and why your previous attempts at activity may not have worked.

Physical activity is a close second to nutrition as a step on the path to healthy living. And it may also reduce your risk of cancer. Throughout this chapter, you'll find out the benefits of physical activity and how this essential daily habit can turn your health around. You may wish to take the informative fitness quiz at the beginning of this chapter to assess your current activity level. It will also help you to choose the right activities for you and guide you toward starting and maintaining an exercise program you'll enjoy.

Take heart, literally! The good news is that even if you start physical activity later in life, you can still get many of the same benefits as if you've been exercising your whole life. So, if you're asking yourself, "When is the best time to start getting active?" The answer is a resounding "Now!"

Where Do You Stand?

Do you wonder just how fit you are right now? Using the short and simple quiz on pages 92–95, you can rate your current fitness level, identify areas where you can improve (which we'll discuss later), and calculate future goals. A word of caution: the quiz is not intended to be a substitute for professional medical advice or consultation, diagnosis, or treatment.

Fit Facts

Physical Activity Lowers Cancer Risk

Physical activity throughout life can help protect against some cancers by burning off excess calories and preventing weight gain, by affecting hormone levels, and by other ways that are currently being studied.

Too many calories and lack of physical activity can lead to excess weight or obesity and to an increased risk for cancers at several sites, including colon, prostate, endometrium, breast (among postmenopausal women), cervix, ovary, and gallbladder. Research has shown that the risk of cancer at many of these sites is reduced in people who exercise. Physical activity may also influence the risk for cancer of the kidney, pancreas, rectum, esophagus, and liver, but more research is needed in these areas.

For breast cancer, physical activity may help regulate hormone levels and reduce the risk slightly. In a recent study, researchers looked at strenuous physical activity during adolescent years and how it affected breast cancer risk later in life. Among women who had not gained weight later in life, those who were active in their teenage years were only about half as likely to develop breast cancer after menopause, when compared to those who were inactive.

But what if you haven't been active your whole life?

There's encouraging news. A study by Dutch researchers found that active women had a 30 percent lower risk of breast cancer when compared to those who were inactive. So what does all this mean? Exercising on a regular basis appears to matter more than the age at which a woman started exercising. If you need some motivation to start, here it is. If you're already active, even better!

Take the Fit Test

Place a check mark next to your current fitness level by answering the following questions. For some of the questions, you may need to estimate what you think your ability is. Be as honest as you can, and don't worry about your results just yet!

1. Cardiovascular capacity: What is your resting heart rate? The best time to determine resting heart rate is soon after waking up. Using a watch with a second hand, place your index and forefingers on a pulse point, such as your neck or wrist, and count the number of beats for one minute.

3 _____ 60 beats/minute or less
2 _____ 60–80 beats/minute
1 _____ 80 beats/minute or more

2. Flexibility: Bend at the waist and touch your toes, without bending your knees. How far can you reach?

3 _____ I can touch my toes or the floor easily.
2 _____ I can barely touch my toes.
1 _____ My fingers are a couple inches above my toes.

3. Strength: How many push-ups can you do continuously? Be sure to use proper form by keeping your back straight and abdominal muscles firm. Women may choose to do a modified form with their knees on the floor.

3 _____ 15 push-ups or more
2 _____ 10–15 push-ups
1 _____ Fewer than 10 push-ups

4. Balance: **Stand on one foot and close your eyes. How long can you hold this position?**

3 _____ 30 seconds or more
2 _____ 15–29 seconds
1 _____ Less than 15 seconds

5. Endurance: **How long does it take you to walk a mile?**

3 _____ 15 minutes or less
2 _____ 15–19 minutes
1 _____ 20 minutes or longer

6. Aerobic capacity: **If you were to walk up four flights of stairs, how winded would you feel?**

3 _____ I can speak easily.
2 _____ I usually need to catch my breath before I speak, but I recover quickly.
1 _____ I'm winded and breathing heavy. It takes a few minutes for me to catch my breath.
0 _____ I need to take a couple of breaks to get to the top. I'm too winded to talk.

(continued on page 94)

(continued from page 93)

7. Activity level: On average, how would you rate your activity level?
(Possible scenarios are in parentheses.)

3 _____ Extremely active (I have a physically active job and I exercise regularly.)

2 _____ Active (I am active at my job; I exercise regularly.)

1 _____ Average (I am physically active two to three days a week or on an irregular basis.)

0 _____ Inactive (I have a desk job and I do not exercise.)

8. Commitment: On average, how many times per week do you participate in an activity (other than an everyday activity) that raises your heart rate?

3 _____ 5 times or more per week

2 _____ 3 or 4 times per week

1 _____ 1 to 3 times per week

0 _____ I don't do anything to raise my heart rate.

9. Motivation: How important is it to you to increase your fitness level and improve your health?

3 _____ Very important; I make it a part of my day.

2 _____ Important; I need to do more.

1 _____ Somewhat important; I know I should do more.

0 _____ Not important; I don't really care, or I have good excuses not to do anything.

Count and Tally Your Answers:

_____ 3   _____ 2   _____ 1   _____ 0

What Your Answers Mean

If you answered 2 or 3 to most questions: You're on the right track! You know how important physical activity is to your health, and it is an established part of your lifestyle. Keep up the good work and continue reading for suggestions and tips to keep your motivation high.

If you answered 1 or 2 to most questions: You're in the middle of the road—you feel strongly about some areas of physical activity, but you need some consistency in your exercise regimen. You may be "hot and cold" in terms of participating in regular physical activity, and you may need to find better ways to motivate yourself. Read further to learn about how much physical activity you should be doing, how to get started, and tips and suggestions for maintaining a regular program of physical activity.

If you answered 0 or 1 to most questions: It's not too late to get moving! You should incorporate more activity in your lifestyle. Don't worry—you're certainly not alone. Over 60 percent of American adults get less than the recommended amount of physical activity per day. The good news is that you only need thirty minutes per day of moderate to vigorous activity to get into better shape and improve your fitness level. You might also need some tips on getting started and suggestions for maintaining your level of physical activity. Keep reading to find out more!

NOTE: This quiz is intended to be used for informational purposes only. Scoring and results are not based on scientific research.

Researchers don't fully understand why physical activity may lower the risk of breast cancer or why weight gain may counteract that effect. Some cancers, such as those of the breast, are responsive to estrogen and other hormones in the blood. One explanation is that physical activity may reduce the levels of these hormones; whereas, extra body fat leads to an increase in the body's production of estrogen, which could cancel out the beneficial effects of physical activity. Additional research is needed to determine how often and how much physical activity is needed to lower the risk, as well as if the intensity of activity plays a role.

There also appears to be a connection between physical activity and colon cancer. Researchers have found that people who are physically active have about half the risk of developing colon cancer compared to people who are sedentary. This may be related to the fact that physical activity stimulates movement through the bowel, reducing the length of time the bowel lining is exposed to potentially harmful substances.

All in all, active people come out the real winners in studies that look at the beneficial effects of regular and moderate physical activity. We'll define what regular and moderate activity means for you and show you some clever ways to work activity into your day.

The Hidden Benefits of Physical Activity

Regular physical activity provides a number of benefits other than reducing your risk for cancer. These benefits, in and of themselves, are reason enough to figure out ways to put activity into your daily routine.

- **Reduces your risk for other major health problems:** Regular physical activity reduces your risk of developing heart disease, diabetes, and high blood pressure. It also indirectly reduces the risk of stroke by lowering blood pressure and increasing "good" cholesterol levels.

- **Builds strong bones:** Physical activity strengthens bones and reduces the risk of osteoporosis in women by increasing bone density. For all adults, being active builds healthy muscles, bones, and joints and reduces the risk of fractures.

- **Prevents back pain:** Activity can help prevent back pain by increasing muscle strength, flexibility, and posture, which are also beneficial for reducing the risk of injury, boosting coordination, and increasing productivity.

- **Controls your weight:** Regular physical activity aids in maintaining weight, controlling weight gain, and reducing the risk of becoming overweight or obese. A more muscular body is more efficient at burning fat and keeping it off.

- **Helps you manage stress:** Studies show that exercise enhances mental health, including reducing the incidence and severity of anxiety and depression and improving mood, attitude, and self-esteem. In other words, exercise enables you to reduce and manage stress levels better.

- **Boosts your immune system:** Regular and moderate physical activity enhances the work of your immune system, which in turn can have a positive effect on your health.

Physical activity may benefit certain people in surprising ways as well. Women who exercise vigorously while trying to quit smoking are twice as likely to remain smoke-free and gain about half the weight of those who do not exercise, according to a study in the *Archives of Internal Medicine*. People who exercise regularly also report fewer sleep-related problems.

Other health benefits—increased flexibility, muscular strength, and endurance—are side effects of fitness. Physically active people are better able to carry out daily activities, less likely to suffer from back pain, and enjoy enhanced coordination and balance. This translates into invaluable long-term advantages that include a reduced chance of disability and falls as you age.

Top 20 Reasons to Exercise

1. Strengthens heart muscle

2. Decreases risk for heart disease and heart attack

3. Improves circulation and oxygen/nutrient transport throughout the body

4. Helps lose weight and keep it off

5. Improves breathing efficiency

6. Strengthens and tones muscles and improves appearance

7. Helps prevent back problems and back pain

8. Improves posture

9. Strengthens bones and helps reduce risk of osteoporosis

10. Strengthens the tissues around the joints and reduces joint discomfort and arthritis if appropriate exercise is selected and properly performed

11. Decreases risk for several types of cancer

12. Improves immune function

13. Maintains physical and mental functions throughout the second half of life

14. Increases self-confidence and self-esteem

15. Boosts energy and increases productivity

16. Improves sleep

17. Helps create a positive attitude about life

18. Relaxes the mind and the body as well as reduces anxiety and depression

19. Increases resistance to fatigue

20. May lengthen lifespan

Reprinted from *Physical Fitness: Guidelines for Success* by permission of JoAnn Eickhoff-Shemek, Ph.D., and Kris Berg, Ed.D.

Adults Need Recess Too

Now that we know why we should exercise, let's look at the reasons why we don't. The evidence is overwhelming that Americans are not active, and that's why the Office of the Surgeon General has taken such a great interest in what might be a nationwide epidemic of inactivity.

As schoolchildren, we looked forward to recess. It was a break from reading and math. We went to playgrounds to play kickball or tag. Recess for our children is no longer the game-filled twenty minutes we remember. Many physical education (PE) classes have been cut for lack of funds, and also to sandwich more classroom time into a busy school day. In the work world, our breaks are often quick dashes to a food-filled vending machine, a quick cup of coffee, or no break at all.

Never mind the late-night comedians who joke about couch potatoes and their children (known as "tater tots"), physical inactivity has become a serious problem over the past fifteen years, nearly to the point of becoming a national crisis. The Office of the Surgeon General has reported that more than half of all Americans are not regularly physically active in their leisure time.

Adults Are Watching the World Grow Round

Leisure-time physical activity among adults varies by age, gender, race, and education level. The Centers for Disease Control and Prevention (CDC) conducts yearly surveys in several areas to assess general health trends in America. These interesting facts are among the findings of the most recent surveys.

- Men are more likely to participate in moderate leisure-time physical activity than women. (See page 121 for a definition of moderate activity.)

- People tend to gain weight after marriage.

Who Plays?

Adults

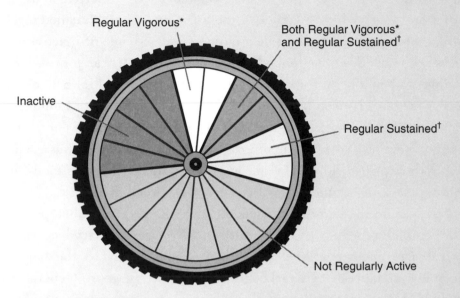

Regular Vigorous*

Both Regular Vigorous*
and Regular Sustained†

Inactive

Regular Sustained†

Not Regularly Active

* *Regular Vigorous – 20 minutes 3 times per week of vigorous intensity*
† *Regular Sustained – 30 minutes 5 times per week of any intensity*
Source: CDC 1992 Behavioral Risk Factor Survey

Reprinted from *1992 Behavioral Risk Factor Survey*. National Center for Chronic
Disease and Prevention and Health Promotion, Centers for Disease Control
and Prevention, U.S. Department of Health and Human Services.

- Young adults (eighteen to twenty-four years old) are more likely to
  engage in leisure-time physical activity than older adults (seventy-five
  years and older).

- College graduates (with sixteen or more years of education) are more
  likely to participate in leisure-time activity than adults with less than
  a ninth-grade education.

- White (non-Hispanic) adults are more likely to be physically active
  than American adults of other racial and ethnic groups.

Even though physical activity is widely accepted as good for overall health and well-being, Americans are increasingly less active. More adults in the United States are overweight than ever before. We're less active due in large part to a greater number of sedentary jobs, especially for those of us who sit in front of our computers all day and move a mouse around our desktop. We're not active in our work, and labor-saving devices at home mow our yards, wash our dishes, open our garage doors, and turn on our TVs and change the channels. Driving has long since replaced walking or biking as a way to get to the local "convenience" store. And leisure time is more often spent in front of the TV or computer, instead of on a bike or family walk.

Children and Young Adults Need to Get Out More

Life has changed. Children no longer walk to school or walk home from school. They often stay after school in child-care programs until working parents pick them up and drive them home. At home, with homework out of the way, many kids turn on the TV, the video games, or the computer, and spend the rest of the evening instant messaging their friends or talking on the phone while lying on their beds.

For many children and adolescents, electronic interaction has replaced many activities that used to involve physical activity, and the

Did You Know . . . ?

One in four adults in the U.S. is not active at all.

More than 60 percent of U.S. adults do not meet the recommended levels of physical activity.

The populations that are the least active include women, African Americans and Hispanics, older adults, and the less educated.

Physical activity decreases with age.

only body part getting any physical exercise are fingers, mouths, eyes, and ears. Television watching now occupies the greatest amount of leisure time in childhood. Physical activity declines even further during adolescence when driving a car becomes a rite of passage, and the bike and in-line skates lie unused in the garage.

It's easy to think about encouraging children to get outside and skateboard or ride a scooter, but those activities are difficult if you live in an unsafe neighborhood, somewhere with high traffic, or simply have no time or daylight left after dinner and homework.

Weekend soccer tournaments, Little League, and T-ball are great activities, but they involve precious family time driving to and from practices and regular games. Busy working parents spend weekends behind the wheel chauffeuring kids to numerous activities but getting less activity themselves. Sometimes the best thing for a parent is not to take a folding chair and newspaper to the kids' baseball practice but to spend that hour walking around the field. Parents who drop kids off at the community recreational center for swimming lessons might consider taking a walk while their child practices.

Getting on the Right Track

"Society, of course, doesn't make exercise easy," according to Paul Ribisl, Ph.D., Chairman of the Department of Health and Exercise Science at Wake Forest University. "You can't find jobs today that require physical activity," he pointed out. "We've been so clever at taking physical activity *out* of our lives." We only need to consider the TV remote control or garage door opener for proof. Most Americans sit all day at work and move only their mouths and their fingers.

"We were given the gift of time and blew it," said Dr. Ribisl. "We've taken the drudgery out of housework and occupations, but we're too foolish to know that the time that was saved should be spent on family, friends, self-enrichment, and exercise. Our machine only works if you exercise it."

Yet we still complain about not having enough time. Only 10 to 20 percent of Americans make time to exercise at recommended levels—a vital component in weight loss and overall good health.

The whole idea behind health promotion programs in the community, at work, through your recreation center, and in some churches is gradual behavior change. All are designed to move you along the stages of change (as discussed in detail in Chapter 1) from just thinking about taking a walk to actually building a walk into your daily routine (or almost daily).

What would it take to move you from the stage of precontemplation (not even thinking about activity) into the stage of contemplation (knowing you need to begin an activity) and then into action (see Introduction)? If you don't go through the stages in progression, chances are you may easily become derailed. It's too big a leap to go from not even thinking about changing a behavior to the action stage.

A heart attack can be a huge motivator for people whose doctors prescribe exercise to reduce the risk of another heart attack. But, like any behavior change, needing to exercise when your life clearly depends on it may still not get you on the treadmill. It's a tough habit to start, even when your life is on the line, according to researchers in the National Exercise and Heart Disease Project. They found that it was difficult for people to maintain an exercise program even after suffering a heart attack.

Nobody said this stuff was easy.

Predicting Success and Staying on Track

The common get-fit-quick scenario goes like this: you look in the mirror and realize you should start exercising. Or, your doctor suggests that your current sedentary ways might pose some health problems for you. So you join a nearby fitness center and with all good intentions, you begin an exercise program. Within several months, you stop exercising. (We offer several common excuses and action steps in the next section.)

A year later you do it all over again. What went wrong here?

Here's what really predicts whether you'll be successful in your exercise endeavors, according to Jim Annesi, Ph.D., Director of Wellness Advancement for the Metro Atlanta YMCA.

- The amount of social support you receive from your spouse, a partner, your family, friends, or other exercisers.

- Your ability to set goals, to conduct positive self-talk, and to manage your new program.

- Your ability to tolerate *perceived* physical discomfort (some people incorrectly assume that exercise should be painful).

Physical gains may not be evident during the first three to six months. Simply getting activity into your schedule is the goal. Once this regular behavior becomes part of your routine, you'll start to see progress physically and mentally. Dr. Annesi estimates that only about 30 percent of new exercisers (and those who are trying again to develop an exercise habit) will continue to exercise for the long-term.

If you accept progress in small steps, and you equate your exercise to feeling great (you're feeling less tired, rejuvenated, sleeping better, and so on), then your chances for continued success are heightened. Whatever your reasons for continuing to exercise, the effects are reinforcing, and you'll keep coming back for more. At that point, you will have reached the "zone" or action stage, and you're feeling great about it.

Excuses, Excuses, Excuses ... What's Yours?

Until regular activity becomes a habit, you'll find it much easier to come up with excuses not to exercise. Weight increases with age until it levels off between the ages of fifty and sixty. Physical activity, on the other hand, usually decreases as you age. So you are often less active at a time in your life when you need it most. Whatever your age, your weight, your job, your situation, you'll find some reason not to exercise. Do any of the following excuses sound familiar?

"I Don't Have Time"

> *Exercise does not take time out of your life. It puts life into your time.*
> —LINDA MAXWELL

Not having enough time is the number one excuse people give. A common misconception is that exercise or physical activity has to be time-consuming because you have to fit it into your schedule or make time in your already hectic day, but most people can find twenty minutes here and there, and that's all it takes.

What's your answer to this question: How much TV do you watch daily? Sacrificing some TV time is a small price to pay for better health. Better yet, use TV time to walk on a treadmill, lift hand weights, or walk in place as you watch your favorite program. As a beginner, all you need is thirty minutes or more on five or more days of the week. And you don't have to do it all at once—you can space out your activity in twenty-minute segments at different times during the day.

Working Americans often use the "no time" excuse because they simply haven't figured out how to work physical activity into an eight-hour-plus workday.

You don't have to go to a gym to be active. Physical activity in small amounts throughout the day is better than none at all. Twenty minutes here or there—walking, gardening, or vacuuming the house after dinner—that's it. No showers. No sweat. But if you do get in a thirty- to forty-minute period of moderate physical activity, you'll lower your blood sugar, blood pressure, and cholesterol, according to one study. The benefits just keep on working.

Employers are recognizing the importance of activity and the return on investment in health care costs and productivity if their employees are active. That's why more and more companies are adding onsite fitness centers or organizing walking and other activity groups. Check into wellness activities in your workplace.

Your action step: Make an appointment with yourself. Put exercise on your to-do list and do it.

"It's Too Expensive"

Few people know how to take a walk. The qualifications are endurance,
plain clothes, old shoes, an eye for nature, good humor, vast curiosity,
good speech, good silence and nothing too much.
—RALPH WALDO EMERSON

If going to a fitness club or a gym is not your style or out of your budget, you can still get a healthy amount of physical activity on your own. You don't have to join an expensive gym or buy equipment or special clothes to become physically active. Those late-night infomercials touting the latest equipment to tighten your tummy can be tempting, but are you getting something you will use in the long run? Some people find these machines helpful, but you don't have to buy all sorts of exercise equipment to get in shape. What you really need you already have. You don't need an ab-anything to work your abdominal muscles. Simple crunches, done properly, are ideal.

Many activities such as walking, swimming, or dancing cost little or nothing. You just need a decent pair of shoes and someplace to go. Some employers even pay part of the cost if you join a nearby fitness center. Or, you can step along with the fitness programs on the exercise channel.

Your action step: Rent an exercise video at your neighborhood library or video store, or tape an early-morning exercise program and play it back before dinner.

"It's Always the Same Old Thing"

If you think you have to do the same activities over and over again to get your recommended amount of physical activity, think again. You will be more inclined to stick with your exercise program if you vary your activities. Athletes call it cross-training, and this technique really works. Plus you'll get the added benefit of strengthening more muscles in different ways.

Simply use a little creativity. Do you like to garden? Do you like to play basketball or softball? Do you have chores around the house, such as mowing the lawn, vacuuming, painting, or even walking the dog? These are all forms of physical activity. Minutes spent doing these activities count toward your thirty minutes of activity each day.

For people who are already active, try walking a different path or walk your regular route only go the other direction. Take a water aerobics class instead of your usual step routine. Sign up for a martial arts class or in-line skating. If you're a morning exerciser, try an evening workout.

Your action plan: Resolve to try something new and different.

"I'm Too Fat"

People who are overweight are usually not active, yet these people often benefit the most from moderate physical activity. Most overweight people who begin an exercise program see almost immediate results in their weight loss efforts, physical abilities, and energy levels. An added advantage of physical activity is that even if you are overweight, but active, your risk of developing cancer may be lower. The key to exercising if you are overweight is to *take it slowly* in the beginning. If you have concerns, physical limitations, or a serious medical condition, talk to your doctor before starting. Certain exercises, such as water-based activities, may be ideal for you.

Some movement is better than none. For example, a 150-pound person burns five calories per minute while walking. Compare that to the one calorie you burn sitting on the couch. Even if you get up to change channels on the TV instead of using the remote, you've become aware of the importance of movement, and you'll begin to add more activity to your everyday life.

Your action plan: Add one activity to your day.

"I'm Too Old"

You have to stay in shape. My grandmother started walking five miles a day when she was sixty. She's ninety-seven today and we don't know where she is.
— ELLEN DEGENERES

Whether you're forty, sixty, or even eighty years old, your age should not discourage you from being physically active. You can become physically active at any age, and movement can reduce the disabilities that commonly accompany aging. If you're younger, being active now will help you to maintain an active lifestyle well into your "golden" years. Those older than sixty-five may need longer periods of time to adapt to an exercise program, but both the healthy and frail elderly can make significant improvements in strength, muscle mass, and flexibility through resistance and strength training.

Your action plan: Age is a just state of mind, but start off slowly if you've been inactive for a while.

"I'm Too Tired"

Sure it's tough to be active when you feel as if you don't have any energy. But consider this: regular physical activity can actually increase your levels of energy. Active people say they feel as if they have more energy, increased concentration, and renewed vigor. This is probably because of a more efficient heart and greater oxygen circulation in the body.

When you're active, you sleep better. A recent study showed a strong correlation between regular physical activity (at least once a week) and reduced risk of sleep disorders. Daytime drowsiness was also reduced.

Your action plan: Replace that afternoon or after-dinner nap with a short walk.

"I'll Hurt Myself"

Most healthy people can safely start a physical activity regimen if they start slowly. Injuries happen when you do too much, too soon, if you don't warm up and cool down, or if you avoid stretching exercises. Injury is a frequent reason that stops regular exercise. So when you do start to become active, reduce your risk of getting hurt by *gradually* working up to your desired activity level.

Warm up to a walk with a casual stroll for a block or two (or walk slowly a few minutes on the treadmill), then start moving a little more and a little faster. Do the same with running. Start with a walk. Cool down the same way by powering down. Most organized exercise classes build in warmups and cool downs. If they don't, do it yourself.

Your action plan: Be kind to your body and work up to a workout.

"Sweating Isn't Cool"

Actually, sweating *is* cool. Your body is cooling itself off. And for most vigorous activities, sweating is an unavoidable consequence. You don't have to run a marathon to get the benefits of exercise. How much you sweat doesn't measure how vigorous the activity is, so don't feel that you need to really push it to get any benefit. Your heart rate is a much better measure of progress and keeps you in that moderate zone (see page 127).

Activities such as walking, biking, or climbing stairs do not necessarily imply "breaking a sweat," and you can scatter these activities throughout your day. As you become more accustomed to exercising, you may want to increase the amount of time and energy that you spend being active.

Wear light, not tight, clothing that is comfortable and airy to help your body stay cool. Just because you're exercising doesn't mean you have to invest in a large supply of tight workout clothes, especially if you don't feel comfortable in that type of clothing. Dress in layers and start peeling off jackets and sweatshirts as your body warms up.

Your action plan: Change your view of exercise from heart-pounding sweating to active movement in daily activities.

"But My Friends Don't Exercise"

It can be difficult to stay physically active when your friends and family are doing something else, like sitting in a lawn chair watching you wash the car. Why not use your new exercise program as a means to spend time with them, and for all of you to become more physically active together? By getting family and friends active, everyone can benefit from mutual encouragement and companionship. You'll also be less likely to stop being active. The alternative is to find friends who share your zest for activity. And you might meet some on the trails, or in the gym or wellness center.

Your action plan: Ask your spouse, a friend, neighbor, coworker, or child to join you in an activity you can both do together.

Reasons why . . .	
People stop exercising once they've started	Injury or illness
	Smoking
	Perceived barriers—health, weight, age
	Lack of trails, parks, or sidewalks
	Excessive television watching
	Bad weather
	Boredom and lack of variation
	Unsafe neighborhood
People continue to exercise	Having a friend or family member join them
	Confidence and enjoyment
	Low to moderate physical activities
	Goal setting and self-monitoring
	Physician recommendation
	Health benefits
	Trying new activities
	Self-esteem and encouragement from within

The Seven Myths About Exercise and Why You Shouldn't Believe Them

You've heard them all: *No pain, no gain. You can't be fat AND fit.* And the ever popular: *I'm afraid I'll look too muscular or bulky.*

Like urban legends circling the Internet, these myths about exercise make no sense when you understand the mechanics of exercise and why it works. Sad to say, many people use these myths as excuses not to exercise. Let's look at the big myths about exercise and put them to rest once and for all.

Myth 1: "I started exercising, but I didn't lose any weight. So I quit."

If you are within your weight recommendations or are underweight, you may not notice any weight loss. In fact, your appetite may increase to offset the calories you're burning. In some cases, weight gain comes in the form of muscle mass, not fat. If nothing else, you're in better shape, and there's a lot to say for that. Don't let the scale measure whether your activity is working.

Physical activity provides many benefits other than weight loss. In addition to possibly lowering your risk for cancer, diabetes, cardiovascular disease, and osteoporosis, you may also achieve relief from stress and depression, sleep better, and increase your muscle tone. In other words, you'll look better and feel great, even if you don't lose weight.

Myth 2: "Muscle weighs more than fat, and I don't want to gain weight."

It is true that muscle weighs more than fat. It's denser and more efficient (in other words, muscle is more metabolically active than fat). Moderate physical activity and light strength training boost your metabolism and increase your muscle mass so that you burn calories more efficiently. More muscle means a higher metabolism, which can lead to weight loss. Unless you're intentionally trying to "bulk up" through activities such as heavy weightlifting or bodybuilding, chances are you're not going to gain much weight in your muscles. And remember, you'll still be getting rid of excess fat. Again, your scale is not the best way to measure your progress. Judge by how you feel (and how your clothes fit).

Myth 3: "Exercising makes me hungrier, so I eat more."

Because metabolism increases with exercise, digestion occurs at a faster rate, which can leave you feeling hungry again. Dieting has the opposite effect of physical activity—it actually lowers your metabolism.

If weight loss is your goal, the combination of fewer calories and more physical activity is the best way to achieve that goal. Depriving yourself of necessary nutrients may leave you feeling weak or lightheaded, so use common sense to determine when and how much you should eat.

A study published in the *Journal of the American Medical Association* found that nearly 70 percent of American adults are trying to lose weight or maintain their weight. The reason many fail is because they are not following the recommended, time-tested safe guidelines of eating less and exercising more.

Myth 4: "You know what they say: no pain, no gain."

Who says you have to suffer to get in shape? Gain comes slowly, without pain, as your body starts to use the muscles in your body. You may have some muscle aches at first, but that may be because you're using muscles that haven't been active for a while. Moderately intense physical activity provides many of the same health benefits as vigorous exercise. If you don't overdo it, your gain can be painless.

Myth 5: "Middle-age spread is unavoidable."

You may notice subtle weight changes starting sometime in your mid-twenties to late thirties and eventually leveling off between the ages of fifty and sixty. As your metabolism slows with age, you, like most adults, may continue to eat the same amount. And those extra calories need to go somewhere. Although so-called middle-age spread may seem inevitable around your "middle," physical activity can counteract this by boosting metabolism and increasing muscle mass, which helps burn more fat and calories, even as you age.

Myth 6: "Fit and fat? It's not possible."

It is possible. Overweight people can be quite fit. Regardless of weight, people who are physically active on a regular basis have a greatly reduced risk of premature death, and possibly of developing cancer, when compared to those who are not active. Even if weight loss is your primary goal, just being active is a huge step to better health. You don't have to choose to lose weight before beginning an exercise program. Make exercise an essential part of your overall weight loss plan.

Myth 7: "Lifting weights makes women too muscular and bulky."

Testosterone levels in women are too low to build large, masculine muscles (except for those women who intensely lift heavy weights). Strength training is especially important for women because it increases their bone density, helping to reduce the risk of osteoporosis. In addition to toned and firm muscles, women also enjoy greater strength and better balance.

Researcher Miriam E. Nelson, Ph.D., from Tufts University's School of Nutrition Science and Policy, found that a year of high-intensity strength training, just twice a week, helped preserve bone density in postmenopausal women while improving strength and balance. With exercise and strength training (and without drugs), women in Dr. Nelson's studies achieved these results.

- Regained bone density, thus reversing osteoporosis

- Became stronger—in most cases even stronger than when they were younger

- Improved balance and flexibility

- Ate as much as ever but grew leaner and trimmer

- Became energized and 27 percent more active

With proper exercise, you can boost metabolism and melt away fat. Because muscle is metabolically active and fat is not, when you increase your muscle mass, you're able to burn more calories, even when at rest. No one in the studies complained about building bulky muscles. A mirror check may show a shapelier figure.

Let's Get Physical

Before You Get Moving

How often have you heard that you should talk to your doctor *before* you start an exercise program? The truth is that your doctor should be talking to *you* about an exercise program, and research is showing that counseling by your primary care doctor can be effective—especially for women. Counseling by the doctor at regular physician visits plus educational materials encouraged people in the study group to exercise.

Your doctor may have some helpful recommendations regarding the types and level of activities that you can participate in. If you experience any out-of-the-ordinary aches or pains or shortness of breath, let your doctor know. He or she will also want to know if there have been any other changes in your health after you've started your exercise program.

Before you slip on your tennis shoes and jogging pants, should you see or talk to a doctor? Most adults probably don't need to see their doctor before starting a *moderately* intensive physical activity program. Use common sense when it comes to starting physical activity. You may be able to do any activity you want as long as you start off slowly and increase your activity level gradually.

On the other hand, speak with your doctor or health care team first if you are a man over forty years old, a woman over fifty years old, or if any of the following conditions or situations applies to you.

* Heart or lung condition

* High blood pressure

- Faintness, dizziness, or loss of balance

- Pregnancy

- Asthma

- Diabetes

- Taking medications that may interfere with your ability to exercise

- Overweight or obesity (twenty to thirty pounds over normal)

- Bone or joint problems, including arthritis or osteoporosis

- Temporary illness, such as the flu

- Out of breath after mild exertion

- Lower back pain

Can Physical Activity Be Dangerous?

Many people are concerned about the risk of injury and even death while exercising before starting a program of regular physical activity. Because injury is a major reason why people stop being active, it's important to make sure you can perform your activities safely. Most injuries occur when people take on too much physical activity, too soon. Don't attempt to do too much in an effort to burn more calories or get into shape faster. Rather, listen to what your body tells you.

Although sudden bursts of *strenuous* physical activity can trigger a heart attack in normally sedentary people who have heart disease, the chance of a heart attack during or after intense exertion is very small—about one in 10,000. This risk is probably much lower for moderate activity. More important, the risk is decreased nearly 100 percent for people who exercise at least five or more times a week. The key is to *start slowly*.

How Fit Are You?

Fitness is a combination of factors, including strength, flexibility, and endurance. In simple terms, being fit means having the strength and energy to do everyday activities without extra effort. That might mean being able to pick up something from the ground, carrying your groceries easily, or climbing a flight of stairs without having to stop and catch your breath. Ultimately, being physically fit enables you to do what you want to without limitations.

Remember the quiz you took at the beginning of this chapter? It should give you a basic idea of where you stand. Now would be a good time to review your answers. If you marked any answer with either 0 or 1 for any question, try to incorporate an activity into your routine that would increase your score in that area. You'll probably find that it will help in other areas as well. For example, your goal may be to walk or jog a mile in thirteen minutes. As you work toward your goal, your heart will also be strengthened, thus lowering your heart rate.

In many cases, working toward cardiovascular fitness can also improve balance, coordination, flexibility, and strength. Stretching before physical activity improves flexibility, and strength training using light weights increases muscular fitness.

It's usually commitment and motivation that people have the most difficulty with. But if you can increase your activity, the rest will fall into place.

Where to Begin

Many health care professionals, personal trainers or fitness instructors, and sports medicine specialists can estimate fitness levels by performing a few simple tests. Fitness assessments are often free, or at least available, to members of a gym, health club, or YMCA. If an assessment is available to you, take a baseline measurement of these elements. Then, a year later, do it again. Many assessments are scored by computer, so you can see a graphic representation of your current status and progress over time.

Professional fitness assessments usually consider some of the following measurements and factors when calculating your fitness status.

- Resting heart rate

- Resting blood pressure

- Age

- Weight and height (used to calculate body mass index or BMI, see page 81)

- Body fat measurements (using calipers)

- VO_2 maximum—your body's maximum capacity (or volume) for carrying oxygen

- Flexibility—using criteria such as the Sit-and-Reach Test, touching your toes, reaching your hand down your spine, or squatting

- Strength—using the number of completed push-ups or sit-ups without stopping

- Endurance—using time it takes to walk or run one-mile course, or perceived effort needed to walk up a flight of stairs

- Your current amount and level of physical activity

Take the Next Step

The ACS recommends that men over the age of forty, women over the age of fifty, and people with chronic illnesses or at risk of heart disease consult with a health care professional before starting any form of physical activity. Your doctor, nurse, or physician assistant can also respond to your questions or concerns about the types of physical activity you can perform and should be notified if you notice changes in your health after becoming more physically active. Wherever you live and work you'll find agencies and organizations that are your best allies in the fight for a healthier you (see Resources).

How Much Is Enough?

Gardening requires lots of water—most of it in the form of perspiration.
—LOU ERICKSON, English author

So how much physical activity do you need before you will start to see benefits? As we mentioned in the last chapter, the ACS considers physical activity an important part of its guidelines for cancer prevention, recommending that all people adopt a physically active lifestyle.

There are still many unanswered questions about the optimal intensity (how hard you exert yourself), duration (how long you do it), and frequency (how often you do it) of physical activity needed to reduce cancer risk. Based on the best current evidence available, the ACS recommends the following.

- **Adults** should engage in at least moderate activity for **thirty minutes or more** on **five or more days of the week**. It's important to note that forty-five minutes or more of moderate to vigorous activity on five or more days per week may further reduce your risk of breast, colon, and other cancers.

If you are less active than recommended by these guidelines, you should gradually increase the intensity, duration, and frequency of physical activity. A good rule of thumb is to increase your activity level by no more than 10 percent in duration or frequency per week. Stretching and warm-up should be part of each exercise session to reduce risk of injury.

- **Children and adolescents** should engage in **at least sixty minutes per day** of moderate-to-vigorous physical activity for **at least five days per week**.

Such activities should include sports and fitness activities at school and at home. To help achieve activity goals, daily physical education programs and activity breaks should be provided for children at school, and television viewing and computer game time should be minimized at home.

Moderate activities are those that make you breathe as hard as you would during a brisk walk. You should be slightly out of breath, but still able to talk in complete sentences. You may choose from a variety of other activities in addition to walking. These might include calisthenics (gymnastic-type activities), jogging, swimming, gardening, yard work, housework, and dancing. Remember, it's important to choose activities that you enjoy.

A step aerobics class may be of moderate intensity for someone who's fit and uses a two-step bench. On the other hand, for someone who has never done a step class, the activity may in fact be quite vigorous at first with just the platform and no added risers.

Variation on a New Theme

If you have been inactive in the past or are just beginning a physical activity program, a gradual increase to thirty minutes per day of moderate to vigorous physical activity on at least five days per week will provide substantial cardiovascular and weight control benefits.

Some experts suggest that physical activity does not need to be completed all at once to be beneficial. Many of the same benefits seen with vigorous activities can be achieved through moderate-intensity activities if the total amount of activity is the same. Adults should burn at least 150 calories per day during their moderate to vigorous physical activity to gain the health benefits associated with this activity, but it doesn't appear that this needs to be done all at one time.

If you're just starting out, you may find it helpful to keep a journal of your activities. Write down what you did and for how long. Keep track of all of your daily activities and see how easily they can add up to thirty minutes or more.

What Is Moderate Activity?

The amount of activity you choose will depend on duration, intensity, and frequency. You will notice that you can spend less time doing more vigorous activities (such as those toward the bottom of the list) than those that require less energy. Most people do not do these activities on a daily basis, so it is important to be aware of other ways to increase your daily activity levels.

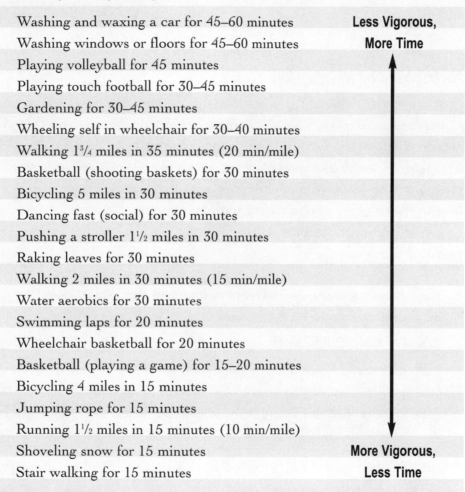

Washing and waxing a car for 45–60 minutes

Washing windows or floors for 45–60 minutes

Playing volleyball for 45 minutes

Playing touch football for 30–45 minutes

Gardening for 30–45 minutes

Wheeling self in wheelchair for 30–40 minutes

Walking 1³/₄ miles in 35 minutes (20 min/mile)

Basketball (shooting baskets) for 30 minutes

Bicycling 5 miles in 30 minutes

Dancing fast (social) for 30 minutes

Pushing a stroller 1¹/₂ miles in 30 minutes

Raking leaves for 30 minutes

Walking 2 miles in 30 minutes (15 min/mile)

Water aerobics for 30 minutes

Swimming laps for 20 minutes

Wheelchair basketball for 20 minutes

Basketball (playing a game) for 15–20 minutes

Bicycling 4 miles in 15 minutes

Jumping rope for 15 minutes

Running 1¹/₂ miles in 15 minutes (10 min/mile)

Shoveling snow for 15 minutes

Stair walking for 15 minutes

Less Vigorous, More Time

More Vigorous, Less Time

The amount of physical activity is influenced by its duration, intensity, and frequency. The same amount of activity can be obtained in longer sessions of moderately intense activities (such as brisk walking), or in shorter sessions of more strenuous activities (such as running).

Adapted from *Physical Activity and Health: A Report of the Surgeon General,* U.S. Department of Health and Human Services, Centers for Disease Control and Prevention, National Center for Chronic Disease Prevention and Health Promotion, The President's Council on Physical Fitness and Sports, 1996.

And the idea that "more is better" still applies, as the ACS guidelines reflect. Although you can get substantial health benefits from thirty minutes of activity a day, doing more is even better for you. If you are already active for at least thirty minutes on most days of the week, try adding a few more minutes or more intense activities over time, eventually working up to forty-five minutes a day.

Start Slowly to Stay on Track

After you've received the OK from your doctor (if necessary), prepare a simple exercise plan. Think of activities you would enjoy and that you can do comfortably. For example, maybe you've been meaning to plant a garden, or you think you'd enjoy an aerobics class. Choosing activities that you take pleasure in, while being realistic at the same time, will improve your chances of sticking with an exercise program.

Consider several factors when choosing physical activities for your personal fitness plan.

- High-impact activities with frequent jumping and heavy pounding can be uncomfortable and can cause injuries. Biking, cross-country skiing, walking, and swimming are low-impact and easier on the joints.

- Activities that require a lot of skill, such as tennis or golf, can be discouraging at first. Try to be realistic in estimating your skill level. If it is an activity that you really want to pursue, work toward advancing your fitness and skill level.

- Another factor to keep in mind is the season. Studies show that physical activity is directly proportional to the weather. Not surprisingly, when it is cold or rainy out, people generally exercise less frequently. Don't let this keep you from your plan! Be creative and have alternatives for unpleasant days, such as walking in the mall instead of outside.

Which Exercise Is Right for You?

Activity	Pros	Cons
Walking	Can be done almost anywhere. Excellent beginner activity. Minimal stress on joints. Develops and maintains aerobic fitness for most adults.	May not be intense enough for the highly fit to reach target heart rate range.
Jogging/Running	Requires no special equipment except proper shoes. Can be done almost anywhere.	May stress joints. Safety issues when done on streets and uneven surfaces.
Swimming	Excellent overall conditioner. Minimal stress on most joints.	Need a pool.
Bicycling/ Stationary Cycling	Exercises large muscles in legs. Minimal stress on most joints. Can be done indoors.	Outdoor: safety issues. Indoor: need equipment.
Aerobic Dance/ Step Aerobics	Excellent overall conditioner if properly designed. Music and group exercise make it enjoyable.	Requires instruction. High impact can stress joints.
Rowing	Exercise upper and lower body muscles. Minimal stress on joints if done properly. Effective for aerobic and muscle fitness.	Need equipment.
Stair Climber	Exercises large muscles in legs. Minimal stress on joints.	Need equipment.
Rope Jumping	Can be done almost anywhere. Inexpensive.	Difficult to sustain unless fairly fit. Stresses joints. Skill required for effectiveness.

Reprinted from *Physical Fitness: Guidelines for Success* by permission of JoAnn Eickhoff-Shemek, Ph.D. and Kris Berg, Ed.D.

Include a schedule as part of your exercise plan. Write down your goals (and whether or not you achieve them). It can be an effective way to keep track of your progress and continue your level of physical activity. Try to get in twenty minutes or more at least three days a week at first, and gradually at least thirty minutes on at least five days. Simply increase the time and intensity as the weeks pass. Remember that these intervals can include several short periods of activity in a day, so jot down these times and activities on your exercise calendar.

Your Personal Fitness Plan

The best piece of advice for beginners is to *start slowly*. This is important in two different contexts. First, in your personal fitness plan, start with activities you know you can handle and increase the time and intensity over weeks to months. Resist the temptation to do too much, especially as you first start to become active. Allow your body to adjust to the increasing effort that physical activity requires.

Second, each time you exercise, be sure to warm up properly. Warming up is important for everyone engaging in physical activity. After your muscles have had some time to adjust to activity—about three to five minutes—stop and stretch the muscles to help prevent soreness and strains. A warm muscle is stretched more easily than a cold one. It's a good idea to include stretching *before* increasing your activity level to prevent injury at the outset, and *after* an activity to reduce soreness.

"Trick" your subconscious by allowing yourself small successes. The goal here is to set up the task so that you can't possibly fail. Start with goals that are ridiculously easy, so you'll be sure to succeed. For example, walking twenty-seven minutes on the treadmill when you planned on thirty may be considered a failure in your mind. But if you vow to walk five minutes on the treadmill, how can you fail?

Beginner's Rules for Physical Activity

1. If you are a man over age forty or a woman over age fifty, or have been sedentary for some time, see or talk to your doctor to get the "green light" before you begin, especially if you are managing a chronic condition.

2. Make a personal physical activity fitness plan that includes the type of activity, when, how long, with whom, and so on. Set easy goals at first and begin slowly.

3. Dress comfortably in loose clothing, wear appropriate footwear, and dress for the weather.

4. Warm up for three to five minutes.

5. Stretch thoroughly.

6. Begin your activity at a low to moderate intensity level. Doing an exercise longer is more beneficial than doing it faster. Slow down or stop if you feel any discomfort.

7. Cool down by walking slowly and stretching again. Proper stretching can lessen achy muscles later on.

8. Review your plan and commit to the next time you intend to be active.

Keeping the Beat

Aerobic activity is usually the basis of most physical activity plans. You can choose any moderately intense physical activity that raises your heart rate for thirty minutes or more. Aerobic activities include brisk walking, jogging, swimming, aerobic dance, racket sports such as tennis, in-line skating, skiing, using aerobic equipment such as stair steppers, ellipticals, or treadmills, and even power yoga. There are several ways to make sure you are exercising at a safe level.

Take the Talk Test. If you are unable to carry on a conversation during physical activity, you are working too hard. Slow down and take a breather. Continue when you are able. Stop if you are breathless, dizzy, lightheaded, or nauseated.

Know Your Zone. As you become accustomed to the challenges of regular physical activity, try to maintain your heart rate at approximately 50–75 percent of your maximum heart rate. This is the target heart rate zone. Use the following chart to determine your target zone. Look for the category closest to your age and read across the line. For example, if you are forty-four years old, your target heart rate zone is 88–131 beats per minute.

Check your pulse to determine if you are within your target heart rate zone. First, count the number of beats at your wrist or neck for fifteen seconds. Multiply this number by four to obtain the beats per minute. If your pulse is faster than your target heart rate, slow down—you're exercising too hard. If it is slower, try to increase your activity level a little.

If you are just beginning, aim for the 50 percent level. As you improve, work toward 75 percent of your maximum heart rate. If your target heart rate zone seems too difficult, do what is the most comfortable for you. You'll improve with time.

Start your actual activity phase at a moderate intensity. As you increase your heart rate, be aware of how you feel. If you feel any discomfort, lightheadedness, or nausea, slow down or stop until you feel better and are ready to try again. If you experience more serious symptoms, such as chest pain, talk to your doctor before continuing.

Normal body signs during physical activity include a faster heart rate, rapid and deeper breathing, and perspiration. You should still be able to

Age	Target Heart Rate Zone 50–75%	Average Maximum Heart Rate 100%
31–40 years	93–138 beats per minute	185
41–50 years	88–131 beats per minute	175
51–60 years	83–123 beats per minute	165
60+ years	78–116 beats per minute	155

Reprinted from *Physical Activity and Weight Control* (NIH Publication No. 96-4031), Weight-control Information Network, National Institute of Diabetes and Digestive and Kidney Diseases (NIDDK), a part of the National Institutes of Health, U.S. Public Health Service.

carry on a conversation. As your fitness level improves, you can increase the duration and intensity of your activity to increase your cardiovascular fitness even further. You will soon notice that it takes you longer to feel winded and fatigued.

Survival of the FITTest

The acronym FITT is a simple way to remember the variables you can manipulate to change your workout or increase your level of activity.

F = frequency (how often you are physically active)
I = intensity (how hard you exercise, either by perceived exertion or target heart rate)
T = time (how long you are physically active)
T = type (what type of physical activity you choose)

When starting your program of physical activity, all the FITT principles will make a difference. Some trainers call this the "training effect." After a couple of weeks your body will adjust to those levels, and you will need to increase one or more of the FITT principles to continue to see results. This is especially true of weight loss plateaus. In order to improve your cardiovascular ability, fitness level, and strength, your body will have to be pushed beyond what it is used to, even if it's only a little. Over time your body will become more and more efficient, like a well-oiled machine.

Another advantage of the FITT principle is that it adds variety to your physical activity. For example, if you regularly bike around your neighborhood, try walking instead. It will work different muscles, and you will burn more calories as your body adjusts to the different activity. To keep the "training effect" going, change any of the FITT variables every four to six weeks.

Fitting Activity into Your Day

Your day is already packed. You're probably thinking, "How am I going to find another thirty minutes for physical activity, even in small segments?" Try to look for opportunities to add a little activity to your day. Remember that small changes can make a big difference in achieving substantial health rewards and reducing the risk of cancer and chronic diseases. Here are some ways to add more activity to your daily routine.

- Take a family walk around the neighborhood after dinner.

- Take a bike ride.

Sample of a Physical Activity Plan				
Date	Frequency	Intensity	Time	Type
3/4–4/1	M, W, F	Brisk, 1 mile	13 minutes	Running
4/8–5/20	M, W, F	Brisk, 1½ miles	15 minutes	Walking
5/27–6/10	M, W, F	Brisk, 5 miles	26 minutes	Biking
7/15–8/19	Su, T, W, Th	Fast, 2 miles	25 minutes	Walking

- Rake the grass or leaves instead of using a blower.

- Pull weeds in the yard.

- Do squats, lunges, crunches, push-ups, or stretches while watching TV.

- Play active games with the kids, such as jump rope, hopscotch, tag, and so on.

- Walk during your lunch break.

- Park your car farther away from the entrance to the mall or your worksite.

- Get off the bus or subway a stop earlier and walk the extra distance.

- Use the stairs instead of the elevator.

- Walk or bike to the store instead of driving.

The Next Time (and the Next Time...)

Look at your exercise plan to see when you've scheduled your next activity period. Mentally prepare and commit to it. Don't dwell on the rest of the week or month! Think short-term! If you're concerned about your goals as a whole, you'll only feel overwhelmed and exasperated. Physical activity will become a part of your everyday way of life if you allow it to become a habit. Old habits are hard to break. New ones are just as hard to start.

Staying Motivated

Take steps to better your chances of keeping up your physical activity program. If your motivation and commitment appear to fade over time, try incorporating one or more of the following ideas into your exercise plan.

- **Convenience** — Most people do not stick to a physical activity program unless it's convenient. Determine how you can make physical activity convenient by looking at your environment and personal schedule. Perhaps there is a park near your home or office where you can walk or run. Consider joining a gym or fitness center on a short-term agreement to make sure you make it a habit (especially if a one-year commitment seems overwhelming right now). But if getting to that workout center puts you in rush hour traffic for an hour, you're better off going home to exercise. If you've been considering investing in home exercise equipment, see if you can rent before you buy, or find an inexpensive unit at a garage sale.

- **Partner(s)** — Exercising with others (including your dog) is so enjoyable for some people that it encourages them to continue being physically active. The physical activity becomes secondary to the social interaction, and everyone gets into better shape!

- **Personality** — If you like being in a group of people, group sports such as softball or volleyball might be the best activity for you. Bowling and golf will give you that social connectedness, but not necessarily any aerobic benefit. Go for it anyway. If you'd rather be on your own, bicycling, swimming, or jogging could be a better fit.

- **Schedule** — If you drag out of bed in the morning, consider exercising in the evening. Likewise, if you're a morning person, plan to exercise when you wake up. Some people claim that getting a workout done first thing in the morning makes them feel energized and as though they've accomplished something positive for the day. But it doesn't matter *when* you schedule your activity, just get out there and do it.

- **Variety** — They say it's the spice of life and in the case of physical activity, it's definitely a motivating factor. Trying new activities not only strengthens different muscles, it also teaches fresh training techniques. You can get renewed inspiration by varying your exercises a little, listening to (different) music or books on tape, or opting for a change of scenery.

- **Specificity**—Rather than having general goals like "getting into shape" or "exercising more," choose concrete goals such as walking twenty minutes on Tuesdays and Thursdays, and doing stretching exercises five minutes each morning.

- **Be successful**—No one likes to continue doing something if they always fail. Set easy goals, succeed at those goals, and raise the bar. Successes, no matter how small, increase motivation. And steady motivation nurtures good habits.

- **Celebrate**—Be your own best cheerleader and rejoice in your successes. Reward yourself when you reach a goal. Do something active with your body just because you can.

- **Motivate yourself**—Try visualization techniques to help your motivation. Imagine yourself in shape and how it feels. Create a vision of yourself feeling fit, rather than focusing on being out of shape.

- **Do something**—You're dreading thirty minutes of exercise, so you abandon it altogether. This happens to many people. The best way to overcome this feeling is to change your goal for the day—walk for fifteen, even ten minutes. Do what you can and don't worry about it. Consistency is the key, and something is better than nothing.

- **Be realistic**—Expect setbacks and prepare for obstacles. Things like time, illness, or bad weather may occasionally get in the way. Don't get discouraged, just accept the inevitable and move on.

- **Take a break**—You're burned out and all you can think of is crashing on the couch. Do it. Take a day or two and reenergize your enthusiasm.

Bumps in the road are a part of life. Just avoid letting yourself off the hook altogether. Make a firm plan to start back up and stick to it.

The approach you take—whether you plan time for activity out of your day or use everyday opportunities to increase your activity level—doesn't matter. What matters is that you have decided to make fitness and physical activity a regular part of your life.

CHAPTER 4

Everything Under the Sun

A perfect summer day is when the sun is shining, the breeze is blowing,
the birds are singing, and the lawn mower is broken.
—JAMES DENT, English author

In outer-space terms, the distance from here on Earth to anywhere "out there" is enormous. It takes our space probes years to reach other planets in the solar system. But if you're a light ray coming from the sun, you can make it to Earth in just eight minutes. And there's always a steady stream of light rays headed our way from the fiery-hot center of our solar system.

Other than the atmosphere around the Earth, nothing else stands in the way of those rays of light until they reach you. In other words, think of your skin—your body's first line of defense—as being eight minutes away from the sun. Damaging ultraviolet (UV) rays travel the ninety-three million miles from the sun in just eight minutes to inflict their harm directly on your skin. Unless, of course, you protect yourself.

Harmful sun rays cause skin cancer—the most preventable, most common form of all cancers. In fact, skin cancer is about as common as all other forms of cancer *combined*. Knowing what we know about the role of the sun in causing skin cancer, and knowing that we can prevent most cases, it's hard to believe that the incidence of melanoma, the most serious form of skin cancer, is actually on the rise. One American dies of skin cancer every hour.

We have work to do in making people aware of greatest outdoor risks and smartest ways to enjoy the outdoors safely. In this chapter we'll discuss what we do know. We'll look at the skin—what it's made of, what can go wrong with it (and what sunlight has to do with this process), and what you can do to protect yourself and your family from the most common of all cancers.

What Do You Know About the Sun and Skin Cancer?

Take the Sun Smarts Quiz and test your knowledge about sun sense. It may be that what you think you know is not backed by scientific evidence. This chapter discusses common myths about harmful rays from the sun, tanning beds, some surprising information on skin color, and sun protection. But first, some basics.

Take the Sun Smarts Quiz

Do you agree or disagree with these statements? What do you know about sun safety, and are you following through in your daily life? Mark yes or no in the space provided, and then read on for related information.

_____ **I can stay in the sun for as long as I want if I'm wearing sunscreen.**

You've heard the message before. Sunscreens are very useful in reducing the risk of skin cancer, but they don't provide total protection from ultraviolet rays. The best way to protect yourself is to seek shade and limit your time in the sun during the midday hours when the sun is at its strongest. Cover up with a shirt and hat, use generous amounts of sunscreen with a sun protection factor (SPF) rating of 15 or higher, and remember sunglasses for eye protection.

_____ **I don't sunbathe, so there's no way I could get skin cancer.**

Sun exposure can increase your risk of skin cancer, but it's not the only cause. Of course, people who spend a lot of time in the sun are at highest risk for certain types of skin cancers. But, occasional exposure (such as on the weekends or on vacation) to strong sunlight seems to actually *increase* the risk for melanoma—the less common, but more serious form of skin cancer. If you have a family history of melanoma, you may be at greater risk and should take care to protect yourself from the sun.

_____ **Waterproof sunscreen will protect me even after swimming or sweating.**

Read the label on the sunscreen. Water resistant sunscreens may only last for eighty minutes of swimming and/or sweating. If indicated on the label, some sunscreens may protect you for longer periods of time, but be sure to reapply as necessary. The Food and Drug Administration (FDA) has banned the use of the word *waterproof* on sunscreen packaging because no sunscreen will protect you indefinitely if you're swimming or sweating.

_____ **I should put sunscreen on my newborn baby so my baby will be safe in the sun.**

Sunscreen is not recommended for children younger than six months old. Keep infants in the shade and protected with comfortable clothing (especially a hat) and avoid exposure to the sun.

_____ I do not need to protect myself on cool or cloudy days.

The temperature doesn't matter—the ultraviolet rays do. Ultraviolet rays are most intense when the sun is high in the sky. Use the shadow test— if your shadow is shorter than you are, the sun's rays are the strongest. Ultraviolet rays can penetrate clouds, so it's important to take precautions even on hazy, cloudy, and winter days.

_____ The only way for me to protect myself from skin cancer is to stay indoors.

Outdoor activity helps maintain your physical and emotional well-being. Simply limit your time in the sun during the midday hours and protect yourself when going out. Also, you don't have to be outdoors to be exposed to the sun's harmful rays. Many people get sunburned while in the car. While riding in a car, you might apply sunscreen especially to your face and hands and wear long sleeves and sunglasses.

_____ Getting _some_ sun is good for me.

The key word here is _some_. Although people often associate a suntan with good health and vitality, a tan is actually a sign of damage to the skin by UV rays. It's true that the body uses sunlight to produce vitamin D, but getting enough vitamin D is generally not a health problem. Your body stores what you need. Skin cancer is the problem, and staying out of the sun is your best defense.

_____ My chances of getting skin cancer are small.

One in five Americans develops skin cancer. Do you want to take that chance?

_____ **Having a "base" tan will protect my skin from being damaged.**

A base tan offers no protection from the damaging effects of the sun. A tan is a sign of damage. In many cases, people who get a base tan often plan on more sun exposure in the near future. Tanning beds, which were once thought to be safer than the sun, may actually increase your risk of developing melanoma.

On Top of It All

What is the largest organ in the human body? You may not realize it, but it's the skin. It takes up more space than the heart, lungs, or even the liver. The skin is also one of the most important organs because it covers and protects the whole body from injury, serves as a barrier between microbes (such as bacteria) and internal organs, and prevents the loss of too much water and other fluids. The skin regulates body temperature and helps rid the body of excess water and salts. Certain receptor cells in the skin communicate with the brain so that you can feel temperature, touch, and pain.

More Than Skin Deep

The skin actually has three layers called the epidermis, dermis, and subcutis. What you see and think of as skin is the top layer called the epidermis. This is where the most common types of skin cancer forms. The two major cell types here are the squamous cells, which form the outer layer, and the basal cells, which lie below the squamous cells. Basal cells continually divide to form new squamous cells, which replace older squamous cells that wear off of the skin surface. Melanocytes are also present in the epidermis. These skin cells produce the protective pigment called melanin, which helps protect the body from the harmful rays of the sun.

The middle layer of the skin is called the dermis. It contains hair follicles, sweat glands, blood vessels, and nerves that are held in place by a protein called collagen, which gives the skin its resilience and strength.

The last and deepest layer of the skin is called the subcutis. The subcutis and the lowest part of the dermis form a network of collagen and fat cells, which helps the body conserve heat.

When you hear about first-, second-, and third-degree burns, this description refers to these three layers of skin, from the outside in. A first-degree burn would involve the epidermis; whereas, a third-degree burn would be much more severe and involve all three layers to the subcutis.

How Skin Tans

When melanocytes in the epidermis are exposed to too much light, they release a pigment called melanin. It is melanin that gives a tan or brown color to the skin and helps protect the deeper layers of the skin

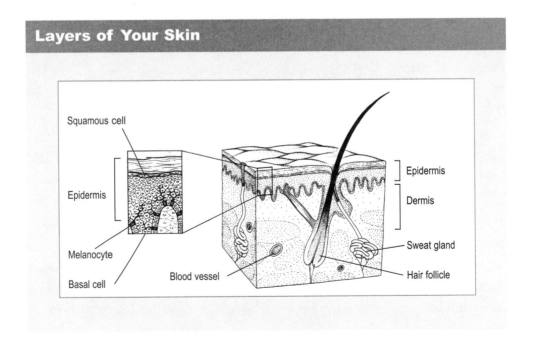

Layers of Your Skin

Squamous cell

Epidermis

Melanocyte

Basal cell

Blood vessel

Epidermis

Dermis

Sweat gland

Hair follicle

from the harmful effects of the sun. Whether you burn or tan depends on your skin type, the time of year, and the amount of sun exposure. The following table classifies skin types by susceptibility to sun exposure.

Skin Type	Tanning and Sunburning History
I	Always burns, never tans, sensitive to sun exposure
II	Burns easily, tans minimally
III	Burns moderately, tans gradually to light brown
IV	Burns minimally, always tans well to moderately brown
V	Rarely burns, tans profusely to dark
VI	Never burns, deeply pigmented, least sensitive

Reprinted from *Choose Your Cover*, Centers for Disease Control and Prevention, National Center for Chronic Disease Prevention and Health Promotion, Division of Cancer Prevention and Control, 2000.

People with skin Types I and II are at the highest risk for skin cancer as a result of excessive sun exposure, but skin cancer can occur in anyone. Think about your history of sun exposure. Do you tan easily or burn? Determine your skin type from the table and keep this in mind as we discuss the sun's effects and prevention techniques.

Moles and Freckles

Most people have moles and freckles, and almost all of them are harmless. Moles are not usually present at birth but begin to appear in children and teenagers. On a cellular level, they are actually a clustering of melanocytes. Once a mole has developed, it will usually stay the same size, shape, and color for many years. The medical term for a mole is a nevus. Moles may occur anywhere on the body. They may eventually fade away in older people.

Freckles are tan or brown spots that appear over time on sun-exposed areas of skin. They are common in people with lighter skin types. Freckles may be more prevalent in summer months, when exposure to the sun is higher. They are an indication of skin that is easily damaged by the sun.

Both moles and freckles may indicate an increased risk for a specific type of skin cancer called melanoma. We'll talk about how to tell the difference between a melanoma and an ordinary mole in detail later in this chapter, when we discuss how to examine your skin.

Exposing the Sun

Ultraviolet radiation is a stream of invisible high-energy rays coming from the sun that can damage DNA, the genetic material of cells, both in the skin and eyes. Although it is part of sunlight, UV radiation is not visible to the naked eye. The amount of UV rays you are exposed to depends on the strength of the light, the amount of time you're exposed to it, and whether or not your skin is protected.

So just how does UV radiation cause cancer? Some forms of high-energy radiation, including UV rays, can damage DNA at a cellular level. This damage can make DNA less able to control how and when a cell normally grows and divides. Changes in DNA, called mutations, seem to be a necessary part of the development of cancer, although it probably takes more than just one mutation in most cases. Some people are born with DNA mutations inherited from their parents, which make them more likely to develop cancer.

This explains why one person may be more likely to develop skin cancer than another, even if exposed to the same amount of UV rays. Unfortunately, no tests can measure who is more at risk. Until a reliable test can be developed, we all need to be careful about our exposure to the sun.

Even if you don't develop skin cancer, other problems may occur from getting too much sun. The obvious and most common problem is painful sunburn. It is, literally, a burn—the same type you could get from a fire or extremely hot water, but sunburn usually covers more of your body.

Over time, excessive sun exposure can lead to premature aging of the skin, giving it a wrinkled, leathery appearance. The risk of cataracts (clouding of the lenses of the eyes) and other forms of eye damage is greater with exposure to UV radiation. And finally, a little known fact about sun exposure is that it also suppresses the immune system. And, after being in the sun, certain infections such as chicken pox and cold sores can become worse.

UVA or UVB—Is One Better or Worse?

Ultraviolet radiation is actually divided into three wavelength ranges.

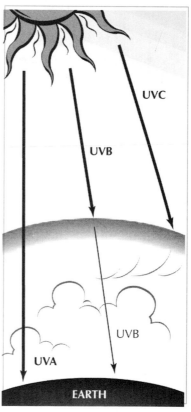

- **UVA** rays are not absorbed by the ozone layer. They are involved in the aging of cells and produce some damage to DNA.

- **UVB** rays are partially absorbed by the ozone layer (see below). They are mainly responsible for direct damage to DNA and are thought to cause most skin cancers.

- **UVC** rays do not reach the Earth because they are completely absorbed by oxygen and ozone in the atmosphere, so they pose no risk to humans.

Reprinted from *The Sun, UV, and You: A Guide to Sun-Wise Behavior*, (EPA430-K-99-035), U.S. Environmental Protection Agency, 1999.

UVA and UVB are the two types of ultraviolet radiation that reach us from the sun. Although UVA and UVB rays make up only 1/10,000,000th of the sun's wavelengths, they are primarily responsible for the damaging effects of the sun on the skin. Scientists now believe that both contribute to skin damage, including skin cancer. *There are no safe UV rays.*

The amount of UV radiation that reaches the Earth depends on a number of factors. The UV Index, discussed in the next section, is a good indication of the intensity of UV radiation on the Earth's surface. Take each of these factors into account when you plan on spending time outdoors anywhere and not just at the beach or in the summer.

- **Closer to the equator.** The intensity of the sun is naturally stronger at the equator because of its location directly overhead. Not only do the sun's rays have less distance to travel, but the ozone layer is also thinner in the tropics.

- **Higher up.** Ultraviolet rays are stronger at higher altitudes because there is less atmosphere to absorb the damaging radiation. Your risk of overexposure is greater the higher you go, which explains why skiers and other winter sports enthusiasts on mountains must do more to protect their skin.

- **Time of day.** The sun is at its highest point in the sky around noon. At this time UV light has less atmosphere to travel through and less distance to travel. In contrast, the sun's rays travel at an angle early in the morning and late in the afternoon, thereby reducing the intensity of damaging UV light.

- **Time of year.** The sun's angle to the Earth changes with the seasons, resulting in changes in UV intensity. UV rays are strongest in late spring and early summer.

- **Weather.** UV rays can reach you even on cloudy days. Although UV levels are reduced on cloudy days, it is possible to burn your skin even if the cloud cover is thick. Overcast days are especially dangerous because many people feel they are safe from the sun's harmful effects, so they don't bother to protect themselves.

- **Mirroring.** The sun reflects off many surfaces, including water, sand, concrete, grass, and snow. UV light can also reach below the water's surface. It's important to be aware of reflection even in shaded areas.

- **Ozone layer.** The ozone layer is in a region of the upper atmosphere called the stratosphere. It absorbs most UVB and all UVC radiation coming from the sun, but it does not absorb UVA radiation. The ozone layer has become thinner due to the release of ozone-depleting substances widely used in industry. The thinner ozone has allowed more of the sun's ultraviolet radiation to reach the Earth.

Measure Exposure Risk with the UV Index

To increase awareness of the damaging potential of UV radiation, the Environmental Protection Agency (EPA) and the National Weather Service developed the UV Index, sometimes called the solar warning index. It predicts the probable intensity of UV radiation reaching the Earth's surface during the sun's highest peak (usually around noon).

The UV Index is predicted daily for fifty-eight cities, based on local conditions. Check your local news, weather reports (especially if you live in a sunny area, such as Florida or Arizona), and radio stations or local newspapers and community web sites.

The UV Index is expressed as a number, ranging from 0 to 10+, and indicates the amount of UV radiation reaching the Earth's surface around noon each day. The UV Index is valid only for about a thirty-mile radius from the city, and, as with any forecast, local variability in cloud cover and other factors may change actual levels experienced. But it can

Using the UV Index

The UV Index can help you be aware of the level of UV radiation exposure expected on a given day. As a result, you can use simple sun protective behaviors to reduce your lifetime risk of developing skin cancer and other sun-related illnesses. What follows is a description of each UV Index level and tips you can use to help be prepared.

0 to 2: Minimal A UV Index reading of 0 to 2 means minimal danger from the sun's UV rays for the average person:

- Most people can stay in the sun for up to one hour during the hours of peak sun strength, 10 A.M. to 4 P.M., without burning.

- People with very sensitive skin and infants should always be protected from prolonged sun exposure.

3 to 4: Low A UV Index reading of 3 to 4 means low risk of harm from unprotected sun exposure. Fair-skinned people, however, might burn in less than twenty minutes:

- Wear a hat with a wide brim and sunglasses to protect your eyes.

- Use a sunscreen with an SPF of at least 15 and wear long-sleeved shirts and long pants when outdoors.

5 to 6: Moderate A UV Index reading of 5 to 6 means moderate risk of harm from unprotected sun exposure. Fair-skinned people might burn in less than fifteen minutes. Apply a sunscreen with an SPF of at least 15. Wear a wide-brim hat and sunglasses to protect your eyes:

- Use sunscreen if you work outdoors and remember to protect sensitive areas like the nose and the rims of the ears. Sunscreen prevents sunburn and some of the sun's damaging effects on the immune system.

- Use a lip balm or lip cream containing a sunscreen. Lip balms can help protect some people from getting cold sores.

7 to 9: High A UV Index reading of 7 to 9 means high risk of harm from unprotected sun exposure. Fair-skinned people might burn in less than ten minutes. Minimize sun exposure during midday hours, from 10 A.M. to 4 P.M. Protect yourself by liberally applying a sunscreen with an SPF of at least 15. Wear protective clothing and sunglasses to protect the eyes:

- When outside, seek shade. Don't forget that water, sand, pavement, and grass reflect UV rays even under a tree, near a building, or beneath a shady umbrella.

- Wear long-sleeved shirts and trousers made from tightly woven fabrics. UV rays can pass through the holes and spaces of loosely knit fabrics.

10+ Very High A UV Index reading of 10+ means very high risk of harm from unprotected sun exposure. Fair-skinned people might burn in less than five minutes. Outdoor workers are especially at risk as are vacationers who can receive very intense sun exposure. Minimize sun exposure during midday hours, from 10 A.M. to 4 P.M. Apply sunscreen with an SPF of at least 15 liberally every two hours:

- Avoid being in the sun as much as possible.

- Wear sunglasses that block 99 to 100 percent of all UV rays (both UVA and UVB). Some reduction in blue light also might be beneficial but colors should not be severely distorted.

- Wear a cap or hat with a wide brim, which will block roughly 50 percent of UV radiation from reaching the eyes. Wearing sunglasses as well can block the remainder of UV rays.

Adapted from *Stay Healthy in the Sun* (EPA430-K-98-004), U.S. Environmental Protection Agency, 1998.

still give a useful estimate and serve as a reminder to take precautions against UV exposure.

The EPA has devised general guidelines about what to do to protect yourself from overexposure to UV radiation. Use the table to determine your exposure level based on the UV Index for your city—today—and be guided by the protective actions you can take.

Even though all people are at risk for the dangers of UV radiation, the UV Index is calculated for a person who burns easily (Type II skin; refer to the chart on page 139 to determine your skin type). The higher the UV Index number, the greater your risk for exposure to UV radiation and the less amount of time before skin damage occurs.

Skin Type Determines Risk, Not Race

In short: Everyone is at risk. Everyone's skin and eyes are susceptible to sun damage. Although people with light skin are more susceptible, darker skinned people, including African Americans and Hispanic Americans, also can be affected. The question is not what racial or ethnic group may be less affected by the sun, the question for you is this: What is your skin type?

Referring to the skin type table on page 139, The Skin Cancer Foundation reported on a study in which participants represented whites, Asians, Native Americans, Pacific Islanders, and African Americans. Among each of these racial and ethnic groups, researchers from the FDA and the National Cancer Institute (NCI) found that each group includes people with a wide variety of skin types. According to one FDA investigator, whites range from Type I to IV; Asians II to V; and African Americans IV to VI. Therefore, we can make no assumptions about sensitivity to UV radiation within each group.

People with darker skin have more melanin, the naturally protective pigment, and they tan more easily than others. Melanin in the skin helps to block out damaging rays to a certain extent, which is why darker skinned people burn less easily. But contrary to popular belief, people with darker skin are not completely protected from sun damage and skin cancer. In fact, in the FDA study, UV exposure was found to temporarily suspend melanin production in every subject — no matter what skin type. Melanin may offer less protection in the days immediately after initial sun exposure, according to the principal investigator from NCI.

Those with lighter skin are more likely to burn. Too much sun exposure in a short period results in sunburn. Sunburn causes skin redness, pain, and swelling. Symptoms of a more serious sunburn include blistering, fever, chills, upset stomach, and confusion, and may require medical attention.

Beware and Use Care

Extra care should be taken to protect babies and children from the sun. Studies show that sunburns as a child or teenager may increase the risk for developing melanoma and other skin cancer later in life.

You need to be aware of your sun exposure and take extra care to protect yourself in the sun if you have any of these risk factors.

- Lots of moles, irregular moles, or large moles

- Were previously treated for skin cancer

- Work indoors all week and then try to catch up on your tan on weekends

- Live or vacation in tropical or subtropical climates

- Usually burn before tanning

- Have fair skin, freckles, or blond, red, or light brown hair

- Have a family history of skin cancer, especially melanoma

- Live or vacation at high altitudes (ultraviolet radiation from the sun increases 4 to 5 percent for every 1,000 feet above sea level)

- Spend a lot of time outdoors

- Have had an organ transplant

- Have certain diseases, such as lupus, that make you more sensitive to the sun

- Take certain medications and herbal supplements that increase your sensitivity to the sun, such as:

    antibiotics, such as tetracycline

    nonsteroidal anti-inflammatory drugs, such as ibuprofen

    phenothiazines, (major tranquilizers and antinausea drugs, e.g., Compazine)

    sulfa drugs (e.g., Bactrim)

    tricyclic antidepressants (e.g., Elavil)

    thiazide diuretics (e.g., Lasix)

    sulfonylureas (e.g., Glyset)

    medications that reduce immunity (e.g., chemotherapy agents)

    St. John's Wort, an herbal used for depression

If you are taking any medications, over-the-counter drugs, or herbal or dietary supplements, ask your doctor, nurse, or pharmacist if any of these products might affect your sensitivity to sunlight.

Just Like the Sun, Only Worse

Many people believe that the UV rays given off by tanning beds and booths are harmless. This is not true. Tanning lamps emit UVA rays and frequently emit UVB rays as well. Both UVA and UVB rays can cause serious skin damage. Because of these dangers, many health experts advise people to avoid sunlamps for tanning.

There is growing evidence that tanning beds may actually increase a person's risk of developing melanoma, the most serious form of skin cancer. This is an area of active research. A Swedish study published in the *British Journal of Cancer* suggests that tanning beds, once thought to be safer than the sun, may be associated with a nearly twofold increase in the likelihood of developing this potentially deadly skin cancer. The risk may be even higher in young people. People thirty-five years old and younger who used the beds regularly had a melanoma risk eight times higher than people who never used tanning beds. Even occasional use among that age group almost tripled the chances of developing melanoma.

Some people also turn to self-tanning lotions. Unlike the sun, the darker color on your skin from sunless tanning products produces no damage. But the darker color does not provide any added sun protection. Consider why you feel you have to change the color of your skin at all. There really is no such thing as a "healthy" tan.

Uncovering Skin Cancer

Cancer of the skin is the most common of all cancers, accounting for about half of all cancers in the United States. The good news is that it's one of the most preventable types. More than one million cases of very curable nonmelanoma (basal cell or squamous cell) skin cancer are found in this country each year. The exact number of people who develop non-melanoma skin cancers each year is not known because doctors do not always report these cases to cancer registries. There are, however, about 2,000 deaths from nonmelanoma skin cancer each year.

Melanoma is another story. The lifetime melanoma risk for the overall United States population is about 1.4 percent (that's about 50,000 people a year, or about one out of every seventy-five people). An estimated 7,400 people die each year from melanoma.

Most skin cancers are a direct result of sunlight exposure. More than 90 percent of them develop on sun-exposed skin: face, neck, forearms, and hands. Many of these cases are the nonmelanoma variety.

Because melanomas develop differently and can be more serious, they are often separated from these less serious forms of skin cancer.

Nonmelanoma Skin Cancers

Nonmelanoma skin cancers are the most common cancers of the skin. The two most common types of nonmelanoma skin cancers are basal cell carcinoma (BCC) and squamous cell carcinoma (SCC). Both basal cell and squamous cell cancers are found on sun-exposed parts of the body, and they appear because of lifetime sun exposure.

What Makes You More Likely to Develop a Nonmelanoma Skin Cancer?

As mentioned before, a risk factor is something that increases your chance of getting a disease. Some risk factors, such as smoking, can be modified. Others, such as your age or race, can't be changed. The following are known to be risk factors for nonmelanoma skin cancer:

- **Too much exposure to strong sunlight:** The sun is the main source of UV radiation. People who are often exposed to strong sunlight without protection have a greater risk of developing nonmelanoma skin cancer. People who live in areas with year-round, bright sunlight have a higher risk. For example, the risk of nonmelanoma skin cancer is twice as high in Arizona as it is in Minnesota. Spending a lot of time outdoors for work or recreation without the protection of clothing, hats, and sunscreen also increases the risk. Tanning lamps and tanning booths are other sources of UV radiation that may produce a greater risk of nonmelanoma skin cancer.

- **Fair skin:** The risk of skin cancer is much higher for anyone with fair skin than it is for people with darker skin, no matter what your race or ethnic background. This is because the skin pigment called melanin, which is found in greater quantity in darker-skinned people, offers some protection from UV radiation. People with fair (light-colored) skin that freckles or burns easily are at especially high risk.

- **Being male:** Men are twice as likely as women to have basal cell cancers and three times as likely to have squamous cell cancers of the skin.

- **Chemical or radiation exposure:** Exposure to arsenic, a heavy metal used in making some insecticides and naturally found in water in some areas, increases the risk of developing nonmelanoma skin cancer. Workers exposed to industrial tar, coal, paraffin, and certain types of oil may also have an increased risk for nonmelanoma skin cancer (see Chapter 8). In addition, people who have had radiation treatment have a higher risk of developing nonmelanoma skin cancer in the area that received the treatment.

- **Certain long-term severe skin problems:** Nonmelanoma skin cancers are more likely to develop in scars from serious burns, areas of skin over severe bone infections, and skin damaged by certain diseases, although this risk is generally small. Certain types of treatment involving UV light, given to some patients with psoriasis (an inflammatory skin disease), can increase the risk of getting squamous cell skin cancer and perhaps other skin cancers as well.

- **Reduced immunity:** People with weakened immune systems are more likely to develop nonmelanoma skin cancer. For example, people who have had an organ transplant often take medicines that weaken the immune system to keep the body from rejecting the organ. This may increase their risk of developing skin cancer.

- **Certain inherited conditions:** A very rare, inherited condition known as xeroderma pigmentosum reduces the skin's ability to repair damage to DNA caused by sun exposure. People with this disorder develop many skin cancers, sometimes beginning in childhood. Another rare condition, basal cell nevus syndrome, is present at birth and can cause multiple basal cell cancers. Most, but not all, cases are inherited.

Basal Cell Carcinoma

Basal cell carcinomas (sometimes referred to as BCC) arise from basal cells in the lowest layer of the epidermis (see page 138). About 75 percent of all skin cancers are basal cell carcinomas. They usually begin on areas exposed to the sun such as the head and neck. Basal cell carcinoma was once found mostly in middle-aged or older people. It is now also being seen in younger people, who might be spending more time in the sun.

Fortunately, basal cell carcinoma is slow growing. It is highly unusual for a basal cell cancer to spread to distant parts of the body. However, if a basal cell cancer is not treated, it can grow into nearby areas and invade the bone or other tissues beneath the skin. This can be a serious problem with such cancers on the face, especially around the eyes.

After treatment, basal cell carcinoma can come back in the same place on the skin. New basal cell cancers can also pop up on other areas of skin. People who have had one basal cell cancer are more likely to develop a new skin cancer within the next five years.

Squamous Cell Carcinoma

Squamous cell carcinomas (sometimes referred to as SCC) begin in the upper part of the epidermis and account for about 20 percent of all skin cancers. They usually appear on sun-exposed areas of the body such as the face, ears, neck, lips, and backs of the hands. They can also begin within scars or skin ulcers elsewhere on the body.

Squamous cell carcinomas are more likely than basal cell carcinomas to invade tissues beneath the skin and are more likely to spread to distant parts of the body. Even so, very few squamous cell skin carcinomas spread to lymph nodes or other organs.

Precancerous Skin Conditions

Actinic keratosis (the plural form, keratoses), also known as solar keratosis, is a precancerous skin condition caused by overexposure to the sun. Actinic keratoses are slow growing. They usually do not cause any symptoms or signs other than patches on the skin; however, they are a warning that the skin has been damaged by the sun. It is possible, but not common, for actinic keratoses to turn into squamous cell cancer. They also frequently go away on their own but may come back.

Melanoma Skin Cancer

Malignant melanoma writes its message in the skin with its own ink and it is there for all of us to see.
—Neville Davis, M.D.

Melanoma is a cancer that begins in the melanocytes (see page 138). Other names for this cancer include malignant melanoma, melanoma skin cancer, and cutaneous melanoma. Because most melanoma cells still produce melanin, melanoma tumors are often brown or black.

Melanoma most often appears on the trunk of the body in fair-skinned men and on the lower legs in fair-skinned women, but it can appear anywhere on the body, including the iris (the colored part of the eye). Having darkly pigmented skin lowers the risk of melanoma but does not eliminate it. People with darker skin can develop this cancer on the palms of the hands, soles of the feet, and under their fingernails and toenails, which only underscores the importance of having your doctor examine your nails without nail polish.

How Common Is Melanoma?

Melanoma is much less common than basal cell and squamous cell skin cancers, but it is far more serious. Melanoma accounts for about 4 percent of skin cancer cases, but causes about 79 percent of skin cancer deaths. Although melanoma is almost always curable in its early stages, it is much more likely than basal or squamous cell cancer to spread (metastasize) to other parts of the body.

The American Cancer Society (ACS) estimates that about 53,600 new melanoma cases will be diagnosed in the United States in 2002, and this number continues to rise each year. About 7,400 people in the U.S. are expected to die of melanoma during 2002. Since 1930, the incidence of malignant melanoma has risen 1,800 percent. Since 1973, the number of new cases for melanoma has more than doubled, and the number of deaths caused by melanoma has increased by about 44 percent. It is one of the fastest growing types of cancer in the United States. Death rates from melanoma are increasing most rapidly among white men aged fifty years and older.

What Makes You More Likely to Develop Melanoma?

Melanoma has several risk factors, many of which are similar to those for other skin cancers. It is important to remember, though, that while certain factors may increase your risk, they do not necessarily cause the disease to develop. Many people with risk factors never develop cancer, while others with this disease have no known risk factors. The main risk factors for developing melanoma include the following:

- **Moles:** As introduced earlier in this chapter, a mole or nevus is a non-cancerous skin tumor. Moles are not usually present at birth but begin to appear in children and teenagers. People with lots of moles (more than 200 moles, or more than fifty if under the age of twenty), and those who have some large moles (greater than ¼ inch), have an increased risk for melanoma. See pages 167–170 to learn how to examine your skin.

- **Fair skin:** The risk of melanoma is much higher for people with fair skin than for those with darker skin. This is because the melanin in darker skin offers some protection from UV rays. But people with darker skin types can also develop melanoma. Anyone with red or blond hair and fair skin that freckles or burns easily is at especially high risk.

- **Family history:** The risk of melanoma is greater if one or more close relatives (mother, father, brother, sister, child) have been diagnosed with melanoma. Around 10 percent of all people with melanoma have a family history of melanoma. But this means that 90 percent *do not* have a family history.

- **Immune suppression:** People who have been treated with medicines that suppress the immune system, such as organ transplant patients, have an increased risk of developing melanoma.

- **Too much exposure to ultraviolet (UV) radiation:** People with too much exposure to light from the sun or from tanning beds are at greater risk for all types of skin cancer including melanoma. However, unlike other forms of skin cancer where the risk seems to be related to the total dose of UV exposure over a lifetime, melanomas are more common in those with a history of high-dose, short-term exposures. Therefore, people who had severe sunburns, especially as children and teenagers, have been found to be at increased risk.

- **Age:** Although about half of all melanomas occur in people over the age of fifty years old, young people (ages twenty to thirty) can also have melanoma. In fact, melanoma is one of the most common cancers in people younger than thirty.

Prevention: Something New Under the Sun

There is good news: skin cancer can be prevented. The challenge, however, lies in changing the attitudes and behaviors that increase a person's risk of developing skin cancer.
—David Satcher, M.D., Ph.D., former U.S. Surgeon General

Head for cover! It's one of the best things you can do to reduce your risk of skin cancer. In fact, about 80 percent of skin cancers could be prevented if we protect ourselves from the sun's rays. Simply put, the best way to lower your risk of melanoma and other skin cancers is to avoid too much exposure to the sun and other sources of UV light. It's as easy as slip, slop, slap, and wrap!

Be Safe While the Sun Shines

So you have the sunscreen labeled SPF 30, maybe even 45, in your beach bag. That's a good start, but putting on the right amounts throughout the day is a must to prevent sunburn, and to lower your risk of getting skin cancer. Sunscreen use is very important, but it's not the only tool necessary to reduce your risk of developing skin cancer. Wise sun protection also involves clothing, hats, sunglasses, and seeking shade whenever possible, say dermatology experts. The more you know, the more you can safely and enjoyably spend time outdoors, reducing your risk of overexposure. Practicing sun safety all year long includes the following strategies:

Look for Shade in the Middle of the Day

The simplest and most effective way to limit exposure to ultraviolet light is to avoid being outdoors in sunlight too long. This is particularly important in the middle of the day between the hours of 10 A.M. and 4 P.M. when ultraviolet light is most intense. That's daylight savings time. Adjust those hours to 9 A.M. and 3 P.M. during standard time. When the sun is overhead, you are more likely to burn. Gauge the sun's intensity by your shadow. If your shadow is shorter than you are, the sun is directly over your head. Not all sunlight is direct. Sunlight can reflect off water, sand, concrete, boat decks, and snow and can reach below the water's surface. UV rays can reach you even on cloudy days.

Slip on a Shirt — Slap on a Hat

You can protect most of your skin with clothing, including a shirt and a hat with a broad brim that shades your face, neck, and ears. Newer hat styles have fabric flaps that can cover your ears and neck. Straw hats are not recommended unless they are tightly woven. A loosely woven straw hat can let light in. Baseball caps don't protect your ears or neck. Long-sleeved shirts, long pants, and clothing made from dark fabric with a tight weave generally provide the best sun protection.

Slop on Sunscreen

Broad-spectrum sunscreens (covering both UVA and UVB) with an SPF of 15 or more should be used on areas of skin exposed to the sun. Be particularly attentive when the sunlight is strongest (between the hours of 10 A.M. and 4 P.M.). And don't forget your lips. Use lip balm also with an SPF of 15 or greater. Some lipsticks contain a sunscreen.

How to Choose and Use the Right Suncreen

Sunscreen is just one part of a comprehensive sun protection program. Do not use sunscreen to extend your time in the sun. Use it along with clothing, a hat, and sunglasses.

Sunscreen now comes in more varieties than ever. Consider several of the following features in choosing and using a product that will give you the best sun protection.

- Look for combined ingredients that block both UVA and UVB, the two most damaging forms of UV radiation. Scientists have long known UVB is the principal cause of sunburn and skin cancer, and more recently it has been shown UVA can compound the damage to cells caused by UVB and give skin a wrinkled, leathery appearance.

- Sun protection factor in sunscreens lets you gauge how long the lotion can protect your skin from UVB rays (a standardized measurement system for UVA radiation hasn't been adopted yet). An SPF of 15 blocks out about 93 percent of UVB, while an SPF of 30 blocks out approximately 97 percent. SPF numbers generally range from 2 to 30 or higher, but just because the SPF numbers are higher doesn't mean the protection is greater.

- Sunscreen products will be required by the FDA to have uniform labels by December 2002 to help consumers make wise decisions about sun protection. Here's what you can expect:

  Manufacturers will not be able to use unsupported, misleading, or confusing terms such as *all-day protection, waterproof, sunblock,* and *visible and/or infrared light protection.*

Like the warnings on packs of cigarettes, sun products will carry a warning statement too. Products will have a "Sun Alert" statement such as: "Limiting sun exposure, wearing protective clothing, and using sunscreens may reduce the risks of skin aging, skin cancer, and other harmful effects of the sun." The message is that sunscreens do not protect against sunburn or repeated exposure to the sun.

In addition to required sun protection factor testing, there will be a new SPF category called "30+" for values above 30.

- To help protect your skin, find the right kind of sunscreen for the activity you're doing, no matter what time of year. Experts recommend year-round use of sunscreen. If you plan to stay in the water, choose a product that doesn't need to be reapplied after every dip in the pool. You need to reapply sunscreen at least every two hours. For outdoor activities, manufacturers have products available with sun protection and insect repellant.

- Always follow the manufacturer's directions. Most recommend applying sunscreen generously to dry skin twenty to thirty minutes before sun exposure so your skin has time to absorb the chemicals. When applying it, pay particular attention to your face, ears, hands, and arms, and generously coat the skin that is not covered by clothing. Apply it at frequent intervals after that—again, every two hours or immediately after swimming or strenuous activity. If you're wearing insect repellant or makeup, sunscreen should be applied before those products. Some makeup contains sunscreen, but only the label can tell you. Makeup, including lipstick, without sunscreen does not provide sun protection.

- How much is enough? One ounce of sunscreen, about a palmful, is considered the amount needed to cover the exposed areas of an adult's body completely.

Always follow directions when applying sunscreen. To work best, sunscreen should be applied before you go outside, used generously on all sun-exposed skin, and reapplied every two hours. A one-ounce application (a palmful of sunscreen) is recommended. Many sunscreens wear off with sweating and swimming and must be reapplied for maximum effectiveness. Use sunscreen even on hazy days or days with light or partial cloud cover because the UV light still comes through.

Sunscreens work by absorbing, reflecting, or scattering the sun's rays, according to the Centers for Disease Control and Prevention. The chemicals in the sunscreen interact with your skin to protect it from UV rays.

Researchers have found that many people use sunscreens so that they can stay out in the sun longer. Staying out longer while using sunscreen just means that you'll end up getting the same amount of UV light as you would otherwise, which won't reduce your risk. Sunscreen will not prevent skin cancer; it just reduces the amount of UV light exposure to the skin. All excessive sun exposure, which shows up on the skin as a burn or a tan, is unhealthy.

The American Academy of Dermatology recommends that you use sunscreen every day if you are going to be in the sun for more than twenty minutes. So just walking outside to pick up the newspaper from the driveway or to check your mailbox is a good time to get a few rays without sunscreen. But small trips here and there add up. Most people underestimate the amount of time they spend in the sun. The National Safety Council says most of us are exposed to nineteen hours of incidental sun exposure per week.

Wrap on Sunglasses

Wearing sunglasses protects the lids of your eyes as well as the lens. Wrap-around sunglasses and ski goggles provide the best protection for the eyes and the skin area around the eyes. Look for sunglasses labeled as blocking 99 percent or 100 percent UVA and UVB. Tags also sometimes read "UV absorption up to 400 nm" or "absorbs UV up to 400 nm," which indicates protection from UVA and UVB.

Avoid Other Sources of UV Light

As mentioned earlier in this chapter, the use of tanning beds and sun lamps is hazardous because the ultraviolet radiation they deliver can be damaging to the skin. There is growing evidence that they may increase your risk of developing skin cancer. Avoiding tanning beds and sun lamps is highly recommended.

Take Extra Precautions

Some medications and fragrances can make your skin more sensitive to the sun, a condition called photosensitivity. Photosensitivity can lead to a variety of reactions upon exposure, from skin that burns more readily to hives, itchy rashes, and even blistering or scaling of skin. Sunscreen does not protect the skin from photosensitivity reactions. Ask your pharmacist or doctor about medications and supplements you are taking, and, if necessary, avoid the sun as much as possible especially when it is its hottest, and be more careful by covering your skin and eyes when out in the sun.

Kid Stuff: Rubbing It In

Young people need to know that the risk of getting skin cancer later can be greatly reduced if they start protecting their skin from the sun now.
— JEFFREY P. KOPLAN, M.D., M.P.H., Former Director of
the Centers for Disease Control and Prevention

Take special care with children, since they tend to spend more time outdoors than adults and can burn more easily. Although many of the sun's worst effects do not appear until later in life, recent medical research has shown that it is very important to protect children and teenagers from overexposure to UV radiation. The majority of most people's sun exposure occurs before the age of eighteen, and studies increasingly suggest a link between early exposure and skin cancer as an adult.

Parents play a crucial role in protecting the health of their children. Parents should guard their children against excess sun exposure by using plenty of sunscreen and reapplying it every two hours. Better yet, keep your children out of the sun during harsh midday hours. Go to the swimming pool in the morning or late afternoon.

Keep children younger than six months out of direct sunlight and minimize their sun exposure. Use hats, clothing, and shading to protect small babies from the sun, rather than sunscreen, whenever possible.

Encourage children six months and older to play in the shade, have them wear protective clothing, and reapply their sunscreen often. As they become more independent, older children can be educated about sun safety and overexposure. It is important, particularly in high sun-exposure areas of the world, to get children in the habit of protecting their skin with clothing, hats, sunglasses, and sunscreen whenever they go outdoors and may be exposed to large amounts of sunlight. This advice, however, is often difficult to follow in school, for example, when children go outside for recess or on school-supervised field trips.

In a 1998 nationwide telephone survey by the ACS, nearly three-fourths of youth between the ages of eleven to eighteen stated that they became sunburned in the summer. Of those who were burned, 38 percent reported using sunscreen with an SPF of 15 or higher before getting the sunburn. Although girls are more likely than boys to use sunscreen, they are also more likely to get sunburned from sunbathing and to use a tanning bed.

A recent study published in the *Journal of the American Medical Association* shows sunscreen may be effective in protecting children from developing moles on the skin, especially for children with freckles, which could mean a decrease in the risk of melanoma later on in life.

Getting to Know You

Everyone can play a vital role in finding skin cancer early. As part of a routine cancer-related checkup, your doctor should check your skin carefully.

You can improve your chances of finding precancerous skin conditions, such as actinic keratosis—a dry, scaly, reddish, and slightly raised lesion—and skin cancer by examining your skin regularly, preferably once a month. The earlier you identify potential problem spots and see your health care team, the greater your chances for a simple and successful treatment. A critical aspect to skin cancer prevention is identifying abnormal moles and skin problems.

How to Examine Your Skin

Self-examination is best done in a well-lit room in front of a full-length mirror. Some people find that the best time to examine their skin is after a shower or bath. A handheld mirror can be used for areas that are hard to see. A spouse or other partner may be able to help you with these examinations, especially for those hard-to-see areas like the lower back or the back of your thighs. Skin cancers, especially melanomas, can pop up anywhere. All areas of your body should be examined, including the scalp, ears, palms and soles, under nail beds, and back.

The first time you inspect your skin, spend a fair amount of time carefully going over the entire surface of your skin. Follow the step-by-step instructions on page 164 to examine your skin.

The American Cancer Society recommends a cancer-related checkup, including a skin examination, every three years for people between twenty and forty years old and every year for anyone aged forty and older.

How to Examine Your Skin

The illustrations below will help you notice a suspicious lesion that may be skin cancer.

Examine your face, especially the nose, lips, and mouth, and the front and back of the ears. Use a hand mirror, floor-length mirror, or both to get a clear view.

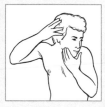

Thoroughly inspect your scalp, using a blow dryer and mirror to expose each section to view. Get a friend or family member to help, if you can.

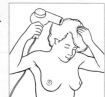

Check your hands carefully: palms and backs, between the fingers, and under the fingernails. Continue up the wrists to examine both the front and back of your forearms.

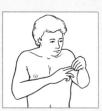

Standing in front of a full-length mirror, begin at the elbows and scan all sides of your upper arms. Don't forget the underarms.

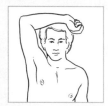

Next focus on the neck, chest, and torso. Women should lift breasts to view the underside.

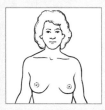

With your back to a full-length mirror, use a hand mirror to inspect the back of your neck, shoulders, upper back, and any part of the back of your upper arms you could not view earlier.

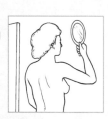

Still using both a hand mirror and a full-length mirror, scan your lower back, buttocks, and backs of both legs.

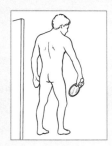

Sit down; prop each leg in turn on a stool or chair. Use a hand mirror to examine the genitals. Check the front and sides of both legs, thigh to shin, ankles, tops of feet, between toes, and under toenails. Examine the soles of feet and heels.

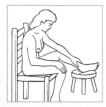

Tricks of the Trade: The Tools You May Need

- Well-lighted room

- Two mirrors—one full-length and one handheld

- Blow dryer (to part the hair on your scalp)

- Two chairs or stools

- A spouse, friend, or family member

The first self-exam is important for two reasons. By going over your body thoroughly, you may notice potential trouble spots that should be seen by a doctor. You will also become familiar with the pattern of moles, blemishes, freckles, and other marks on your skin so that you'll be able to notice any changes as time goes on.

Look for changes in size, texture, shape, and color of blemishes or a sore that does not heal. Anything unusual (crusting, scaling, oozing, or bleeding) may be a warning sign of skin cancer. The skin may also feel itchy or tender. Of course, there are many harmless causes for skin lesions. If you're unsure about something that looks suspicious, see your doctor.

More than half of all newly reported melanomas are detected by the patients themselves, according to a study at Johns Hopkins. But doctors spot them earlier in more treatable stages. The researchers said every doctor visit is an opportunity for a skin check. So ask your doctor to take a look, even when you're there for another reason.

A dermatologist (a doctor who specializes in treating skin diseases) can actually map your skin and note on paper (or even photograph) any areas to watch during the next examination. This way you and your doctor have a record of your moles and their size and locations and the date. Then if you find something and wonder just how long it has been there, you can check the record.

Both nonmelanoma and melanoma skin cancers usually appear on the skin (although melanomas can arise in other areas, such as the eyes or mouth). Most skin problems do not turn out to be cancer, but only tests done by a doctor can tell for sure whether a growth on the skin is cancerous (or precancerous). Below we describe the signs and symptoms for nonmelanoma and melanoma skin cancers.

Look at the Surface

Nonmelanoma skin cancers are the most common cancers of the skin (see pages 150–153). What do these skin cancers look like? They can look like a variety of marks on the skin. They most often appear on sun-exposed areas of the body, such as the face, ears, neck, trunk, and arms but may appear anywhere on the body. The key warning signs are a new growth, a spot or bump that's getting larger over time, or a sore that doesn't heal within three months.

- *Basal cell carcinomas* often appear as flat, scaly, red areas or as small, raised, shiny, waxy areas that may bleed following minor injury. For example, you might accidentally nick one when shaving your face or legs. They are hard to the touch. The borders of these cancers are often described as "pearly"—they are bumpy and are raised higher than the rest of the lesion. You might also see one or more irregular blood vessels, or blue, brown, or black areas.

- *Squamous cell carcinomas* may appear as growing lumps, often with a rough surface, or as flat, reddish patches in the skin that grow slowly. They may be scaly or crusty and over time may become open sores.

- *Actinic keratoses* are small (usually less than one-quarter inch across), rough spots that may be pink-red or flesh-colored. Usually they develop on the face, ears, back of the hands, and arms of middle-aged or older people with fair skin, although they can arise on other sun-exposed areas of the skin. People with one actinic keratosis will usually develop many more. Some actinic keratoses and other skin conditions that could become cancers may have to be removed; however, you and your doctor should regularly check others for changes that could indicate cancer.

Other types of nonmelanoma skin cancers are rare and not detailed here, but a qualified doctor should be able to identify any suspicious areas you may have. Nearly all basal cell and squamous cell cancers that are detected early and treated promptly are cured. Treatment is usually removal and analysis under a microscope. In a simple office procedure, your doctor will numb the area and remove the suspicious area with a scalpel or a special biopsy tool.

Know Your Moles

Most people have moles, and almost all moles are harmless. But, certain types of moles have an increased risk of developing into a melanoma. Although sun exposure plays a role in its development, melanoma can appear on any area of the body, even places where the skin has never been exposed.

People with lots of moles and those who have some large moles have an increased risk for melanoma. If you have suspicious looking moles, your doctor may monitor them closely with periodic examinations, or may remove them if they have certain features that suggest they may be changing into melanoma. Routine removal of many moles is not generally recommended as a way to prevent melanoma. For people with many moles, careful periodic examination by a dermatologist, in combination with monthly skin self-examination, is recommended.

So how can you tell a normal mole from one that is or could become cancerous?

- **A normal mole.** A normal mole is generally an evenly colored brown, tan, or black spot on the skin. It can be either flat or raised. It can be round or oval. Moles are generally less than six millimeters across (that's about ? inch, or the width of a pencil eraser). A mole can be present at birth, but it is much more likely to appear during childhood or young adulthood. Several moles can appear at the same time, especially on areas of the skin exposed to the sun.

- **An abnormal mole.** One type of mole that increases the risk of melanoma is the dysplastic nevus or atypical mole. Dysplastic nevi (nevi is the plural of nevus) look a little like normal moles, but also typically look a little like melanoma. The moles can appear in areas that are exposed to the sun, as well as in those areas that are usually covered, such as the buttocks and scalp. They are often larger than other moles and may have an irregular (not round) border. They may also have some slight variations in color. Some people have many dysplastic nevi.

  Dysplastic nevi often run in families. A person who has family members with dysplastic nevi has about a 50 percent chance of developing these nevi. Someone with one or more dysplastic nevi and with at least two close relatives with melanoma has a 50 percent or greater risk of developing melanoma. Moles that are not dysplastic or congenital (present at birth) are unlikely to turn into a melanoma skin cancer.

- **Birthmarks (congenital moles).** Moles present at birth are called congenital melanocytic nevi. The average lifetime risk of developing melanoma may be about 6 percent for people with congenital melanocytic nevi, but this risk is affected by the size of the nevus. People with large congenital nevi have a greater risk, while the risk is less for those with small nevi.

Know Your ABCDs

Almost everyone has moles. In fact, the average person has about twenty-five. Most moles are perfectly harmless, but a change in any mole is a sign that you should show it to your doctor.

The ABCD rule is a simple, easy-to-remember guide to the warning signs for melanoma. Melanoma may appear without warning, and it may begin in or near a mole or other dark spot in the skin. That's why it's so important to know the color, size, and location of the moles on your body, so you'll recognize any changes. Unlike basal cell and squamous cell cancers, which don't usually spread to other parts of the body, colonies of melanoma cells can spread and reach vital internal organs and grow. These are much more difficult to treat if not detected early.

Be on the look out for any changes in your moles and notify your doctor about moles with any of the following features.

A is for **ASYMMETRY:** One half of a mole or birthmark does not match the other.

B is for **BORDER IRREGULARITY:** Normal moles are round or oval. With melanoma, the edges are irregular, ragged, notched, or blurred.

C is for **COLOR:** The color is not the same all over and may have differing shades of brown or black, or sometimes patches of red, white, or blue.

D is for **DIAMETER:** The area is larger than six millimeters (that's ¼ of an inch, or about the size of a pencil eraser) or is growing larger. In recent years, doctors are finding smaller melanomas between three and six millimeters.

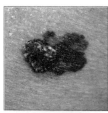 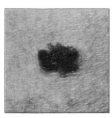 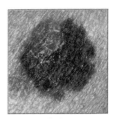 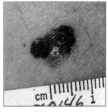

| Asymmetry | Border Irregularity | Color | Diameter |

The most important warning sign for skin cancer is a spot on the skin that is *changing* in size, shape, or color over a period of a month to years. You might see pigment spreading from the border into surrounding skin. The mole may change in sensation and become itchy, tender, or painful. You may see scaliness, oozing, or bleeding, or the appearance of a bump on the surface.

Some melanomas do not fit the ABCD rule, so it is particularly important to be aware of any changes in your skin and see your doctor. Don't wait for your annual appointment. Although melanoma can be deadly, if it's detected early, it is almost 100 percent curable.

Prevention Before Detection

With simple changes in behavior and attitude, skin cancer may be highly preventable, and someday may even become uncommon. The real hope for the future lies in prevention and early detection. You can be your skin's best friend by becoming familiar with how your skin normally looks and feels, and by taking precautions to reduce your risk of skin cancer. Clearly, most skin cancers can be prevented by avoiding overexposure to the sun and to other sources of UV radiation, and when outdoors by protecting your skin with clothing, a hat, sunscreen with an SPF of 15 or higher, and sunglasses.

CHAPTER 5

Break Away from the Pack

"Nonsmoking section, please." One day the American Cancer Society (ACS) hopes that this will be an obsolete phrase as more cities across the country adopt cigarette smoking bans in restaurants. Smokers are increasingly being forced to make special arrangements to smoke since we have become aware of the dangers. The harmful effects of smoking have become a part of our collective consciousness. Just about everyone knows that smoking is unhealthy. We've come a long way baby! But don't skip ahead just yet. What you may not know is how much you are at risk for lung cancer from secondhand smoke, even if you are not a smoker. Or maybe if you are a smoker, you're looking for more motivation to cut down or quit.

Whether you are a nonsmoker, smoker, live with a smoker, or know someone who smokes, this chapter is for you. Here you'll learn the health effects of tobacco on yourself and others, as well as how you can reduce the risk of cancers associated with tobacco use. We explain options for quitting smoking as well as the keys for success.

The Truth About Tobacco

Cigarettes are killers that travel in packs.
—Unknown

Cigarettes kill more Americans than alcohol, car accidents, fires, suicide, AIDS, homicide, and drug abuse *combined*. Tobacco use is, quite simply, the most preventable cause of premature death in our society. Even the tobacco industry has finally admitted that tobacco use is harmful to your health.

The good news is that cigarette smoking in adults in the United States has dropped from 42 percent in 1965 to less than 23 percent today. Even better news is that more than 75 percent of adult Americans do not smoke; but a lot of people, nearly 25 percent of them, still smoke. That's almost one in every four Americans. And a lot of people (430,700 a year) still die from smoking and its effects. Let's take a closer look at the truth about all forms of smoking and tobacco use, including the search for a "safe" cigarette.

Cigarettes

*We accept that the best judgment of all the evidence
is that smoking causes lung cancer.*
—NICK BROOKES, Chairman and CEO
of Brown & Williamson Tobacco Company

Cigarette smoking accounts for the majority of tobacco use in the United States. There is overwhelming evidence that cigarette use is linked to lung and other cancers. The facts about smoking and cancer are alarming.

- **Lung cancer causes far more deaths than any other cancer, in both men and women.** Lung cancer is one of the most difficult cancers to treat. It is very hard to detect when it is in the earliest, most treatable stage. It can hide for years without causing any symptoms. In most cases, by the time it's found, the cancer has already spread to other parts of the body. Less than 15 percent of people with lung cancer will live longer than five years.

- **Lung cancer, fortunately, is a largely preventable disease.** About 87 percent of lung cancer deaths are related to smoking. Men who smoke are more than twenty times more likely to die from lung cancer, and women who smoke are twelve times more likely to die from it. Groups that advocate nonsmoking as part of their religion, such as Mormons and Seventh-Day Adventists, have much lower rates of lung cancer and other smoking-related cancers.

- **Lung cancer is not the only cancer caused by smoking.** Smoking is also linked with cancers of the mouth, throat, esophagus, pancreas, cervix, kidney, and bladder. Recent studies have indicated that smoking is also associated with cancers of the stomach, liver, colon and rectum, and with a form of acute leukemia as well.

Cigarette Smoking and Cancer

Major Cause of These Cancers	Contributing Cause to These Cancers
Lung	Bladder
Larynx (voice box)	Pancreas
Oral cavity (lip, tongue, mouth)	Uterine
Pharynx (throat)	Cervix
Esophagus	Kidney
	Stomach
	Liver
	Some leukemias
	Colon and rectum

- **Cancer is not the only disease caused by smoking.** Smokers are at increased risk for heart and lung diseases, and a host of other problems, which are explained further in this chapter (see pages 184–187).

The Search for the "Safe" Cigarette

Smoking low tar and nicotine cigarettes is the equivalent of
jumping out of the 29th floor of a building rather than the 31st.
—KENNETH WARNER AND JOHN SLADES, American Journal of Public Health

Some people think that switching from high-tar and high-nicotine cigarettes to those with lower tar and nicotine content makes smoking safer, but this is not always true. When people switch to lower tar and nicotine brands, they often smoke more cigarettes or more of each cigarette to get the same nicotine dose as before. A low-tar cigarette can be just as harmful as a high-tar cigarette when taking deeper puffs, puffing more frequently, or smoking cigarettes to a shorter butt length. Even if smokers who switch to lower tar brands do not make these changes to compensate, the health benefits are insignificant when compared to the benefits of quitting completely.

Menthol cigarettes are not safer than nonmenthol brands and may even be more dangerous. These brands contain enough menthol to produce a cool sensation in the throat when smoke is inhaled. About 28 percent of all cigarettes sold in the United States are menthol. About 76 percent of African-American cigarette smokers smoke menthol cigarettes as compared to 23 percent of whites.

People who smoke menthol cigarettes can inhale more deeply or hold the smoke inside longer than smokers of nonmenthol cigarettes. This may partially explain why African-American smokers, who statistically smoke fewer cigarettes a day (but more menthol cigarettes), are more likely than white smokers to die from smoking-related diseases such as lung cancer, heart disease, and stroke.

Some tobacco companies are test-marketing cigarettes that they claim have fewer toxins than other brands. These so-called light cigarettes provide smokers with false assurances that they are reducing their risks, when in fact they are not safe. Research has shown that smoking light cigarettes commonly results in smokers taking in more harmful substances—not fewer—as they smoke more cigarettes and inhale deeper to get the nicotine their bodies crave. "Calling these cigarettes 'less toxic' than others doesn't mean they're less likely to give you cancer," said Ron Todd, M.S. Ed.D., Director of Tobacco Control for the ACS.

Simply put, there are no safe cigarettes.

WARNING: There is no safe tobacco product. The use of any tobacco product—
including cigarettes, cigars, pipes, and spit tobacco; mentholated, "low-tar,"
"naturally grown," or "additive free"—can cause cancer and other adverse health effects.
—Centers for Disease Control and Prevention

Clove Cigarettes

Clove cigarettes, also called kreteks, are a type of tobacco product imported from Indonesia. They contain 60 to 70 percent tobacco and 30 to 40 percent ground cloves, clove oil, and other additives. Users often have the mistaken notion that smoking clove cigarettes is safer than smoking tobacco or marijuana, but they pose all the same health risks as cigarettes.

Flavored Cigarettes

Flavored cigarettes, often called bidis (or beedies), are imported mainly from India. They are sold in tobacco specialty stores, and frequently in health food stores. They have become popular with teenagers in the past few years. This may be due in part to the fact that they come in a variety of candy-like flavors, such as strawberry, vanilla, root beer, and grape, and they are often less expensive than regular cigarettes.

Even though bidis contain less tobacco than regular cigarettes, recent studies have found that bidis have higher levels of nicotine, tar, and carbon monoxide because the bidi is wrapped in an unprocessed tobacco leaf. In addition, because they are thinner than regular cigarettes, they require about three times as many puffs per cigarette. Bidis pose the same health risks as regular cigarettes. The truth is that bidis are just cigarettes with a sweet façade.

Many younger smokers prefer both flavored and clove cigarettes. They are nearly ideal in design as a "trainer" cigarette for capturing young people as smokers. The false image of these products as clean, natural, and safer than conventional cigarettes seems to attract some young people who may not otherwise start smoking.

Spit Tobacco

If flavored cigarettes are not attractive enough to young people, then surely the role models in baseball dugouts across the country are. Why is it the TV cameras always catch your favorite slugger, catcher, or first baseman chewing and spitting?

Spit (also called smokeless) tobacco is available in two different forms: snuff and chewing tobacco.

- Snuff, a fine grain tobacco, comes in cans or pouches. Users take a "pinch," "dip," or "quid," and place it between the lower lip or cheek and gum and suck on it.

- Chewing tobacco comes in pouches in the form of long strands of tobacco that, when used, are commonly called "plugs," "wads," or "chew."

Spit tobacco is never a safe alternative to smoking. Spit tobacco can have several harmful effects on your health. It contains nicotine, the same addictive drug found in cigarettes and it can lead to serious problems with your gums and teeth, as well as to chronic bad breath.

But the most serious health effect of spit tobacco is an increased risk of cancers of the mouth and throat. Cancers of the mouth occur several times more frequently among dip users than among non-tobacco users, and the risk of cancer of the cheek and gums may increase nearly fifty-fold among long-term snuff users. Spit tobacco may also play a role in cardiovascular disease and high blood pressure.

Cigars

A cigar is defined as a roll of tobacco wrapped in a tobacco leaf or in any substance containing tobacco (as opposed to a cigarette, which is wrapped in paper). Cigars come in different sizes. Some (called cigarillos) are as small as a cigarette, while others are much larger. It is not unusual for some premium brands to have as much tobacco in one cigar as is found in a whole pack of cigarettes.

The allure of a "fine cigar" has shaped public perception and misinformation about them. Cigars have long been associated with wealth, social prestige, and celebrations, such as the birth of a son or daughter. In recent years, they have become more popular than ever, fueled in part by the efforts of the tobacco industry to glamorize cigars and the willingness of movie stars and athletes to be paid and photographed smoking cigars. Especially for women, the industry seems to have tapped into an impulse among some to be slightly outrageous, to do something a little over the line, to be liberated from old restrictions and stereotypes. While the reasons people smoke cigars are varied, that fact is, like cigarettes, cigars can become addictive. And like cigarettes, cigars cause lung cancer.

Many people mistakenly believe that cigar smoking is less harmful than cigarette smoking. This is because while almost all cigarette smokers inhale, most cigar smokers do not. For those who do not inhale, the smoke does not reach the lungs in the same quantity as it does in cigarette smokers. However, for cigar smokers, the risk of death from lung cancer is still at least three times higher than the risk for nonsmokers.

Cigar smokers with a history of cigarette smoking, however, are more likely to inhale. Those who do inhale have an increased risk of death from lung cancer, eleven times greater than that of nonsmokers. And unfortunately, an emerging trend among cigar companies is the alteration of the pH values of their products, which makes them easier to inhale. That same curing and fermenting process further enhances the flavor yet increases the levels of harmful ingredients.

But the risks for those who inhale don't stop at lung cancer. Compared to nonsmokers, cigar smokers who inhale deeply are six times more likely to die from oral cancer, twice as likely to die from esophageal cancer, and thirty-nine times more likely to die from cancer of the larynx. They also face more than twice the risk of death from pancreatic cancer and more than three times the risk of death from bladder cancer compared to nonsmokers.

Pipes

Certainly a pipe, then, must be less harmful, so the reasoning goes. Similar to cigar smoking, pipe smoking is often associated with higher social status or with being well educated (think of the college professor stereotype). But pipe smokers face many of the same risks as do cigarette and cigar smokers.

A pipe is usually made of wood, marble, or clay with a mouthpiece at one end and a "bowl" at the other end where tobacco is tamped into it. As is true of other forms of tobacco use, smoking a pipe is not a healthy alternative to smoking cigarettes. A study published in the *Journal of the National Cancer Institute* shows that cigar and pipe smokers who smoke at a rate comparable to cigarette smokers have a similar risk for developing lung cancer.

Like cigar smokers, most pipe smokers do not inhale. However, they are still at an increased risk for lip, mouth, and tongue cancers. Because it is virtually impossible to avoid inhaling smoke totally, these smokers are also increasing their risk of lung cancer. The risk is higher among smokers who smoke both cigarettes and pipes (or cigars), and for smokers who switch to pipes (or cigars) after years of cigarette smoking.

Marijuana

Many of the cancer-causing substances in tobacco are also found in marijuana. Marijuana cigarettes contain more tar than tobacco cigarettes. Pot smokers inhale deeply and hold the smoke in the lungs to trigger the intoxicating effects. Marijuana cigarettes are also smoked all the way to the end where the tar content is the highest.

The connection, if any, between marijuana and lung cancer has been hard to prove because it is not easy to gather information about the use of illegal drugs. On top of this, many marijuana smokers also smoke tobacco cigarettes. This makes it difficult to know how much of the risk is from tobacco and how much may be from marijuana. Medical reports, however, suggest marijuana may cause cancers of the mouth and throat.

Who's at Added Risk and Why?

The risk for dying of lung cancer is twenty times higher among women who smoke two or more packs of cigarettes per day than among women who do not smoke.
—Women and Smoking: A Report of the Surgeon General, 2001

For women and young people, the use of tobacco products poses unique risks. Even though men are more likely to smoke than women, approximately 23 million adult women in the United States currently smoke cigarettes. And although all fifty states prohibit the sale of cigarettes to minors, now-banned smoking icon Joe Camel deceived far too many of America's teens into thinking that smoking is cool. At least 4.5 million adolescents (aged twelve to seventeen years old) also smoke, of which at least 1.5 million are girls.

You don't see the Marlboro Man on TV anymore (ironically, the actor who originally portrayed him died of lung cancer). In fact, you don't see any TV advertising for smoking products, and such ads are also banned in many sports venues. Nonetheless, even animated children's films continue to be loaded with tobacco or alcohol use in the story plots, without any reference to the potential negative consequences. And the good guys use tobacco and alcohol as frequently as the bad guys, according to research published in the *Journal of the American Medical Association*.

Women Are on the Line

Tobacco use among women has been shown to increase the risk of cancer, heart and lung diseases, and reproductive disorders. More than 160,000 women die each year from these smoking-related diseases. Approximately 66,000 women die each year from lung cancer alone, which has far surpassed breast cancer as the leading cause of cancer deaths among women, even though women fear breast cancer far more. The lung cancer death rate among women has increased by more than 600 percent over the last fifty years, reflecting an increasing number of women who began smoking after World War II, and is continuing to rise. Nearly 90 percent of these deaths are due to smoking.

Most deaths from heart disease and stroke in women are in those past menopause; however, smoking increases the risk more in younger women than in older women. Some studies suggest that smoking cigarettes dramatically increases the risk of heart disease among younger women who are also taking birth control pills.

Nearly 13 percent of pregnant women smoke throughout their pregnancy. Pregnant women who smoke are more likely to have a miscarriage, stillbirth, pre-term delivery, or a lower birth-weight baby. There is also a direct relationship between smoking during pregnancy and death among newborns and sudden infant death syndrome (SIDS).

Tobacco use by mothers also affects children after birth. Breast milk of women who smoke has been found to contain nicotine. Mothers in the U.S. who smoke at least ten cigarettes a day can worsen, or even cause, asthma among their children by exposing them to secondhand smoke. Exposure to secondhand smoke also increases a child's risk of pneumonia, bronchitis, and fluid in the middle ear.

Some Young Adults Just Can't Say "No"

Every day in the U.S., more than 6,000 adolescents try their first cigarette, and more than 3,000 become daily smokers. Think about it: When was the last time you met someone who started smoking as an adult?

Most people begin smoking between the ages of ten and eighteen. Peer pressure and curiosity are the major influences that encourage kids to experiment with smoking. Also, children with parents who smoke are more likely to begin smoking than those who have nonsmoking parents as role models. Young people often have a hard time understanding that the decisions they make now about smoking and using tobacco products will affect their overall health many years down the road.

Nearly 35 percent of high school students and about 15 percent of middle school students report being users of some form of tobacco (cigarettes, cigars, or spit). Young people use cigarettes more than any other form of tobacco—nearly one-third of high school students are current cigarette smokers.

The younger people start smoking cigarettes, the more likely they are to become strongly addicted to nicotine, and the higher their risk of lung cancer. For most smoking-related cancers, the risk of developing cancer rises as the person continues to smoke.

There are other health implications to smoking as a young person as well. Studies clearly show that cigarette smoking causes heart disease and stroke in adults. Early signs of these serious diseases can be found in adolescents who smoke. Also, teenage smokers suffer from

In the U.S., the Percentage of ...

- Adult smokers who started smoking when they were seventeen or younger ~80%

- Adolescent smokers who wish they had never started smoking — 70%

- Adolescent daily smokers who thought they would not smoke in five years that are still smoking five to six years later — 75%

- High school students who have tried cigarette smoking — 70%

- High school students who have smoked a whole cigarette before the age of thirteen — 25%

- Male high school students between the ages of twelve and seventeen who have used some form of spit tobacco — 20%

- High school students who had smoked cigars or cigarillos on at least one of the past thirty days — 18%

- High school students currently using chewing tobacco or snuff ~14%

- Middle school students who had smoked cigars or cigarillos on at least one of the past thirty days — 6%

shortness of breath, faster heart rate, reduced lung function, and overall poorer health.

Children and adolescents who participate in school sports are less likely to be smokers. On the other hand, young people who smoke are more likely to use other drugs, get in fights, carry weapons, suffer from mental health problems such as depression, attempt suicide, and engage in unprotected sex.

Hidden Dangers in Secondhand Smoke

It is now clear that disease risk due to inhalation of tobacco smoke
is not limited to the individual who is smoking.

—C. EVERETT KOOP, M.D., former U.S. Surgeon General

So maybe you've never smoked, or you quit a long time ago. Does this mean you're free of the increased risks that smokers have?

Unfortunately, no. If you've ever entered a smoke-filled bar, restaurant, home, or workplace, or ridden in the car of a smoker, then you have breathed most of the same harmful, cancer-causing chemicals in smoke. As an involuntary smoker—a nonsmoker breathing the smoke from others, as well as smoke from burning cigarettes—you are at increased risk. Smoke from others is also called environmental tobacco smoke, passive or involuntary smoking, and secondhand smoke.

Your risk of developing disease depends on the amount of tobacco smoke to which you are exposed. As an involuntary smoker, you inhale less tobacco smoke than an active smoker because the smoke mixes with the air around you. But the Environmental Protection Agency estimates that secondhand smoke causes about 3,000 lung cancer deaths each year in nonsmoking adults and impairs the respiratory health of hundreds of thousands of children. And exposure to cigar smoke is even worse. Secondhand smoke from cigars contains many of the same poisons and cancer-causing agents as does cigarette smoke but in higher concentrations and greater amounts because cigars often burn longer and give off more smoke.

If there are smokers in your family, your chances of dying from lung cancer are as much as 30 percent higher than if you lived in a family of nonsmokers. Involuntary smoking also causes heart disease, aggravates asthmatic conditions, and impairs blood circulation. Keep this in mind when checking out in-home day care centers and providers.

Increased Risk from Other People's Smoke

- Overall, nonsmoking wives of husbands who smoke have a 30 percent increased risk of lung cancer compared with women whose husbands don't smoke.

- Nonsmokers exposed to twenty or more cigarettes a day at home have twice the risk of developing lung cancer.

- Passive smoking is estimated to cause approximately 3,000 lung cancer deaths in nonsmokers each year; of those, about 800 occur as a result of exposure to secondhand smoke at home and 2,200 from exposure in work or social situations.

- Children of smokers have greater chances of developing illnesses such as colds, bronchitis and pneumonia, asthma, chronic coughs, ear infections, and reduced lung function.

These are the results of studies that have focused on people who live with smokers; if you live with just one smoker, you are at risk for lung cancer.

Quitting for the Health of It

To Your Health!

Health concerns usually top the list of reasons why people want to quit smoking. Nearly everyone knows that smoking can cause lung cancer, but few people realize it is also a risk factor for many other cancers. The risks of developing different kinds of cancers and chronic illnesses depend on the amount you smoke each day, the age you started smoking, and the number of years you've smoked. Roughly translated, the sooner you quit, the better your health will be. *And it's never too late to quit.*

Nature gives us just one pair of lungs. They must last a lifetime, playing a central role in breathing—about eighteen times a minute, every minute of the day. Normally, you don't even think about breathing. But with a bad chest cold, chronic bronchitis, or emphysema, you may suddenly become aware of how precious each breath is. Aside from lung cancer, smoking increases the risk of respiratory diseases such as emphysema and chronic bronchitis.

Smokers also have twice the risk of dying from heart attacks as do non-smokers. And smoking is a major risk factor for peripheral vascular disease, a narrowing of the blood vessels that carry blood to muscles in the arms and legs. Smoking has effects on the immune system. In fact, a study published in the *New England Journal of Medicine* shows that smokers are four times more likely than nonsmokers to contract near-fatal blood infections or meningitis from the same bacteria that cause pneumonia. Male smokers are also more likely to suffer from problems with impotence.

And then there are the effects that you—and everyone else—can see: premature wrinkling of the skin, bad breath, unpleasant smelling clothes, hair, house,

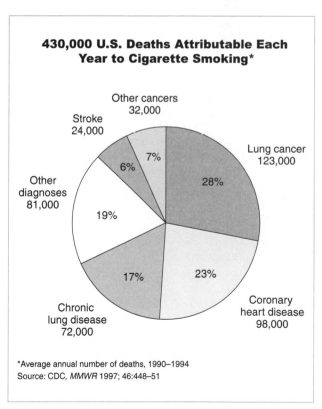

430,000 U.S. Deaths Attributable Each Year to Cigarette Smoking*

Other cancers 32,000

Stroke 24,000

Other diagnoses 81,000

Lung cancer 123,000

Coronary heart disease 98,000

Chronic lung disease 72,000

7%

6%

28%

19%

17%

23%

*Average annual number of deaths, 1990–1994
Source: CDC, *MMWR* 1997; 46:448–51

Benefits You Can See and Those You Can't

The health benefits of quitting smoking are immediate and just keep getting better over time.*
After you've quit smoking for . . .

Twenty minutes:	Blood pressure drops to a level close to that before the last cigarette. Temperature of hands and feet increases to normal.
Eight hours:	Carbon monoxide level in the blood drops to normal.
Twenty-four hours:	Chance of heart attack decreases.
Two weeks to three months:	Circulation improves. Walking becomes easier. Lung function increases up to 30 percent.
One to nine months:	Coughing, sinus congestion, fatigue, shortness of breath decrease. Cilia (small hairs in the lungs) regain normal function, increasing ability to handle mucus, clean the lungs, and reduce infection. Overall energy increases.
One year:	Excess risk of heart disease is half that of a smoker.
Five years:	Stroke risk is reduced to that of a nonsmoker five to fifteen years after quitting.
Ten years:	Risk of lung cancer is half that of continuing smokers. The risk of cancer of the mouth, throat, esophagus, bladder, kidney, and pancreas also decreases.
Fifteen years:	Risk of heart disease is that of a nonsmoker.

* The benefits may be more or less, depending on how heavily you smoked and for how many years.

and car, and yellowing nails. Someone once said that if the effects of cigarette smoking appeared on our skin instead of on our lungs—where it can't be seen—no one would smoke.

Regardless of a smoker's age or smoking history, there are advantages to quitting smoking. Benefits apply to healthy people (because of secondhand smoke) and to those who might already have smoking-related diseases. Your health reasons for quitting might include some of the following.

- People who quit smoking, regardless of age, live longer than those who continue to smoke. And fifteen years after quitting, the risk of death for ex-smokers has returned to nearly the same level as that of persons who have never smoked.

- About half of the people who smoke die from diseases caused by smoking. About half of these die before their seventieth birthday. On average, smokers die ten to twelve years younger and live seven years less than nonsmokers.

- Quitting smoking decreases the risk of lung cancer, heart disease, stroke, chronic lung diseases, and respiratory illnesses.

- Ex-smokers have fewer health complaints, better self-reported health status, and lower rates of bronchitis and pneumonia.

And even among people who have tried and tried again to quit, those periods of not smoking actually help lung function. A study in Finland tracked people over thirty years and found that people who never smoked, those who had smoked and quit, and "intermittent" quitters were better off than continuous smokers.

For the Health of Others

Smoking not only affects your health, but also the health of those around you. Studies have shown that secondhand smoke can cause lung

How many parents sneak a smoke, as if they think their kids don't know what mommy does in the laundry room or what daddy is doing in the garage? Who are you kidding with the mouthwash and room deodorant spray? If you have children, you want to set a good example for them. When asked, nearly all smokers say they don't want their children to smoke, but children whose parents smoke are more likely to start smoking themselves. You can become a good role model for them by quitting now.

cancer in healthy nonsmokers because it contains the same harmful chemicals that smokers inhale. Secondhand smoke can also cause eye irritation, headaches, nausea, and dizziness.

Secondhand smoke poses special dangers to mothers and children. It is associated with SIDS and low-birth weight infants. Smoking by mothers is linked to a higher risk of their babies developing asthma in childhood, especially if the mother smokes while pregnant. Babies and children raised in a household where there is smoking also have more ear infections, colds, bronchitis, and other respiratory problems than children from nonsmoking families. (See pages 183–184 for more information on secondhand smoke.)

This Habit Isn't Cheap Either

The prospect of better health is a major reason for quitting, but there are others as well. Smoking is expensive. It's not hard to figure out how much you spend on cigarettes: multiply the number of packs you smoke per day (be honest) by the cost per pack. Then multiply by 365 days per year. The number may surprise you. Now multiply that by the number of years you have been smoking, and the number will probably astound you.

Multiply the cost per year by ten (for the upcoming ten years of smoking) and ask yourself what you would rather do with that much money. Imagine yourself lighting that money on fire. Smokers also pay more for life and individual health insurance. The actuaries know your risks and figure that into the cost of your premiums.

Changing Perceptions

Like it or not, finding a place to smoke can now be a real hassle. Even outdoors. Outcasts. Smokers huddle together in rain and sleet and cold of night. How often do you see smokers clustered in clouds of smoke in bus stop-like shelters or inside doorways of their office buildings? There is no doubt that smoking is less socially acceptable now than it was in the past.

Although their decisions may not be entirely based on social acceptance, most employers have instituted some type of smoking restriction or even a complete ban on company property, and some employers prefer to hire nonsmokers. Studies show that smoking employees cost businesses more to employ because they are "out sick" more frequently, usually with colds and coughs. Time away from work for smoking breaks leads to measurably lower productivity.

Hotels and motels are offering smoke-free rooms—even to the point that no smoker has ever, theoretically, stayed in that room to leave behind the toxic effects from the smoke. Rental properties more recently have adopted nonsmoking policies for the fire hazards associated with smoking. Landlords may choose not to rent to smokers because maintenance costs and insurance rates may both rise with smokers occupying buildings.

If you're a smoker, your friends may ask you not to smoke in their homes or in their cars. Public buildings, concerts, and sporting events are largely smoke-free. In the purely social realm, smokers may find that their opportunities for dating or romantic involvement, including marriage, are largely limited to other smokers, who comprise only about one-quarter of the population. Smoking preference is commonly stated in personal ads. It's a big deal.

Why It Is So Hard to Quit

To cease smoking is the easiest thing I ever did.
I ought to know, I've done it a thousand times.
—MARK TWAIN

If you've tried to quit using any tobacco product in the past, you know how hard it can be. The ingredient that all tobacco products have in common is nicotine. Nicotine is naturally found in tobacco. It is a highly addictive substance, often compared to heroin and cocaine, and almost always underestimated. The body becomes physically and psychologically dependent on nicotine. Studies have shown that smokers must overcome both of these to be successful at quitting and staying a nonsmoker.

Like many addictive drugs, nicotine creates a permanent tolerance in the body. When an ex-smoker smokes a cigarette even years after quitting, the nicotine reaction may be triggered, quickly hooking the person on the old habit. (See pages 200–201 to learn how to deal with withdrawal symptoms.)

Take the "Call It Quits" Quiz

Not every smoker wants to quit, but 76 percent say they would like to. Most know that smoking is harmful to themselves and others, and these risks are explained later in this chapter. They know it causes lung cancer, heart disease, and other ills. Two-thirds of smokers have tried to quit. If you're among those who've tried, only you know why you weren't successful.

Think about how you use tobacco to get through your daily life. Do you see any patterns? Everyone wants to quit on the first try. But if you tried and you're still smoking, think of the last time as a trial run. Think about the following questions before you try to stop smoking. Smoking is as much a mental addiction as it is a physical addiction. You may wish to discuss your responses with your doctor, a smoking cessation therapist, or an ACS volunteer.

What are your reasons for smoking?

- ❑ Smoking makes me feel better if I'm worried or stressed.
- ❑ Holding a cigarette gives me something to do with my hands.
- ❑ I'm addicted to the nicotine in tobacco.
- ❑ Going for a smoke lets me take a break during the day.
- ❑ Smoking helps me focus and gives me energy.
- ❑ Smoking helps me feel comfortable in social situations.
- ❑ Smoking helps me organize my day.
- ❑ I smoke out of habit.
- ❑ I smoke because I have cravings.
- ❑ Smoking helps me control my weight.
- ❑ I smoke when I'm bored, depressed, or frustrated.
- ❑ Smoking makes me feel accepted.
- ❑ Cigarettes are like a friend to me.
- ❑ I smoke when I am happy or when I want to celebrate.
- ❑ I smoke to reward myself for getting through tough situations.

Other reasons I smoke: _____

_____

_____

If you want to quit, what are your reasons? Check all that apply to you:

- ❑ I want to improve my health.
- ❑ I want to feel better.
- ❑ My doctor recommends it.

❑ I don't want my family and friends to breathe my secondhand smoke.

❑ I want to be able to _____ without getting out of breath.

❑ I want to have a healthy baby.

❑ I want to have more money for _____ instead of cigarettes.

❑ I don't want to be addicted anymore.

❑ I want to stop coughing all the time.

❑ I don't want to smell like smoke anymore.

❑ I want to make my family and friends proud of me.

❑ I want to have more social opportunities.

❑ I'm tired of the inconvenience.

❑ I don't want tobacco to rule my life.

Other reasons: _____

_____

_____

If you've tried to quit, what happened?

• What was good about quitting?

   ❑ I felt better.
   ❑ I saved money.
   ❑ Cigarettes didn't control me.
   ❑ I was proud of myself.
   ❑ Other people were proud of me.

Other good things: _____

_____

_____

- What was hard about quitting?

  ❑ Dealing with cravings for cigarettes.
  ❑ Not knowing what to do with my hands.
  ❑ Quitting for good when others around me were smoking.
  ❑ Giving up certain cigarettes, like the one after lunch, or this one:

  _____

  ❑ Not knowing what to do when I got angry, nervous, or upset.

Other difficult things: _____
_____
_____

- Why did you go back to tobacco?

  ❑ Where were you? _____
  ❑ What were you doing? _____
  ❑ Whom were you with? _____
  ❑ How were you feeling? _____

- If you came across the same situation again, how would you deal with it and NOT smoke? _____

- How do you plan to deal with difficult situations after you quit?

  _____

- When you tried to quit in the past, what helped and what didn't?

  _____

- Whom can you rely on to help you through the tough times? Family, friends, or doctor? _____

- What quit methods did you use? Should you try another way?

  _____

The Keys to Successful Quitting

It is hard to fight any addiction, and smoking is no different. But you can quit! Quitting smoking is a lot like losing weight. It takes a strong commitment over a long period of time. Everyone wishes there were a magic bullet—a pill or method—that would make quitting painless and easy. But that is not the case.

If 45 million people, the number of former smokers in the U.S., can kick the habit, so can you.

How to Quit: It's Your Choice

Smokers often say, "Don't tell me *why* to quit, tell me *how*." There is no one right way to quit, but there are some key elements in quitting smoking successfully. These four factors are crucial.

- Making the decision to quit

- Setting a quit date and choosing a quit plan

- Dealing with withdrawal

- Maintenance or quitting for good

The decision to quit smoking is one that only you can make. Others may want you to quit, but the real commitment must come from you.

Successful cessation may include one method or a combination of methods, including using step-by-step manuals, attending self-help classes or counseling, using a nicotine replacement therapy (nicotine patch or gum), or medications (such as the prescription drug Zyban). Although these methods and stop-smoking aids may be helpful, the bottom line is that you really have to want to quit. Successful quitting is a matter of planning and commitment, not luck.

Nicotine Replacement Therapy

The nicotine patch, gum, nasal spray, and inhalers are also known as nicotine replacement therapy or nicotine substitutes. They are medicines that provide nicotine without the other harmful components of tobacco. They treat the very difficult withdrawal symptoms and cravings that 70 to 90 percent of smokers say is their only reason for not giving up cigarettes. By using a nicotine substitute, a smoker's withdrawal symptoms are reduced, allowing the smoker to deal with the psychological aspects of quitting smoking.

Nicotine replacement therapy only deals with the physical aspects of addiction. It is not intended to be the only method used for helping you quit smoking. Rather, it should be combined with other smoking cessation methods that address the psychological components of smoking, such as a stop-smoking program. Studies have shown that combining nicotine replacement with a program that helps change behavior can double the number of smokers who successfully quit smoking.

The most effective time to start nicotine replacement is at the beginning of an attempt to quit. Often smokers first try to quit on their own, then decide to try a nicotine replacement. Nicotine replacement should *not* be used if you plan to continue to smoke or use another tobacco product. All nicotine replacement therapies produce side effects, but these are rarely severe enough that they must be discontinued. Smokers who are pregnant or have heart disease should consult with their doctor before using over-the-counter nicotine replacement.

When choosing which type of nicotine replacement you will use, think about which method will best fit your lifestyle and pattern of smoking. Consider whether or not you want something to chew or occupy your hands. Are you looking for once-a-day convenience? For example, nicotine patches are convenient and only have to be applied once a day. Nicotine gum is an oral substitute and allows you to control your dosage to help keep cravings at bay. Nicotine nasal spray works very quickly when you need it. Nicotine inhalers allow you to mimic the use of cigarettes by puffing and holding the inhaler.

Nicotine Patches

Also known as transdermal nicotine systems, nicotine patches provide a measured dose of nicotine through the skin. As the nicotine doses are lowered over a course of weeks, the smoker is weaned away from nicotine. Patches can be purchased without a prescription. Several types and different strengths are available. Package inserts describe how to use the product, as well as special considerations and possible side effects.

Nicotine Gum

Nicotine gum is a fast-acting form of replacement in which nicotine is absorbed through the mucous membrane of the mouth. It can be bought without a prescription. For best results, follow the instructions on the package insert.

One advantage to nicotine gum is that it allows you to control the nicotine doses. Also, people with sensitive skin may prefer the gum to the patch. Long-term dependence is one disadvantage of nicotine gum and most doctors recommend limiting its use to six months.

Nicotine Nasal Spray

Nasal spray delivers nicotine quickly to the bloodstream as it is absorbed through the nose. It gives immediate relief of withdrawal symptoms and offers you a sense of control over nicotine cravings. Because it is easy to use, smokers report great satisfaction. It is available by prescription only. Generally, it should not be used for longer than six months, tapering the dose at the end of three months. There is the danger of using more than is needed, so instructions must be followed closely. If you have asthma, allergies, nasal polyps, or sinus problems, your doctor may suggest another form of nicotine replacement.

Nicotine Inhalers

The nicotine inhaler is a plastic tube with a nicotine cartridge inside. When you puff on the inhaler, the cartridge provides a nicotine vapor. Unlike other inhalers that deliver most of the medication to the lungs, the nicotine inhaler delivers most of the nicotine vapor to the mouth. With the nicotine inhaler, a smoker may feel like they are substituting some of the behavioral aspects of smoking. It was introduced in 1998 and is available only by prescription.

Other Methods of Quitting
Prescription Medications

Bupropion (Zyban) is a prescription antidepressant in an extended-release form that reduces symptoms of nicotine withdrawal. This drug affects chemicals in the brain that are related to nicotine craving. It can be used alone or together with nicotine replacement. Studies show that Zyban can help keep weight gain down. Early evidence suggests that it may be more effective to combine nicotine replacement therapy with Zyban than use either one alone. In one study, Zyban helped 49 percent of smokers quit for at least a month. In the same study, 36 percent of nicotine patch users were able to quit for a month. When both methods were used, 58 percent of smokers were able to remain smoke free for over a month. This medication should not be taken if you have a history of seizures, anorexia, heavy alcohol use, or head trauma.

Other medications, such as clonidine and nortriptyline, have the potential to be useful as well; however, they have not been approved by the Food and Drug Administration for use as aids for smoking cessation. More research needs to be done to determine their effectiveness and specific dosing requirements. Unpleasant side effects are also common with clonidine and nortriptyline.

Hypnosis

Some smokers try hypnosis to help them quit. It is used to create a state of restful alertness during which a person enters into a trance-like state, becomes more aware and focused, and is more open to suggestion. In general, hypnosis is not very effective when used alone, but it may be useful as part of a comprehensive program.

Acupuncture

In traditional acupuncture, needles are inserted just beneath the skin at specific locations that are thought to be connected to the function of certain organs or networks of organs throughout the body. For smoking cessation, it often involves the insertion of needles or small staples into the outer ear. Some believe that acupuncture is useful for quitting smoking, but there is little evidence to support its effectiveness. Most research has found that acupuncture is not effective in helping people quit smoking.

Motivational Rewards

Some methods use a system of rewards to motivate people to quit smoking. These systems are designed to provide concrete and immediate rewards to smokers who have just quit. In a typical program, the leader collects a deposit from each participant at the beginning of treatment and refunds a part of this sum at each follow-up session if the person has continued to be smoke-free. Although this system is successful in the short run, the results often don't last after the contract expires.

Aversive Smoking Strategies

Though not widely popular, there are several techniques used to create an aversion to cigarettes. Rapid smoking is one type, which requires smokers to deeply inhale from a cigarette about every six seconds until they become nauseated. This is intended to turn the perception of smoking from enjoyment into displeasure. However, it can produce some serious complications, such as increased heart rate, blood pressure, and carbon monoxide in the blood. Other methods, such as bupropion and nicotine gum, are just as effective and better tolerated. The Office of the Surgeon General reported that this strategy has shown some success when used as part of a comprehensive program, and it may be an option for smokers who have been unable to quit through other methods and who can tolerate aversive strategies.

Smoking Deterrents

Other over-the-counter products, such as those that change the taste of tobacco, stop-smoking diets that curb nicotine cravings, and combinations of vitamins, have little scientific evidence to support their claims.

Set a Quit Date

Once you've made a decision to quit, you're ready to pick a quit date. Pick a specific day within the next month as your Quit Day. Write it down. Tell friends and family about it so you'll be less likely to put it off. If you're thinking about attending a class, look into it now so you'll be ready for that day (see pages 202–203). Do your best to stick to it and above all…don't get discouraged.

Most smokers prefer to try to quit cold turkey—abruptly and totally. They smoke until they decide they are going to quit and then stop all at once, or they may smoke fewer cigarettes for a week or two before their Quit Day. Nicotine substitutes can help reduce withdrawal, but they are most effective when used as part of a stop smoking plan that addresses both the physical and psychological components of quitting smoking.

Another technique smokers might try involves cutting down on the number of cigarettes smoked each day. With this method, the amount of nicotine in the body is gradually reduced. Some people decide to cut out cigarettes smoked with a cup of coffee, or decide to smoke only at certain times of the day. While it sounds logical to cut down in order to quit

The withdrawal symptoms on the left often prompt some of the psychological rationalizations on the right, which can trigger people to start smoking again to boost blood levels of nicotine back to a level where there are no symptoms. Physical withdrawal symptoms usually start within a few hours of the last cigarette and peak about forty-eight to seventy-two hours later. They can last for a few days to several weeks.

Typical physical withdrawal symptoms	Typical psychological rationalizations
• Depression	• I'll just have one to get through this rough spot.
• Feelings of frustration and anger	• Today is not a good day; I'll quit tomorrow.
• Irritability	• It's my only vice.
• Trouble sleeping	• How bad is smoking, really?
• Difficulty concentrating	• Uncle Harry smoked all his life and he lived to be over ninety.
• Restlessness	• Air pollution is probably just as bad.
• Headache	• You've got to die of *something*.
• Tiredness	• Life is no fun without smoking.
• Increased appetite	

In dealing with the physical symptoms of withdrawal, the mind conjures up rationalizations. A rationalization is a mistaken belief that seems to make sense at the time, but is not based on facts. As you go through the first few days without smoking, write down any rationalizations as they come up and recognize them for what they are—messages that can trap you into going back to smoking.

gradually, in practice this method is usually not effective. One problem is that many people begin to taper up, not down, if they start to have cravings.

Dealing with Withdrawal

When smokers try to cut back or quit, the absence of nicotine leads to withdrawal symptoms. Withdrawal is both physical and psychological. Physically, the body is reacting to the absence of the drug nicotine. Psychologically, the smoker is faced with giving up a habit. You'll need to deal with both if you're going to be successful.

If you have been smoking for any length of time, smoking has become linked with nearly everything you do. It takes time and a great deal of mental energy to "un-link" smoking from your daily life. Change your routine so that you no longer associate certain activities and times of the day with smoking. You may even wish to avoid certain people and places where you are tempted to smoke, especially during the first few days. Later on you may be able to handle such situations with more confidence.

Another suggestion for avoiding lighting up is to have gum, hard candy, or crunchy vegetables on hand to substitute for the oral component of smoking. Keep yourself busy and active (and this might be a good opportunity to pick up that hobby or sport). If the craving to have a cigarette becomes intense, take deep breaths and picture your lungs filling with fresh, clean air. Remind yourself why you want to stay quit and the health benefits of being a nonsmoker. As a last resort to lighting up, tell yourself "Wait at least ten minutes." If you delay for a short time, it may allow you to suppress or move beyond the urge to smoke.

Where to Go for Support

There's no need to go it alone. Tobacco users who try to quit on their own tend to have more difficulty staying quit. With so many quitting options than ever for smokers, it's critical to enlist the support of your doctor and other resources. Research shows that adding social support to medication treatment can increase long-term success. Individual and group counseling are both much more effective than strategies that do not include contact. There are hundreds of resources when you're ready to quit—organizations and classes, books, and web sites (see Resources).

At work: call the human resources office where you work; many companies have information about smoking cessation programs. The Great American Smokeout is an awareness campaign that is often held in companies every November. Take part or adopt a smoker for the day if you're a nonsmoker. If your company has an Employee Assistance Program, call the counselors who can direct you to community stop-smoking programs. Your employer might even pay for you to attend, or partially or fully reimburse you.

In the community: a variety of other health-serving organizations and community- and hospital-based groups offer information on how to quit and where to go for help. Support groups are available to provide emotional support, friendship, and understanding.

What to Look for in a Stop-Smoking Group

Stop smoking programs are designed to help smokers recognize and cope with problems that come up during quitting and to provide support and encouragement in staying quit. Studies have shown that the best programs include either individual or group counseling. There is a strong association between the intensity of counseling and the success rate. In general, the more intense the program, the greater the likelihood of success. Intensity may be increased by having more or longer sessions, or by increasing the number of weeks over which the sessions are given. So, when considering a program, look for one that has the following characteristics.

- Session length: *at least* twenty to thirty minutes

- Number of sessions: *at least* four to seven

- Number of weeks: *at least* two

Some communities have a Nicotine Anonymous (http://nicotine-anonymous.org) group that holds regular meetings. This group applies the principles of Alcoholics Anonymous to the addiction of smoking. There is no fee to attend.

The ACS offers telephone services for tobacco users interested in quitting. Contact the ACS at 800-ACS-2345 (http://www.cancer.org) for more information.

There are some programs to watch out for as well. Not all programs are ethical. Be very careful of programs that do any of the following.

- Promise instant, easy success with no effort on your part.

- Use injections or pills, especially "secret" ingredients (nicotine replacement is covered elsewhere).

- Charge a very high fee—check with the Better Business Bureau if you have doubts.

- Are not willing to provide references from people who have taken the class.

You can also talk with your doctor and contact any of the organizations listed in the Resources at the back of this book. They can provide you with current information, advice, and suggestions for ending tobacco use once and for all.

Fears and Concerns About Quitting
Weight Gain

Many smokers do gain some weight when they quit; however, the gain is usually less than ten pounds. For some, a concern about weight gain can lead to a decision not to quit, but the weight gain that follows quitting smoking is generally very small. It is much more dangerous to continue smoking than it is to gain a small amount of weight.

You are more likely to be successful with quitting smoking if you deal with the smoking first, and then later take steps to reduce your weight. While you are quitting, try to focus on ways to help you stay healthy, rather than on your weight. Eat plenty of fruits and vegetables and limit your fat intake. Be sure to drink plenty of water, and get enough sleep and regular exercise. Walking is a great way to add some physical activity to your day, and regular exercise increases your chances of quitting for good.

Stress

Smokers often mention stress as one of the reasons for going back to smoking. Stress is a part of all of our lives, smokers and nonsmokers alike. The difference is that smokers have come to use nicotine to help cope with stress. When quitting, new ways of handling stress must be learned. Nicotine replacement can help to some extent, but for long-term success other strategies are needed.

Exercise is a good stress-reducer. It can also help with the temporary sense of depression that some smokers experience when they quit. There are also stress-management classes and self-help books. Check your community newspaper, library, or bookstore.

Spiritual practices such as prayer and meditation have been used very successfully with other addictions and are an integral part of twelve-step recovery programs. These same principals can be applied to quitting smoking and can help with stress reduction.

Quitting for Good

Remember the quotation by Mark Twain? Maybe you, too, have quit many times before. So you know that quitting for good is the final, and most important, stage of the process. You can use the same methods to stay quit as you did to help you through withdrawal. Think ahead to those times when you may be tempted to smoke, and plan on how you will use alternatives and activities to cope with these situations.

More dangerous, perhaps, are the unexpected strong desires to smoke that occur, sometimes months (or even years) after you've quit. To get through these without relapse, try the following.

- Review your reasons for quitting and think of all the benefits to your health, your finances, and your family.

- Remind yourself that there is no such thing as *just one cigarette* — or even one puff.

- Ride out the desire to smoke. It will go away, but do not fool yourself into thinking you can have just one.

Be Prepared for Relapses — It's All About Trying Again

Quitting is hard, but don't give up! What if you do smoke again? The difference between a *slip* and a *relapse* is within your control. You can use the slip as an excuse to go back to smoking, or you can look at what went wrong and renew your commitment to staying off smoking for good.

Many smokers can expect setbacks or relapses; it's a normal part of quitting altogether. Don't be discouraged if at first you start smoking again. Some smokers try a number of times before they quit for good. Studies show that each time you try to quit, the more likely you will be to eventually succeed. With each try, you learn what helps and what hurts. Any attempt to quit is a step in a healthier direction.

And, there is more good news! One study published in the *Journal of*

Clinical Epidemiology states that even smokers who quit but go back to smoking retain better lung function than smokers who never quit. The same is true for smokers who have tried to quit several times and failed. Remember that most people have to try several times before they finally quit. You learn something each time you try, and each time you try to quit, you are more likely to succeed. You can review your past attempts to quit and identify what worked and what didn't, so you can use your most successful strategies again.

Most relapses take place the first week after quitting, when withdrawal symptoms are strongest and your body is still dependent on nicotine. This will be your hardest time when you'll need to equip yourself with all the resources you have available to get you through this critical period.

Most other relapses occur within the first three months after quitting, when situational triggers, such as a particularly stressful event, occur unexpectedly. People reach for cigarettes at these times because they associate smoking with relaxing. It's difficult to prepare for this kind of situation, so you'll need to recognize it when it first begins. Smoking is a habit, but it's a habit you can break. It's never too late to make a fresh start.

CHAPTER 6

Is Cancer Contagious?

You have freedom of choice, but never freedom from consequence.
—JOHN W. ALSTON, motivational speaker

Infections and cancer? We've known for a long time that certain diseases are caused by infections, but *cancer*?

Only in the last thirty-five years or so have we learned how some cancers in humans can be triggered by infections with certain viruses, bacteria, and parasites—some of which you may never have heard of. This connection between infectious diseases and cancer was hard to find because in many cases it takes years after infection for cancer to become apparent. As a result, researchers, public health officials, and doctors are just beginning to get a handle on how some infections may play a role in the development of cancer.

Choices for a Lifetime

Most people have no problem picturing lifestyle habits such as smoking or overexposure to the sun being related to cancer, but it's tougher to make the cancer connection with infections. Some of these infections can be transmitted by sexual contact. These are especially important because recognizing the specific sexual behaviors that increase your risk of these infections can help you avoid some of them. Other infections related to cancer are spread from person to person in other ways, and some are nearly impossible to avoid.

So far in this book, we've discussed how decisions you make can affect your health, especially your chances of developing cancer. In this chapter we'll look at infections that increase your risk of developing cancer. Because many of these are preventable infections, we will focus specifically on how your choices about sex can also have an effect on your risk for certain forms of cancer. We'll go into some detail about these infections and discuss what you can do to protect yourself from these unwanted microbial guests.

Although the infections described in this chapter can increase your risk of developing certain types of cancer, most people with these infections never develop cancer. The likelihood of developing a cancer may also be influenced by other risk factors. For example, *Helicobacter pylori* infection can increase a person's risk of developing stomach cancer, but that risk is also influenced by smoking and dietary factors, such as high intake of smoked and salted foods and starches and low intake of fruits and vegetables.

The Hidden Epidemic

Sexually transmitted diseases (STDs) are conditions that can be spread or contracted through sexual intercourse or intimate contact. Intimate sexual contact may involve the genitals, mouth, or anus. Some common STDs include chlamydia, gonorrhea, syphilis, herpes, and acquired immunodeficiency syndrome (AIDS). Bacteria or viruses commonly cause STDs. Although most bacterial STDs can be treated with antibiotics, some have developed resistance to medications.

Viruses can cause STDs such as herpes, genital warts, hepatitis C, and AIDS, among others. Although some of these can be controlled with medication or may even go away by themselves without treatment, we do not yet have medicines to cure them.

As we will discuss in some depth in this chapter, some of the cancer-related viruses and bacteria discussed here (such as human T-cell leukemia/lymphoma virus type 1, Epstein-Barr virus, hepatitis C, and *Helicobacter pylori*) are more commonly contracted by means other than sex. And some STDs (such as hepatitis B and AIDS) can also be transmitted by other means, such as by sharing hypodermic needles or during childbirth.

Yet STDs are high on the list of preventable health risks. Each year an estimated 15 million Americans contract one or more STDs. Half of those become infected with diseases that will last their entire lives. Among sexually active people, these diseases occur regardless of age, gender, lifestyle, ethnic background, and socioeconomic status. By learning more about STDs and other infections, you can take precautions to help protect yourself against their serious consequences.

The Sexual Link

> *You cannot escape the responsibility of tomorrow by evading it today.*
> —ABRAHAM LINCOLN

Can sexual activity cause cancer? The answer you want to hear is "No!" Because sexuality has sometimes been seen as "sinful," people who are diagnosed with cancer in certain areas of the body worry that sexual activity has caused their cancer. *For most cancers, there is no link between your sex life and the risk of developing cancer.*

Certain cancers, however, may be linked to sexual activity. *They are not directly caused by having sex, but are related to an infection that is passed from one person to another through sexual contact.* In many cases the roles of these infections are not fully understood. In fact, most people who get these STDs never develop cancer. Perhaps the infection is not the only cause of these cancers. Some people may be more likely to develop cancer because of their age, poor health, heredity, or past experience with other cancer-causing agents. For example, women who smoke cigarettes have an increased risk of developing cervical cancer.

Cancer cannot be passed from one person to another, even through contact as close as kissing, intercourse, or oral-genital sex. Many couples worry that cancer is contagious. News stories about viruses and cancer can also be confusing. Contrary to the myths, a cancerous cell from one person's body cannot simply take root and grow in someone else. Even if a cancer cell were to somehow enter a healthy person's body, the immune system would recognize it as someone else's cell. And because it doesn't belong there, the immune system would destroy it. **Cancer itself is not contagious.**

An In-Depth Look at Viruses: The Unwanted Guests

Viruses are among the simplest of life forms. They are too small to be seen even through an ordinary microscope. All other forms of life (animals, plants, bacteria, fungi) are made up of cells, the basic building blocks of life. Most cells have the ability to copy themselves, thereby splitting into two cells, which is generally how multicelled organisms (like humans) grow. They can do this because they have a genetic "blueprint" (deoxyribonucleic acid, or DNA for short), along with some other parts (proteins) that constantly carry out the plan on the blueprint.

But a virus, which is smaller than a cell, doesn't have these other parts, so it cannot grow or divide on its own. It can only multiply after invading a

Are You at Risk?

Sexual contact is the primary route of transmitting infections that may cause certain types of cancer. You may wish to ask yourself the following questions about your sexual activity and related risk factors to determine if you may be at increased risk for developing a viral-related cancer.

There is no scoring for this questionnaire. Your response does not imply that you will develop cancer as a result of your sexual history. These questions merely serve as a tool for you and perhaps a reminder to get tested if you are concerned about having a sexually transmitted infection.

Implications for each of these questions are discussed throughout this chapter.

_____ 1. Did you begin having sexual intercourse before the age of fifteen?

_____ 2. Do you use a condom during every sexual encounter (anal, oral, and vaginal)?

_____ 3. Do you currently have multiple sexual partners? Have you had many (ten or more) sexual partners?

_____ 4. Are you an IV drug user who has shared a hypodermic needle or used an unsterilized needle?

_____ 5. Are you currently or have you been diagnosed as being infected with hepatitis B or C viruses, HIV, herpesvirus type 8, or human T-cell leukemia/lymphoma virus type 1 (HTLV-1)?

_____ 6. Did you receive a blood transfusion or donate blood prior to 1985?

_____ 7. Do you work closely with blood or blood products?

_____ 8. Do you smoke?

_____ 9. Do you get screened regularly for sexually transmitted diseases?

"host" cell, because it needs the host cell's machinery to reproduce. It does this by inserting its own genetic blueprint (DNA or ribonucleic acid, or RNA for short) into the cell, where it forces the cell to make the building blocks of new viruses. The new viruses eventually break out of the host cell, sometimes killing it in this process. These new viruses are then free to infect other cells in the body or in other individuals, and the cycle continues.

But some types of viruses, instead of killing the cell, leave their DNA or RNA in the host cell as an unwanted guest. Days, months, or even years later, an event (such as stress) can trigger the viral replication process. Some viruses even insert their DNA directly into the cell's own DNA. Not only does this change what the cell does, but in some cases it pushes the cell closer to becoming cancerous.

Viruses can infect animals, plants, and even bacteria. Most viruses are specialized—they infect only one species. Even among viruses that infect humans, there is a lot of diversity. Some can only infect cells in the nose or throat. Others may only be able to get into cells in the lungs, or into certain blood cells. Sexually transmitted viruses can often infect cells in the penis, vagina, or rectum, or enter the bloodstream through tiny breaks in the skin.

Viruses also differ as far as the seriousness of the infections they cause. Some, like the viruses that cause the common cold, are usually only a temporary annoyance. Others may cause no symptoms at all. But some can bring about serious problems, such as a weakened immune system as in the case of HIV. And some may lead to cancer.

Viruses and Cancer

Scientists have known for nearly a century that infectious diseases, and viruses in particular, lead to some cancers in animals. But only recently has this process been confirmed in humans. Seven sexually transmitted viral infections are known to be associated with cancer at this time.

The most familiar sexually transmitted virus is probably HIV. However, the various types of hepatitis viruses affect far more people than HIV, as do some of the less familiar viruses such as Epstein-Barr and human papillomaviruses. Each is discussed in detail along with the types of cancer associated with them.

A few words of caution (and comfort): Although some viral infections can increase a person's risk of getting certain types of cancer, *most people with these infections will never develop these cancers*. It is becoming clear that a

Viruses That Cause Cancer

Virus	Associated Cancer(s)
Human immunodeficiency virus (HIV)	Kaposi's sarcoma (KS), (invasive squamous cell) cervical cancer, non-Hodgkin's lymphoma
Human papillomaviruses (HPV)	Cervical, vulvar, vaginal, penile, and anal cancer
Human T-cell leukemia/ lymphoma virus (HTLV-1)	Adult T-cell leukemia/lymphoma
Human herpesvirus 8 (HHV-8); Kaposi's sarcoma-associated herpesvirus (KSHV)	Kaposi's sarcoma
Epstein-Barr virus (EBV)	Nasopharyngeal cancer, Burkitt's lymphoma, other types of non-Hodgkin's B-cell lymphomas
Hepatitis B virus (HBV)	Liver cancer
Hepatitis C virus (HCV)	Liver cancer

virus may need to be "triggered" by another agent, a so-called cofactor, or some other circumstance before a cancer can develop. And the likelihood of developing cancer may also be influenced by other risk factors, controllable or not.

Even though viral infections that influence cancer risk are contagious, it is important to remember that cancer is not a contagious disease. A healthy person cannot contract cancer from someone else who has cancer. A healthy person can, however, contract an infectious disease from someone who has the disease.

Human Immunodeficiency Virus

HIV belongs to a class of viruses called retroviruses. It is the virus that causes AIDS. Although HIV can be isolated in the lab from nearly all body fluids, tissues, and secretions, it can only be acquired through contact with certain body fluids from another person with the virus.

The virus can be transmitted by injection into the bloodstream (using contaminated needles, for example), by vaginal or anal intercourse, through blood products or organ or tissue transplant, or from mother to child during pregnancy, birth, or breast-feeding. All blood products and donor organs are now routinely screened for the presence of HIV, and the risk of infection through transfusion to someone unknowingly is extremely small.

The virus that causes AIDS is HIV, but it is important to realize that people infected with HIV (especially those who are being treated effectively) do not necessarily have AIDS, which has a specific definition related to decreased immune function. Most people infected with HIV develop AIDS over time, as their immune systems become weaker.

The virus attacks and infects a certain type of T lymphocyte (T cell), which is a type of white blood cell. This attack weakens the body's immune system. When the body is less able to fight off infections, other viruses already in the body may be able to become more active. The body is less able to defend itself against abnormal cells that are growing out of control. Although scientists do not believe that HIV causes cancer directly, the weakened immune system caused by HIV infection may allow some cancers to develop that normally would not.

Aside from cancer, HIV infection can lead to other life-threatening problems, including severe opportunistic infections (so called because they do not normally cause problems in healthy people), loss of appetite and weight, and nervous system disorders such as headaches, nerve pain, and even psychological problems.

Cancers Associated with HIV

The Centers for Disease Control and Prevention has identified certain cancers as AIDS-defining diseases: Kaposi's sarcoma (KS), lymphoma (especially non-Hodgkin's lymphoma and primary central nervous system lymphoma), and invasive cervical cancer. Other forms of cancer that may be more likely to develop in people with HIV infection are Hodgkin's disease, anal cancer, oral cancer, and cancer of the testicles. Of course, people without HIV or AIDS can also have these types of cancer.

About four out of ten people who have AIDS will develop a cancer at some time during their illness. Individuals infected with HIV tend to have cancers that are diagnosed at an advanced stage and do not respond as well to treatment. The relationship between HIV and these cancers is still not completely understood; however, it is believed that the cancers can grow rapidly because these individuals have suppressed immune systems.

Kaposi's sarcoma. Kaposi's sarcoma used to be a rare disease that affected elderly men of Mediterranean or Jewish heritage, organ transplant patients, or young African men. It is a type of cancer that typically causes tumors to develop in the tissues below the skin surface or in the mucous membranes of the mouth, nose, or anus. Kaposi's sarcoma was relatively

Test Your Knowledge about HIV/AIDS

How much you know about the spread of HIV?

1. Worldwide, the most common method of transmission of HIV is

   a.   Intravenous drug use

   b.   Homosexual (same sex) contact

   c.   Heterosexual (opposite sex) contact

   d.   During pregnancy (from mother to child)

2. The fastest growing population of HIV-infected people is

   a.   Homosexual men

   b.   IV drug users

   c.   Heterosexual men

   d.   Heterosexual women

3. Which of the following can spread HIV?

   a.   Insect bites (such as mosquitoes)

   b.   Kissing

   c.   Coughing/sneezing

   d.   Drinking from the same cup/eating off the same plates

   e.   Shaking hands

   f.   Sitting on the same toilet seat

   g.   Using the same telephone

   h.   The water supply

4. HIV is a virus that is easily transmitted from person to person. True or false?

The answers may surprise you:

1. The most common method of HIV transmission worldwide is: c. Heterosexual contact.

Although the majority of cases in the United States have historically been among homosexual men and IV drug users, intercourse between men and women is by far the main means of transmission worldwide. And as HIV has spread into the general population in the U.S., new cases among heterosexual, non-IV drug users have continued to increase.

2. The fastest growing population of HIV-infected people is: d. Heterosexual women.

Originally a predominantly male disease, new HIV/AIDS cases in women have continued to increase in the U.S. in recent years, even as the number of new cases among men has begun to decline. In fact, among the nearly 35 million estimated cases of adults with HIV/AIDS worldwide, almost half are now women. (See the web site of the World Health Organization, http://www.who.int, for more information.)

3. Which of the following can spread HIV? This was a trick question: None of the above.

Over the past twenty years we have come to understand a great deal about HIV, including the fact that it doesn't survive long outside of the body (see next answer). And although the virus is present in different body fluids, the concentrations of virus in many of these are not high enough to be infectious. The best way to protect yourself against HIV infection is through safe sexual practices.

4. HIV is a virus that is easily transmitted from person to person. False.

HIV is actually a rather fragile virus outside of the body, surviving for a few minutes at best on a countertop or other surface. And it cannot be transmitted through the skin. Even when transmitted through contaminated needles, it is not nearly as infectious as some other viruses, such as hepatitis B.

rare before the AIDS epidemic. However, in the early 1980s the incidence of KS increased dramatically. In fact, a cluster of cases of KS among homosexual men was actually partly responsible for recognition of AIDS and eventual discovery of HIV.

In the past twenty years, the majority of KS cases have been associated with HIV infection and AIDS in homosexual men. These cases are referred to as AIDS-related KS. It is now known that KS in people infected with HIV is related to a second viral infection with human herpesvirus type 8 (HHV-8) (also discussed in this section).

Non-Hodgkin's lymphoma. Non-Hodgkin's lymphoma develops in about 4 to 10 percent of people with AIDS. It is the second most common cancer associated with HIV disease, after KS. It is a cancer that starts in lymphoid tissue, which is formed by several types of immune system cells that work together to resist infections. Lymphoid tissue is found in many places throughout the body, including lymph nodes, the thymus (found behind the chest bone and in front of the heart), the spleen (on the left side of the abdomen next to the stomach), the tonsils and adenoids, in the bone marrow, and scattered within other areas such as the digestive system and respiratory system.

Cervical cancer. Over 95 percent of cases of cervical cancer are thought to be related to human papillomavirus (HPV) infection (discussed further in this section). But infection with HIV may increase the chance that an HPV infection will lead to cancer. Therefore, it is very important that women infected with HIV undergo regular screening for cervical cancer.

Women who are infected with HIV are at high risk for developing invasive cervical cancer. Cervical cancer begins as an abnormal growth of the cervical cells called cervical intraepithelial neoplasia (CIN). As the disease progresses, the tumor cells become malignant and break through the thin membrane underneath them, allowing the cells to invade the uterus and become invasive cervical cancer. The term *invasive* indicates that the cancer has spread to neighboring tissue.

Effective treatment of CIN is critical in preventing its progression to invasive cervical cancer. Studies have shown that untreated CIN is more likely to progress to invasive disease in HIV-infected women than in women without the virus. Women with AIDS and invasive cervical cancer have a greater likelihood of the cancer coming back after treatment and a greater likelihood of dying of this disease than HIV-negative women.

Human Papillomavirus

Human papillomaviruses (HPVs) are actually a group of more than eighty types of viruses. They are called papillomaviruses because they tend to cause warts, or papillomas, which are benign (noncancerous) tumors. These warts can appear on the skin, mouth, larynx (voice box), anus, or genital organs. The types of HPVs that cause the common warts that grow on hands and feet are different from those that develop in the mouth and genital area.

Genital papillomaviruses can be passed from one person to another through sexual intercourse and oral or anal sex. They may cause warts to appear on or around the genitals or anus of both men and women. In women, visible warts may also appear on the cervix. An infection with HPV does not always produce warts or other symptoms, so a person may be infected with and pass on HPV without knowing it.

Different strains of HPVs are divided into low-risk and high-risk categories. Low-risk strains are often visible as warts but rarely develop into cancer. High-risk HPV types aren't usually contained in visible warts but have been linked with genital and anal cancers. Both high-risk and low-risk types of HPVs can cause the growth of abnormal cells, called dysplasia, in the cervix.

Although HPV was once considered to be a lifelong infection, recent evidence suggests that the virus is eventually no longer detectable in the body. Researchers are now looking into ways to treat, or even prevent, HPV infection through the use of vaccines and other methods.

Cancers Associated with HPV

Certain specific types of HPV are the principal cause of cervical cancer and have a role in causing some cancers of the penis, vagina, and vulva, and may play a small role in anal and other cancers as well.

Cervical cancer. Although about 95 percent of cervical cancers are related to HPV, becoming infected with HPV does not necessarily mean that a woman will develop cervical cancer. In fact, most women infected with HPV don't get cervical cancer.

Other factors, such as smoking and chlamydial infections (see page 229) have been shown to contribute to HPV-induced cervical cancer. While there are other risk factors that appear to be associated with cervical cancer, most cases are also linked to sexual behavior and contracting HPV. Most women who develop cervical cancer are over the age of fifty, but it can occur earlier, sometimes even before the age of thirty.

Cervical cancer is slow growing and highly curable *if diagnosed early*. The Pap test can be used to identify changes in cells of the cervix caused by HPV infection. (See Chapter 9 for more information on the Pap test and other screening methods.) New tests are now available that can directly identify DNA from HPVs, and identify the exact HPV type causing the infection. HPV testing and typing is not routinely recommended and most health care providers do not use this testing. However, clinical research is underway to determine the role of this test in preventing cervical cancer.

Penile cancer. Infection with HPV is believed by many researchers to be the most important avoidable risk factor for penile cancer, possibly contributing to about half of all cases. The risk factors for men are similar to those for cervical cancer: smoking, multiple sexual partners or sex with someone who has had multiple partners, and having unprotected sex. The large variations in penile cancer rates throughout the world strongly suggest that penile cancer is a preventable disease.

The good news is that cancer of the penis is very rare in North America and Europe. It accounts for only 0.2 percent of cancers in men and 0.1 percent of cancer deaths in men in the U.S. When penile cancer is detected early, treatment is simplest, most effective, and less likely to result in significant side effects or complications.

Vaginal cancer. Infection with HPV also increases a woman's chance of developing cancer of the vagina. Because vaginal and cervical cancer have similar risk factors (such as HPV infection), having a cancer or pre-cancerous condition of the cervix increases a woman's risk of developing vaginal cancer. Vaginal cancer is responsible for about 0.3 percent of female cancers.

Vulvar cancer. The vulva is the external portion of the female reproductive system, consisting of two prominent skin folds known as the labia majora, and two more barely visible, hairless skin folds called the labia minora. Cancer of the vulva (also known as vulvar cancer) can occur on any part of the female external reproductive system but most often affects the inner edges of the labia majora or the labia minora.

The human papillomavirus is thought to be responsible for as many as half of all cases of vulvar cancer in women. Recent studies suggest that vulvar cancer will develop in about one-third to one-half of HPV infection cases. Vulvar cancers associated with HPV infection seem to have certain distinctive features. Women with these cancers are usually smokers and tend to be younger (between the ages of thirty-five to fifty-five years old) than typical vulvar cancer patients. In the U.S., vulvar cancer accounts for about 0.6 percent of all cancers in women. When vulvar cancer is detected early, it is highly curable.

Anal cancer. The human papillomavirus can be transmitted through anal intercourse. Certain types of HPV cause anal warts, some of which can become cancerous. Anal cancer affects women somewhat more than men, and they are more likely to die of the disease. In recent years, the rate of anal cancer among men, particularly homosexual men, has increased. Male homosexuals who practice anal sex are about thirty-three times more likely to have anal cancers than heterosexual men. The exact cause of most anal cancers is not known. However, scientists have found that the disease is associated with a number of other conditions, such as HPV or HIV infection, smoking, and older age.

Anal cancer is rare and many cases can be found early in the course of the disease. Treatment for most cases is very effective, and most people with this cancer can be cured if diagnosed early.

Human T-cell Leukemia/Lymphoma Virus

Human T-cell leukemia/lymphoma virus type 1 (HTLV-1) is a member of the retrovirus family, similar to HIV. The virus is considered rare in the U.S., but it seems to be increasing in some areas. It is found mostly in southern Japan, the Caribbean, Africa, parts of South America, and in the southeastern part of the U.S. in some immigrant populations.

Like HIV, HTLV-1 spreads by sexual intercourse, by injection with a contaminated needle, or from mother to child during pregnancy or birth. The virus is found in breast milk, and it can also be transmitted by transfusion of blood or blood products. However, all donated blood is now routinely tested for HTLV-1, which has greatly reduced the possibility of infection through transfusion.

Cancer Associated with HTLV-1

The cancer associated with HTLV-1 is a rare type of non-Hodgkin's lymphoma called adult T-cell leukemia/lymphoma, which affects the blood and lymph system. It is much more of a health threat in areas where the virus is common. In some areas of Japan, for example, the virus is responsible for about half of the non-Hodgkin's lymphoma cases. But in the U.S., it causes less than 1 percent of lymphomas. Once infected, a person's chance of developing the disease can be about 3 to 4 percent after a long and variable latent period (twenty or more years).

Preventing the spread of HTLV-1 could have a great impact on non-Hodgkin's lymphoma in areas of the world where this virus is common. The same strategies used to prevent HIV spread could also help control HTLV-1.

Human Herpesvirus Type 8

Human herpesvirus type 8 (HHV-8), also known as Kaposi's sarcoma-associated herpesvirus (KSHV), is a member of the herpes family of viruses. It is related to other herpes viruses, such as the viruses that cause chickenpox, cold sores, and genital herpes, as well as Epstein-Barr virus (also called "mono") and cytomegalovirus (CMV). But these other viruses are not the same as HHV-8 and do not cause KS.

It is thought that anywhere from 1 to 25 percent of the U.S. population is infected with HHV-8. The virus is transmitted sexually and may be passed on during pregnancy or birth as well.

Cancer Associated with HHV-8

Researchers are not yet sure how HHV-8 contributes to development of KS—the type of cancer that causes tumors to develop in the tissues below the skin surface and is commonly found in people with HIV. In fact, some researchers are not convinced that it does because this virus can be detected in people without KS or who have no KS risk factors. This observation suggests that HHV-8 infection does not directly cause KS, but can contribute to development of the disease in people who have one or more other conditions (such as HIV infection or whose immune systems are weakened because of an organ transplant).

Almost all people who develop KS have a suppressed immune system. However, the virus is not thought to cause disease in healthy people who are infected.

Some researchers have suggested that HHV-8 is a risk factor for multiple myeloma, although the association is not universally accepted. The virus has been found in the blood of patients with myeloma. This recent discovery needs to be confirmed in additional studies.

Epstein-Barr Virus

The Epstein-Barr virus (EBV) is usually a relatively harmless type of herpes virus that is most commonly associated with infectious mononucleosis, also called mono or the "kissing disease." People with infectious mononucleosis often have fever, fatigue, a sore throat, and occasionally small sores in the mouth. The virus is present in saliva and is thought to be transmitted from person to person through kissing, coughing, sneezing, or the sharing of cups or utensils.

Most people in the U.S. are infected with EBV before the age of twenty, and only about one-fourth to one-third of those infected will develop infectious mononucleosis. Some people have only common cold symptoms, while still others have none at all. Symptoms of mono typically last a few weeks, occasionally as long as a month or two. Thereafter, the virus remains dormant in the body for the rest of a person's life, where it is detectable by a blood test.

Cancers Associated with EBV

Epstein-Barr virus increases a person's risk of developing nasopharyngeal cancer (a type of facial or oral cancer), Burkitt's lymphoma, and some other types of non-Hodgkin's B-cell lymphomas. It is true that, on very rare occasions, EBV may trigger these types of cancers many years after the initial infection. However, this happens in fewer than one in a million people who have the virus in their body.

Nasopharyngeal cancer. Many people infected with EBV develop infectious mononucleosis, but their immune system is able to recognize and destroy the virus, so they recover normally without any long-term problems. In some rare cases, however, the virus interacts with cells in the nose and upper throat, altering their DNA. This can lead to the development of nasopharyngeal cancer many years after the initial infection.

EBV infection alone is not sufficient to cause this condition because this cancer is so rare and because EBV infection is quite common in most parts of the world. The exact cause of most cases of nasopharyngeal cancer is not known. Scientists have found that the disease is associated with certain dietary habits, other acquired infections, and inherited characteristics.

Burkitt's lymphoma. This type of cancer, named after the doctor who first described it, occurs in the lymphatic tissue. The lymphatic system is important for filtering germs, cancer cells, and fluid from the extremities and internal organs. As mentioned earlier, lymphatic tissue is found in many places throughout the body, including lymph nodes, the thymus, the spleen, the tonsils and adenoids, in the bone marrow, and scattered within other systems such as the digestive system and respiratory system.

Burkitt's is a very aggressive type of non-Hodgkin's lymphoma (see pages 225–226) that usually affects children. In areas of central Africa where Burkitt's lymphoma is common, it usually starts as a growing mass in the neck or jaw. In Africa, chronic infection with malaria and EBV are other important risk factors for this disease. Cases in the U.S. are much less common and usually start in the abdomen. Burkitt's lymphoma appears to be related to EBV in nearly all African cases, but in only a small percentage of U.S. cases. The American form of Burkitt's lymphoma is less closely associated with EBV.

Non-Hodgkin's B-cell lymphoma. EBV may be associated with an increased risk of developing other types of lymphoma as well. The majority of lymphomas come from B cells, which are forms of lymphocytes, a type of white blood cell that normally helps the body fight off infections. (T cells are the other type of lymphocyte.) The combination of EBV infection with immune system deficiencies, such as those in people with AIDS or with organ transplants, may increase the risk of developing non-Hodgkin's lymphoma.

Hepatitis B and C

Hepatitis is a general name for several types of diseases that cause inflammation of the liver. Viruses cause the most cases of hepatitis in the U.S. Several viruses are named for their ability to infect the liver, using "hepatitis" followed by a letter from A through E. Other causes of hepatitis include certain toxins, parasites, and immune system diseases.

The symptoms of infection with a hepatitis virus can vary. Sometimes there are no symptoms at all. Other people develop a flu-like illness and a yellowish color in the eyes and skin (called jaundice). In severe cases, hepatitis can lead to liver failure, coma, or even death.

The hepatitis viruses differ in their abilities to infect the liver. Only hepatitis B virus (HBV) and hepatitis C virus (HCV) can cause chronic hepatitis, which can increase the risk of liver cancer and cirrhosis of the liver. Cirrhosis is the irreversible scarring that occurs from chronic liver inflammation.

Hepatitis B virus is more likely to cause symptoms at the time of infection than HCV. However, most people infected with HBV recover completely within a few months, and only a small percentage of people become infected over the long term. People with chronic infections are called "carriers." There are over a million carriers of HBV in the U.S. Those who don't realize they are infected can unknowingly transmit the virus to other people.

In contrast, the majority of the 150,000 people infected with HCV each year will develop chronic hepatitis. There are about 4 million Americans chronically infected with HCV. This disease is so common because the virus was not identified until fairly recently. Blood supplies weren't tested for HCV until 1992, and many people who received transfusions before this time became infected.

Both HBV and HCV are present in body fluids such as semen, blood, saliva, vaginal secretions, breast milk, and in open sores. Routes of transmission include sexual contact, IV drug use, childbirth, and blood transfusions (although this has become very rare since testing began).

Although HBV is the most common cause of viral hepatitis worldwide, a vaccine is now available. Immunization is especially important for those who are at high risk, such as health care workers, sex partners of infected persons, IV drug users, infants born to infected mothers, and any others at risk. The three-shot series for HBV is now routinely given to babies as part of their shots. And many school children who have not been immunized are required in many school districts to receive the shots.

There is currently no vaccine for HCV. Therefore, prevention of HCV infection (and HBV infection in people who have not been immunized) is extremely important.

Cancer Associated with HBV and HCV

Chronic infection with either HBV or HCV is a very important liver cancer risk factor. These infections are responsible for making liver cancer one of the most common cancers in many parts of the world. Fortunately, in the U.S. liver cancer is relatively rare.

Together, HBV and HCV are responsible for a large percentage of liver cancer cases in the U.S. How HCV causes liver cancer is not known; however, researchers believe that it develops in association with chronic liver disease. Most cases of HCV-related liver cancer occur with a history of liver disease, chronic liver inflammation, or cirrhosis for three decades or more. This may suggest that chronic liver disease or inflammation is the primary risk factor, rather than the HCV infection alone.

Men, alcoholics, people with cirrhosis, people over the age of forty, and those infected with HBV or HCV for at least twenty to forty years are at highest risk for developing liver cancer.

Doctors have found that treatment with the drug interferon may prevent the development of liver cancer in people infected with HCV. But, interferon causes significant side effects, such as fatigue, depression, and fevers. Studies of newer forms of interferon and the drug ribavirin are underway.

Recent studies also suggest that HCV may also have a role in the development of some types of non-Hodgkin's lymphomas.

Bacteria and Cancer

Helicobacter pylori

Many researchers believe infection with the bacterium *Helicobacter pylori* is a major cause of stomach cancer. Long-term infection of the stomach with this bacterium may lead to inflammation and damage to the inner layer of the stomach, a possible precancerous change of the lining of the stomach. Patients with adenocarcinoma of the stomach have a higher rate of infection than people without this cancer. *Helicobacter* infection is also associated with some types of lymphoma of the stomach. But the vast majority of people who carry this bacterium in their stomachs never develop cancer.

Nitrates and nitrites are substances commonly found in cured meats, some drinking water, and certain vegetables. They can be converted by certain bacteria, such as *Helicobacter pylori*, into compounds that have been found to cause stomach cancer in animals.

Most ulcers are caused by *Helicobacter pylori*, although certain foods and stress can make ulcers worse. The most common ulcer symptom is burning pain in the stomach. Antibiotics are generally used to treat the infection.

It is not yet known if people without symptoms who have chronic infection of their stomach lining with *Helicobacter pylori* should be treated for this infection. This issue is a topic of current research.

Chlamydia trachomatis

As mentioned earlier, recent studies have linked chlamydial infections with HPV-induced cervical cancer, although further research is needed to confirm this association (see page 220). Chlamydia is a curable STD caused by a bacterium (*Chlamydia trachomatis*). It is one of the most widespread bacterial STDs in the U.S., affecting more than 4 million people each year. The infection may move inside the body if it is not treated. There it can cause pelvic inflammatory disease, which is a serious infection of the female reproductive organs, and epididymitis, which is an inflammation of a part of the male reproductive system located near the testicles known as the epididymis.

You can get genital chlamydial infection during oral, vaginal, or anal sexual contact with an infected partner. Because the infection does not make most people sick, you can have it and not know it.

The symptoms may be mild or not exist at all. Those who do have symptoms may have an abnormal discharge (mucus or pus) from the vagina or penis, or pain while urinating. These early symptoms may be very mild. Symptoms usually appear within one to three weeks after being infected.

The bacterium can cause an inflamed rectum, as well as inflammation of the lining of the eye (known as "pink eye"). It can also infect the throat from oral sexual contact with an infected partner. Antibiotics are generally used to treat the infection.

You can reduce your chances of getting chlamydia or of giving it to your partner by using latex condoms correctly every time you have sexual intercourse.

If you are infected but have no symptoms, you may pass the bacterium to your sex partners without knowing it. Therefore, many doctors recommend that anyone who has more than one sex partner, especially women less than twenty-five years of age, be tested for chlamydial infection regularly—even if they don't have symptoms.

Parasites and Cancer

Certain parasitic worms that can live inside the human body can also increase the risk of developing certain cancers. None of these infections are acquired in the U.S., but they are a concern for people who live in or travel to other parts of the world.

Opisthorchis viverrini is a type of liver fluke has been associated with increased risk of developing cancer of the bile ducts. This infection occurs almost exclusively in East Asia and is rare in other parts of the world. *Schistosoma haematobium* is a parasite found in developing countries of Africa and Asia where it has been associated with cancer of the urinary bladder.

Testing for Infections

The diagnosis of many kinds of infectious diseases usually comes as a surprise. Imagine you have a fever, feel achy, can't eat, have a little diarrhea, and vomit. The flu, you think. You see your doctor. A blood test and medical and sexual history point to hepatitis B.

Medical facilities that can perform testing, other than your doctor, include hospitals, health clinics, or local health departments. Special laboratory tests are used to determine if you are positive for an infection. Most detection tests are performed in the medical setting. But home-testing kits for HIV, for example, can be performed privately and confidentially, and submitted to a lab for analysis.

Some viruses, such as HHV-8, are not tested for at all—simply because they are relatively rare or only occur in association with a specific cancer. In the case of Epstein-Barr virus, nearly 90 percent of the population has been infected without any long-term symptoms. It is only when a person develops one of the cancers associated with the virus—

either because the cancer itself is rare or because the individual has a weakened immune system — that doctors check for a virus.

What You Can Do

An ounce of prevention is worth a pound of cure.
— Henry de Bracton, English author

Although many of the infections discussed here can be transmitted by blood (except HPV), there is good evidence indicating that some can be sexually transmitted. Prevention, therefore, is possible through safe sex practices. If you are sexually active, you can learn how to protect yourself from STDs.

The best way to reduce the risk of cancer related to infections is to avoid known risk factors and certain behaviors whenever possible.

Ways to Reduce Your Risk of STDs

Only one method of preventing STDs is absolutely, positively, 100 percent effective. No sexual contact or activity at all (called abstinence) is the only method that reduces your chance of contracting some infections to zero and significantly lowers the risk for several others. Although abstinence is not for everyone, studies show that at least postponing the beginning of sexual activity in life may help prevent some types of associated cancers from developing later in life. Admittedly, this is a tough message for parents and teachers to convey to a fourteen-year-old whose hormones are singing a much different tune.

The following are general guidelines for the prevention of STDs.

Use Condoms Effectively

Latex condoms protect against the risk of pregnancy, as well as most STDs. Although condoms can reduce the chance of exposure to viruses, they are not foolproof. Learn how to use a condom properly—before engaging in sexual activity. Have one readily available, just in case, and insist on using them for every sexual encounter. Be straightforward and frank about asking a new partner to wear a condom. Ask your partner about prior exposure to STDs or any unexplained physical signs or symptoms.

Until recently, it was thought that the use of condoms could prevent infection with HPV. But recent research suggests that condoms *cannot* totally protect against the infection. This is because the virus can be passed from person to person by skin-to-skin contact with any HPV-infected area of the body, such as genital or anal areas not covered by the condom.

Of course, it is still important to use condoms to protect against HIV and other STDs. Oral sex can be made safer if you wear a condom or if you use an "oral dam," a rubber sheet that fits over a woman's vulva, during oral sex. Ingesting bodily fluids is also not recommended because it is thought that some viruses can be transmitted this way as well.

Choose Your Partners Carefully

Maintain a mutually monogamous relationship (only one sex partner), or limit the number of partners you have. Because many sexually transmitted infections have no signs or symptoms, it's important to remember that either partner could have an STD and not be aware of it. If you are not in a monogamous relationship, limiting the number of sexual partners you have can also reduce your risk.

Inform Your Partners

If you are diagnosed with a viral infection, you can take steps to prevent further transmission of the virus. Most doctors encourage their patients to tell their sexual partners about a newly diagnosed sexually transmitted infection so that the partners can seek medical attention. Local health departments may contact infected people to obtain more information about sexual partners so that they can be tested and treated, if necessary. For most viral diseases, there is no cure and infection is lifelong.

Public health officials take sexually transmitted infections very seriously for two reasons: one, unnoticed symptoms can cause considerable health problems to individuals; and, two, with the proper identification and treatment, the rates of STDs can be reduced. In addition to lower medical costs and better health, fewer STDs could also lead to fewer cases of viral-related cancers.

Get Regular Checkups

Anyone who is sexually active with multiple partners should have regular checkups and tests, even in the absence of visible signs of infection. This is especially essential for women, who often have no symptoms. The American Cancer Society recommends that all women begin yearly Pap tests and pelvic examinations at age eighteen or when they become sexually active, whichever occurs earlier (see Chapter 9). If a woman has had three satisfactorily negative annual Pap test results in a row, this test may be done less often at the judgment of a woman's doctor. But the annual pelvic examination should be continued, regardless of how often the Pap test is done.

Cervical cancer is an excellent example of the importance of routine screenings. The Pap test (named after the doctor who developed it, Dr. Papanicolaou) can identify cancer as well as precancerous conditions. Women whose cancer is found in its early stages have a nearly 100 percent survival rate after appropriate treatment and follow-up.

Pay attention to symptoms that persist even if they seem mild, and be sure to have a general medical checkup as recommended by your doctor. Some of the infections discussed in this chapter, such as viral hepatitis or *Helicobacter pylori*, won't be found by cancer screening tests. But they may be found when your doctor asks about your symptoms and does certain routine blood tests.

Be Sensible

Alcohol and drugs can make you feel less inhibited. They can also impair your judgment and may indirectly lead you into an unsafe sexual encounter without taking all the proper precautions.

Avoid injecting illegal drugs, particularly if needle exchange, sharing a needle, or reusing a needle is involved. If you decide to get a tattoo or body piercing, go to a licensed, professional business where the implements and jewelry are properly sterilized.

It is always a good idea to avoid sharing toothbrushes, earrings, or razors with family and friends.

Wear double disposable gloves if you must touch or clean up blood. This is especially important if you work in a health care setting, if you are a dentist, dental hygienist, or day care employee.

The smartest advice remains the soundest: choose your partners carefully, be sensible about your sexual practices, and have regular medical checkups.

CHAPTER 7

Stress Less, Laugh More,

Your Mind and Body Will Thank You

Life is what happens to you while you're busy making other plans.
—JOHN LENNON

Life happens. You get a flat tire on your way to work; your teenage daughter's boyfriend has a pierced tongue; a friend sends you a computer virus, you open the attachment, and your computer crashes; coffee spills on your freshly ironed pants; someone accidentally mixes a red T-shirt in the white clothes wash; and life goes on. These are the everyday events that stress us.

Then there are the big things: the boss fires you, your marriage is on the rocks, your mother dies, you retire, you have children and get married, not necessarily in that order. Or you get a great new job. Even good things in life can create stress.

Big stress, small stuff—your body responds. Some people are incredibly resilient when it comes to life's little stressors. Other people seem to handily breeze through the serious events. The rest of us bite our nails, lose sleep, worry a lot, or get headaches.

Stress does not cause cancer. But, when we are stressed, we sometimes make unhealthy lifestyle choices, such as drinking more alcohol, exercising less, smoking cigarettes, or eating poorly—all of which are factors that may play a role in the development of cancer. This is where learning how to manage stress comes into play. You can learn how to recognize stress early and deal with it in healthy ways, so you can make better lifestyle choices.

Stress may have a variety of effects on your lifestyle choices and health, but you're still in control. You can refocus your energy with stress-reducing activities, such as progressive muscle relaxation, meditation, or positive imagery.

Of course, it's not as simple as that. This chapter discusses stress in everyday terms and gives you practical advice about stress—how to identify it, control it, and live with it.

Are You Stressed?

*Americans have more time-saving devices and less time
than any other people in the world.*
—Duncan Cladwell

Stress is a natural and unavoidable fact of life. It is not the same for everyone, nor is it always negative. Controlled stress can be stimulating in a positive way. It can increase your level of alertness and help you perform at your best; whereas, prolonged or overwhelming stress may negatively affect your lifestyle choices. It can drive you to grab a fast-food meal, put off exercising just one more day, or reach for that quick beer or cigarette. These unplanned choices in everyday life can soon become habits—habits that you can't live with.

Stress is a completely individual experience; however, the degree of stress in your life depends on a number of factors: your physical health, the quality of your interpersonal and professional relationships, the amount of responsibility you have at work and at home, the number of commitments you make, expectations of and support from other people, and the number of traumatic events or changes that have recently occurred in your life. Most people would say they have experienced serious stress at some point in their lives.

People who are inadequately nourished, get too little sleep, and are in overall poor health have reduced abilities to cope with everyday stresses. Significant life transitions, such as death, divorce, birth, or a new or difficult job situation, also play a major role in the amount of stress experienced.

Assess Your Stress

Doctors, and specifically psychiatrists and psychologists, often assess stress levels in relation to particular life-changing or traumatic events. Major life events—both good and bad such as the loss of a loved one, divorce, unemployment, financial setbacks, marriage, retirement, birth of a child, and moving—can all have an impact on your level of stress. But again, people handle these things differently. The more *perceived* stressful life-changing events you have experienced, the higher the likelihood that you may develop stress-related physical symptoms. By recognizing these symptoms early, you will be able to make better decisions about how to manage stress.

Checklist of Stress Symptoms

The following is a list of stress symptoms associated with work, interpersonal relationships, and health. This tool is intended to be used to identify the signs of too much stress in various aspects of your life. Read each symptom carefully and check whether or not you believe the symptom to be characteristic of you at the present time.

Symptoms at Work

1. I'm having difficulty keeping my mind on my work ____

2. I find myself constantly complaining ____

3. I have suffered a serious loss of motivation ____

4. I feel that things are out of control ____

5. I'm generally bored ____

6. I have been absent more frequently than usual, or I have had a strong desire to excuse myself ____

7. I'm uncertain as to how my work is being evaluated ____

8. I feel increasing pressure from my work (feeling constantly behind) ____

9. I'm experiencing trouble with my supervisor, subordinates, or fellow workers ____

10. I'm confused with regard to my duties ____

11. I feel I have very little decision-making power regarding my job ____

12. I'm taking so much work home that it's interfering with my family life or friendships ____

Symptoms in Interpersonal Relationships

1. I'm told I fail to consider the feelings of people I care the most about ____

2. I'm increasingly preoccupied and unable to listen to others ____

3. I have become restless or increasingly irritable ____

4. I'm emotionally withdrawn and often wish to be alone ____

5. Nothing seems light or funny to me anymore   ——

6. I obtain little joy from social events or vacations   ——

7. I find myself staring at the TV for long periods of time to avoid conversing with others   ——

8. I argue more with family members or close friends   ——

9. I have less contact with others   ——

10. I'm experiencing sexual difficulties   ——

Symptoms in One's Body or Mind

1. I'm unable to sleep or I feel the need to sleep more   ——

2. My eating habits have changed   ——

3. I'm noticing more generalized aches and pains   ——

4. I'm using alcohol, tobacco, or other drugs that affect the way I feel more frequently   ——

5. I have recently broken out with sores, blisters, or rashes   ——

6. I have recently experienced more allergic reactions   ——

7. I constantly worry and feel anxious   ——

8. I'm constantly fatigued and/or uninterested in daily activities   ——

9. I'm experiencing increased headaches, backaches, or ulcer flare-ups   ——

10. I'm experiencing feelings of dizziness, queasiness in my stomach, or tightness in my chest   ——

11. I frequently feel tension in my muscles   ——

Reprinted by permission of Kenneth B. Matheny, Ph.D., ABPP, 1995.

What Stress Can Do to Your Body

- Weaken the immune system, making you susceptible to colds and possibly other diseases

- Reduce concentration, causing poor performance

- Cause weight gain or weight loss

- Cause excessive drinking

- Disrupt sleep (either sleeping too much or unable to sleep), resulting in increased likelihood for accidents

- Aggravate already-existing conditions, such as heart disease, digestive problems, some skin diseases, high blood pressure, arthritis, headaches, and menstrual pain

- Bring on frequent headaches

- Show up as neck or back pain

Lions and Tigers and Bears, Oh My! Stress Takes on Many Forms

It's not what you're eating, it's what's eating you.
—JANET GREESON, PH.D.

When you're stressed, your body produces a measurable physical response. Your heart beats faster, your lungs work harder, blood pressure rises, muscles tense up, and you find yourself on high alert. Researchers describe this vigilant state as the body's fight-or-flight response, supposedly evolving from our primitive ancestors who were on guard against dangers such as saber-tooth tigers.

Today's tigers might be the mere thought of speaking in front of a large audience, or flying in an airplane. Whatever it is in your mind that gets your body keyed up and the adrenalin pumping, that's stress. Adrenaline and some kinds of neurotransmitters (other chemicals in the brain) are released in stressful situations. It's a natural response for intense, threatening situations, and may even help you carry out that presentation before the board of directors, but over a long period of time, extreme stress has been shown to negatively affect health. You may not even know exactly what's stressing you, but your body feels the effects.

Workplace Stress

Stress can arise from everyday responsibilities and obligations. Because work is a large part of daily life, workplace situations are major contributors to stress that often become chronic or prolonged. Stressed-out workers are at greater risk for injury, have reduced concentration, may experience sleepiness, and are absent from work more often due to illness. Sometimes, in rare cases, severe stress on the job leads to hostility, harassment, and violence. According to a survey of over 2,000 American workers, people who described their jobs as highly stressful were more likely to report health problems.

Lack of control or input over workplace circumstances is often cited as a top reason why employees experience stress. Organizations and managers who do not communicate changes or responsibilities clearly often produce feelings of anxiety in their employees. Other stressors include long hours, a great deal of business-related travel, lack of job security, office politics, and disproportionately low pay compared to level of responsibility. Layoffs, reduction in force, downsizing—whatever you call it, the people departing the company are (understandably) stressed. And often the "survivors" left at the company feel stress too, with added workloads, not knowing if they're "next," and wondering why they are still there.

Although you may not realize it, even a good event such as a promotion, a new project, or a positive presentation can bring about stress.

Lifestyle Stress

The home is nostalgically thought of as a safe, comfortable haven—a refuge from the frenetic outside world. Family and home life bring joy, but it can't be denied that they also bring a certain amount of stress. With the rising number of single-parent households, one person is increasingly responsible for raising children, providing meals, working a full-time job, and maintaining a home. Feeling overwhelmed or having too much to do is definitely stressful living.

Stress from the Inside Out

Whether or not a person experiences a high-stress situation with work or another part of life, stress is actually generated internally. It is simply the human response to something that happens on the outside that an individual identifies as "stressful." Worrying over events beyond our control creates anxiety. People who believe that life is not turning out as they think it should or have preconceived ideas about how things should be can experience a great deal of stress. Other states of mind that bring about stress include feeling powerless or unable to handle a situation, fearing the worst could happen, failing to achieve a desired goal, or blaming yourself or others for unfortunate events.

The manner in which you handle stressful situations determines how much stress you might experience. It's only when stress is not properly managed that the negative physical effects appear. And minor symptoms of stress are the early warning signs that situations are getting beyond your control. At that point, if you recognize the signs, you may need to manage your life differently so that stress doesn't overwhelm you.

When Stress Becomes Anxiety

Stress is triggered by an existing identifiable cause, often called a stressor. Anxiety is stress that continues after the stressor is no longer present, and it is often not even associated with a stressful or threatening situation. Anxiety is an emotional disorder characterized by apprehension, fear, and nearly the same physical and psychological symptoms as stress. Chronic feelings of hopelessness, anxiety, and fear will deprive you of accessing healthy coping strategies. So, it is important to pay attention to these emotional signs.

One of the difficult things about anxiety is that you may not always know when you are experiencing it. You may think you are just worried. Before you realize what is happening, you are experiencing serious symptoms of anxiety. Sometimes people may become overly anxious and may no longer cope well with day-to-day life. If this happens to you, it may be a good idea to seek outside help to learn effective ways to cope. Ask your doctor or nurse about your symptoms of anxiety. An assessment can be made to determine the cause of your anxiety and what can be done to treat it.

Stress and Illness

Scientists know that a person's mind and body interact, but these interactions are complex and not well understood. For example, many types of stress activate the body's endocrine (hormone) system that in turn can cause changes in the immune system, which is the body's defense against infection and some kinds of illness. However, the immune system is a highly complex network of cells and organs whose activity is affected by a number of factors, not just hormones. Studies have shown that, under certain laboratory conditions, various types of stress can either stimulate or suppress the immune systems of animals.

About Anxiety

What to Look For:

Panicky feelings

Feeling of losing control

Difficulty solving problems

Feeling excitable

Anger or irritation

Increased muscle tension

Trembling and shaking

Headaches, upset stomach, diarrhea, constipation

Sweaty palms, racing pulse

What to Do:

Talk with your doctor about your anxiety and the possible ways to treat it

Identify the thoughts that may be causing the anxiety

Solve day-to-day problems that are causing you stress

Engage in some pleasant, distracting activities

Seek help through counseling and support groups

Use prayer or other types of spiritual support

Try deep breathing and relaxation exercises several times a day
  (see pages 253–254)

Do Not:

Keep feelings inside

Blame yourself for feelings of anxiety and fear

Call the Doctor:

If you are having trouble breathing, are sweating, and/or feel very restless

If you experience trembling, twitching, and are feeling "shaky"

If your heart rate and pulse have rapidly increased

If you have severe problems with sleeping several days in a row

Stress can affect immune systems in humans, as well as alter how people feel and view the world. Research has shown that people with higher-than-average levels of stress who often feel helpless, hopeless, and out of control tend to be at higher risk for infection. The relationship of psychological factors to infection, however, is not clearly understood. Long periods of stress or depression can lead to poor nutrition that can weaken the immune system and contribute to infection.

Does Stress Cause Cancer?

This is a complex question. Scientists are studying the links between stress and the onset, as well as progression, of certain diseases (such as stress causing a pre-existing condition to worsen). Although studies reported by the National Cancer Institute (NCI) have shown that stress-causing events alter the immune system, so far, **there is no scientific proof to show stress causes cancer.** That said, investigators of several studies have reported an increased incidence of early death, including cancer death, among people who have experienced some of the high-stress events such as the loss of a spouse or other loved one.

We must, however, evaluate any reports with caution. Most cancers become apparent only after they have been growing in the body for a long time—anywhere from two to thirty years. This time period contrasts with the short intervals reported in studies correlating bereavement with subsequent death from cancer. Recognizing the need for continued research on this topic, the NCI is funding a study on the links between emotions and the endocrine and immune systems. So far neither this study, nor any other published study, has provided scientific evidence of a direct cause-and-effect relationship between emotions or stress and cancer.

Is There a Link Between Personality and Cancer?

*It is more important to know what sort of a person has a disease
than to know what sort of disease a person has.*
—HIPPOCRATES

Some researchers have been interested in the link between personality and cancer. For instance, some studies conclude that people who have problems expressing anger are more likely to get cancer. These studies have flaws in the way they were carried out. Most cancer specialists do not believe there is any link between personality and cancer. The disease is too complex to have a single cause. At this time, **there is no scientific proof showing that personality traits will cause cancer**.

This area of research, called psychoneuroimmunology (PNI), however, deserves further study. PNI is the scientific study of the mind and how it affects the body. It specifically investigates associations between the brain, behavior, the immune system, and the onset and progression of disease.

Despite the lack of scientific evidence that stress or a certain personality type causes cancer, it may be fair to say that when people are stressed, they begin making unhealthy choices, such as drinking more alcohol, exercising less, smoking more, and eating poorly. This is why it is important to identify stress early, manage it regularly, and cope with it in positive ways. The suggestions offered in the following section are meant to encourage you to face your stress head-on and develop healthy lifestyle habits.

The Art of Managing Stress

For fast-acting relief, try slowing down.
—LILY TOMLIN

What stresses you out? Driving in traffic? Monthly sales quotas? Kids crying in a restaurant at the next table? Financial pressures? Deadlines,

deadlines, deadlines? Taken alone, a single incident may not show up as a blip on your stress radar, but little incidents throughout the day or week add up.

To begin the process of stress reduction, it's a good idea to first identify sources of stress in your life (see pages 238–239). Jot down an informal account of daily events and activities that drain your time and energy, or trigger anxiety, anger, or a negative physical reaction. Also note experiences that evoke a refreshing feeling, a sense of accomplishment, or a pleasant physical reaction. You may find it helpful to use a wall calendar, Day-Timer, or personal digital assistant for your notes. A simple event description, the day, and the time will serve as a reminder for stressors.

Also note the stress cues in your body. These are the signs your body gives you that something's not quite right. Some common physical cues are blushing, gritting your teeth, tense muscles, shortness of breath, tightness in your chest or throat, clenched fists, racing heart, sweaty palms, or a feeling of fatigue.

Once you recognize your stress cues, you'll be better able to manage the stress, defuse it, and move on.

The stress management techniques offered here are, of course, not intended to replace professional care. For some people it's not as simple as recognizing stress and "dealing with it." There are times in many people's lives when counseling, or even medication, may be extremely helpful. You may find that using coping skills, relaxation techniques, and certain lifestyle choices can help you put your stress into perspective and focus on what's important in life. Certainly, this is easy to say but usually difficult to do, especially if you feel things may be getting out of control. If you feel you're experiencing physical or psychological symptoms that may be related to chronic stress, such as heart irregularities, pain, migraine headaches, or depression, consult a doctor without hesitation. Help is available.

Quick Tips for Stress Relief

- Play often and laugh out loud

- Seek the company of good friends and quality time

- Enjoy balanced meals that don't weigh you down

- Be honest, flexible, and direct

- Make rest and relaxation a regular part of your life

- Express yourself

- Share responsibilities

- Enjoy a hobby

- Live in the present and let go of the past

- Set your own priorities and plan for success

Reorder Your Priorities

We must free ourselves of the hope that the sea will ever rest.
We must learn to sail in high winds.
—HANMER PARSONS GRANT

When it seems you can't juggle one more thing, life circumstances bring you more. Work, family, obligations, commitments—the great American juggling act can be overwhelming.

Check your daily log of stress-producing events. Because it's impossible to eliminate stress completely, your objective may be to reorder your priorities. One big step in reducing stress is to add pleasurable events to your day. This is good news because many stressful situations cannot be easily whisked away or postponed, so making time for recreational activities is as important as getting enough sleep, eating healthy, and exercising. Consider as many enjoyable relief options as possible.

If the stressful situation is work-related and it's impractical to change jobs or reduce your hours, plan a relaxing lunch with friends, a brisk walk, or arrange to take a long weekend. If the stress is at home, make time to get away for an hour or two. Prioritize your tasks by asking yourself two questions: Is this chore absolutely necessary? If so, how soon does it need to get done? Replace activities that you can cut out with those that interest you.

Many people think that special time for personal enjoyment takes away from important obligations and responsibilities (such as that briefcase full of work you brought home from the office). Self-sacrifice is admirable, but not always necessary, and may even be damaging to your health, especially if it makes you irritable, angry, or tired. Having hobbies or personal interests does not make you selfish. On the contrary, these outside interests may make you a more creative and productive person.

Go ahead, take that vacation. Many people save up their vacation time, hold it over, or take the cash and stay on the job. What many don't realize is that vacations may be good for your health. Aside from fleeing work stress, vacations may work their magic by providing opportunities for vacationers to interact with family and friends, and to exercise, suggest some researchers. Of more than 12,000 men in one research study taking place over nine years, those who took regular annual vacations had a lower risk of death from heart attacks than the men who skipped their vacations.

How long to go for, where to go, and what to do may not be important—you don't need a traveler's guide to know that getting away from it all can be revitalizing, especially if you leave the cell phone and laptop behind.

Cope with Stress One Step at a Time

- Avoid expecting too much of yourself and of others. Being critical, disappointed, or frustrated leads to more stress. Expectations and reality are often two very different things. You can't change other people; you can only change how you react to them.

- Set realistic goals. Don't set yourself up for defeat by trying to achieve the impossible. Avoid the role of the "superhero."

- It's OK to say "no." Many of us try to please everyone, but in reality, we can't be everything to everyone. Meeting your own needs before responding to other people is critical for personal fulfillment and happiness.

- Ask for help if you need it, and take on one thing at a time. This will help you avoid being overwhelmed, as well as give you a sense of accomplishment.

- Reverse negative thoughts and situations by focusing on the positive. Envision a positive outcome, and then mentally prepare for it.

- Take time to be alone. Just a few moments of quiet reflection can invigorate your mind and allow for a mental readjustment, if necessary.

Alter Your Reactions

God grant me the serenity to accept the things I cannot change, the courage to change the things I can, and the wisdom to know the difference.
— Reinhold Niebuhr

You can reduce your emotional responses to stress—and even learn to change your behavior to stressful events. For example, the next time you're sitting in impossible traffic, steaming about being late or missing a meeting, look in the rearview mirror. Make up a funny story about the driver behind you and watch a smile appear on your face. A good laugh is like jogging on the inside, and it works.

If a police officer pulls you over for speeding, close your eyes for a moment, take a deep breath, and transport your mind to your favorite spot on earth and, just for a second, be there. Your mind will associate all the powerfully good feelings you felt then and bring them to your present dilemma, and your reaction may be much more calm and controlled—inside and out. (So why were you speeding in the first place?)

Learning to react calmly to a stressful situation can effectively reduce the amount of stress you experience. Successful stress reduction from any technique will not be immediate or result from a half-hearted effort. Chronic stress may require some revolutionary lifestyle changes. And if you are serious about reducing the amount of stress you are experiencing, as well as concerned about the long-term effects to your health, prepare yourself to be open-minded and accepting of different techniques. Think about the way you want to live your life, what level of stress you can tolerate, and then choose which of the following techniques (or combination of techniques) works best for you.

Talk About It

The concept of "getting in touch with your feminine side" is a common satire on open communication and "letting it all out." The fact of the matter is that bottled up feelings can lead to hostility and anger. For some people, sorting out thoughts by direct communication with a trusted individual or writing in a journal can greatly diminish the harmful consequences of stress. Your family and friends want to be part of your life, and if something is bothering you, they may be able to help by providing love, support, and guidance.

Similarly, keep in mind that you may be that trusted individual for someone else: listening, empathizing, and responding are essential for maintaining strong relationships necessary for mutual fulfillment. Research has shown that a network of social support that includes friends, family, support groups, religious associations, and extracurricular activities can help reduce stress.

Listen to Music

When stress pushes your buttons, try pushing the buttons on your CD player, advises Alicia Ann Clair, Ph.D., MT-BC, professor and director of Music Therapy at the University of Kansas. Use gentle music to pace your activities and stimulating music to increase your energy during the times of your day when you need motivation. Some people use music in the early afternoon at work to help them focus at a time when their concentration levels begin to wane. In the late afternoon pressure cooker, Dr. Clair suggests using appropriate music to relax and manage your stress response. She even suggests using music and visualization as part of your ritual before bed to promote a good night's sleep.

Which music is right for you? Dr. Clair says to select music that does not distract you from your primary activities. Music engages your mind and body by entraining your physical and emotional responses—in other words, music brings the mind and body on the same track. Relaxing music slows the tempo of life. Faster tempos lift your mood.

Try a Variety of Relaxation Techniques

There's more to life than increasing its speed.
—Mahatma Ghandi

Relaxation techniques, such as visual imagery, hypnosis, or relaxation exercises, can have a very positive impact on anyone who is stressed, including the person struggling with chronic illness. These types of activities are being organized in conjunction with traditional treatment in many health care institutions today for people with cancer and other illnesses. These are not an alternative to traditional medical treatment, but are in addition to, or "complementary" to, conventional medicine.

There are many different types of relaxation techniques. Choose one that works best for you.

- *Visual imagery* is a relaxation technique that involves mental exercises designed to enable the mind to influence the health and well being of the body.

- *Progressive muscle relaxation* is a technique that increases awareness of how to identify tension in the body and the ability to relax specific muscles groups throughout the body.

- *Deep abdominal breathing* involves learning how to breathe from the lower part of the abdomen. Many people breathe from the chest rather than the abdomen, which is less effective in creating a state of relaxation.

- *Slow rhythmic breathing* begins with staring at an object or a peaceful scene, or closing the eyes, and concentrating on breathing slowly and deeply.

- *Autogenic training* is a technique used to teach the mind and body to respond to positive messages that are repeated to oneself. Autogenic phrases help people to monitor themselves by focusing their awareness on the connection between verbal commands and physical relaxation.

- The *Relaxation Response*, a form of meditation developed by Herbert Benson, M.D., involves sitting comfortably in a quiet place and repeating a word, sound, phrase, or prayer silently.

The Instant Sit Back, Relax Technique for Reducing Stress

- Go through a few simple movements to relieve tension in your body: stretch fully; move your arms over your head; bend your spine; roll your head gently in circles.

- Sit down and slowly close your eyes. Consciously choose to let go. Make this an active decision. Talk yourself into it; tell yourself that this is the most important thing you can possibly do for the next few minutes.

- Push the small of your back into the chair or sofa so that you are sitting up straighter than usual. See how comfortable you can become by letting the chair support you totally. Imagine you are going limp like a rag doll, but keep your head level. Let yourself go and sink as deeply into the chair as you can.

- Exhale deeply. See how deeply and completely you can let your breath out. As the air nears what seems to be the end, try to let out just a little more. This will lessen your tension tremendously. You are not trying to force or control your breath, rather you are letting go, releasing. Inhale deeply through your nose and expand your abdomen, not your chest. You should be able to feel your rib cage dropping each time you exhale through your mouth. Exhaling in this way should feel like a deep sigh. Go ahead. Make a sighing noise. It helps. Do this several times.

- Scan through your body to pick up points of tension, as if you were reading yourself on radar. Concentrate on one area of the body at a time. When you detect tension or discomfort, see if you can think it away. Tell your body to go limp around the point of tension and to release it from your body. Try this scanning technique until you find no more points of tension.

Adopt Healthy Habits

Stressed is desserts spelled backward.

—BRIAN LUKE SEAWARD, PH.D.

If you are stressed out, evaluate the recent choices you may have made: watching TV instead of taking a walk, staying up late and not getting enough sleep, eating fast food, smoking, or drinking more. People under stress often seek relief through self-destructive means, thus carrying on the cycle of stress. A sedentary lifestyle can lead to heart disease, disrupted sleep patterns, and increased tension. Alcohol, nicotine, junk food, and caffeine are called artificial stress reducers because they temporarily often mask the symptoms of stress.

- *Exercise:* It is widely accepted that exercise is an excellent stress reducer. It improves circulation and strengthens the body against infection. Spending time outside or in an active environment can also improve your mood. This book presents much useful information on the value of exercise and its role in disease prevention (see Chapter 3).

- *Diet:* Maintain a healthy diet and regular times for meals (see Chapter 2). Enjoy a diet rich in fruits and vegetables and low in fat, salt, and sugary treats because all are known to contribute to heart disease, diabetes, and other health problems. There is no evidence that vitamins or dietary supplements protect against the effects of stress. Herbal and dietary supplements advertised to "bust your stress" are unproven and possibly harmful. Here's a stress-less tip: Eat breakfast. One study of 126 adults between the ages of twenty and seventy-nine years old found that those who ate breakfast every day felt less stressed, less depressed, and reported lower levels of emotional distress than people who didn't eat breakfast every day.

- *Sleep:* Getting enough sleep is key to reducing stress and revitalizing the mind and body. People who do not get enough restful sleep are often irritable, anxious, and less productive. There is a complex relationship between sleep and the restorative processes in the immune system. Some researchers suggest that a significant loss of sleep (or sleep deprivation) in a normal adult reduces immune system functioning, which could cause a biological response similar to the body fighting off an infection.

Your Safety Net—Ask Your Doctor for Help

You know your stress triggers. You know how your body is responding. Don't dismiss common distress signs such as difficulty sleeping, excessive fatigue, headaches, sour stomach, and recurring colds. These could be signs of a more serious condition, and you may require more than daily meditation, deep breathing, and yoga to get back on track. Medical care may be necessary. Your outward physical symptoms may be telling you something. Taking an aspirin for a daily headache or an antacid for a constantly upset stomach might just mask other, deeper problems.

This is also the case with unmanageable emotional symptoms. If you feel you're having difficulty coping with problems in your life, or are feeling anxious or depressed, consider talking to your regular doctor. He or she may be able to help you sort things out, or can at least point you in the direction of someone who can. Often short-term therapy can help you with stress-related problems and teach you coping mechanisms for future situations. If necessary, prescription medications can be used in tandem with behavioral counseling with very good success. No matter what your situation, or how helpless or hopeless you might feel at times, good help is available.

CHAPTER 8

Living in a Hazardous World

*Life consists not simply in what heredity and environment do to us
but in what we make out of what they do to us.*
—HARRY EMERSON FOSDICK, clergyman

The cancer specialists at the University of Nebraska Medical Center don't see as many patients with cancer caused by asbestos as their colleagues in East Coast cities, where this mineral was used in heavy manufacturing and shipbuilding. At first, no one at the Nebraska medical center in Omaha suspected asbestos-related cancer in a tiny seventy-three-year-old grandmother. But when Myrna Block sought their opinion in 2001, all signs pointed to a very rare cancer called mesothelioma. Exploratory surgery confirmed this most unusual and surprising diagnosis, and that's when the detective work began.

Where had she grown up? Lived? Worked? She had been a schoolteacher, and her husband an industrial engineer. They had been living with their three young children in Buffalo, New York, until his job brought them from the East Coast to Omaha in the 1970s. None of the puzzle pieces seemed to fit until doctors discovered that her husband's occupation, not hers, might have been the cause for her cancer. She revealed that her husband had worked at a company that used asbestos as lining for industrial fittings they manufactured in the 1960s—more than thirty-five years ago.

Bingo! He carried home the tiny fibers on his clothing and body and in his hair. Because she had close contact with him, and washed his clothes, she was exposed almost as intimately to the cancer-causing asbestos as if she herself had worked at the plant. The fibers had lain dormant in her body for decades, only to trigger one of the rarest and deadliest forms of cancer caused by an outside substance.

Life in a Bubble

Unlike cancers caused by personal choices, such as smoking or unhealthy diet, some cancer risks are out of our control or unknown at the time, as in this example. There certainly must be cancer-causing materials we don't even know about yet. But the good news is that we do know about many you might encounter at home, at work, at your doctor's office, and in the world around you.

Some exposures are inevitable, while others can be avoided, or at least reduced.

We certainly can't and won't live in a bubble. It's time to discover what you need to do, or not do, to protect yourself and your family. After reading some background information about cancer-causing chemicals and radiation, you should know the details about environmental risks, which of them are genuine concerns, which you can safely ignore, and which scientists are still not sure about.

This chapter focuses on how we determine whether or not something in our environment causes cancer. We'll discuss some of the better-known cancer-causing agents, as well as what you should be aware of. We'll also touch on some controversial, but unproven, causes of cancer. And along the way we'll give you some tips for reducing your risk.

Environmental Causes of Cancer

Strictly speaking, your "environment" is the combination of circumstances, physical conditions, and outside influences surrounding you. You may have heard of the "nature versus nurture" debate and the question of which is more important in our development as human beings. Some of our traits are inherited (nature), while others may be a product of our interactions with the world around us (nurture). The general consensus is that both are important for determining who we are.

Cancer can be thought of in the same way. Scientists generally agree that most cancers arise because of a combination of the genes we inherit from our parents and some outside influences. The key is in identifying exactly what these genetic and outside (environmental) factors are. Put another way, any factor that is not inherited as part of your genetic makeup is environmental.

When the average person talks about environmental factors, he or she is usually referring to pollution of the air or water. To cancer epidemiologists, environmental factors are anything and everything other than your genetic predispositions. These factors include ones related to our habits and lifestyle decisions, as well as exposures in our workplace and in the general environment. Environmental factors known to be related to cancer include smoking, poor diet, lack of exercise, certain infections, and sunlight. In fact, an estimated three-fourths of all cancer deaths in the United States are thought to arise from these types of outside environmental factors. Many of them are lifestyle related and involve personal choice, as discussed earlier in this book.

To put this chapter in perspective, the remaining environmental risks—exposure to occupational and industrial hazards and pollution—are thought to account for fewer than 10 percent of all cancer cases.

Take the Safety Quiz

Many of us are concerned about the world around us and take precautions intended to protect ourselves from hidden dangers. Do you really know which of these exposures increase cancer risk and which are thought to be harmless? Which precautions might lower that risk and which are inconveniences or expenses without any likely benefit? Consider these examples.

_____ **Have you had your house tested for radon?**

You probably should. Radon causes thousands of preventable lung cancer deaths every year. Radon can be found in any home whether it's new or old, insulated well or not, or has a basement or a concrete slab.

_____ **Do you wash fruits and vegetables to rinse off pesticides that were applied in the field? Or do you buy organically grown produce for assurance that chemicals were not used in the growing process?**

Washing your food is probably not necessary, but there is no harm in it—it might also reduce risk of infections. There is no need to buy "organic" produce, although it is fine for people who are concerned about pesticides.

_____ **Are you careful about the products you keep under your kitchen sink? Do you use and dispose of household cleaning products with caution and care?**

These are reasonable precautions, but ordinary use of common household products is not likely to have a significant impact on cancer risk.

_____ **Have you installed a water filtration system, or do you buy bottled water or use a filtered water pitcher?**

Usual filtration systems do not remove arsenic, the most significant carcinogen in drinking water (see pages 291–292 for more information on arsenic). Some types of filters do remove substances (such as lead) responsible for other health problems, as well as improve the taste of the water.

_____ Do you use a hands-free headset with your cell phone?

There is no evidence that cell phones increase cancer risk, but hands-free phones are certainly safer while driving. Since cell phones have not been around long, we can't say for certain whether an association with health problems will be discovered until years from now. The type of radiation involved with cell phones indicates that a link to cancer is extremely unlikely.

_____ Do you dye your hair? Have you considered using temporary hair dye instead of permanent?

There is probably no risk or minimally increased for users, but hair dye is certainly not a necessity so people who are concerned can follow steps outlined in this chapter.

_____ Do you use underarm antiperspirants or talcum powder?

There is no risk from antiperspirants. However, some evidence suggests talc use may increase ovarian cancer risk. Inhaling talc can cause lung problems. Cornstarch is safer, for those who want to use a powder.

_____ When dining out, do you reach for those pink or blue packets of artificial sweetener?

Most evidence indicates that there is no risk, but people who are still concerned can avoid or limit use of these products.

_____ Do you work in a high-risk occupation, that is, with chemicals known or suspected to be carcinogens? Do you follow appropriate precautions?

Appropriate precautions include using a mask, wearing protective clothing, and showering immediately after work. This is very important advice for workers in these occupations.

Q&A About Cancer-Causing Substances

What Is a Carcinogen?

Scientists realized more than one hundred years ago that some chemicals and forms of radiation could cause cancer. Certain infections can also lead to cancer (see Chapter 6). It is now known that cancer occurs as a result of several changes that take place within the cell. The process that changes normal cells into cancer is called carcinogenesis. The chemicals and other exposures that bring about these changes and increase the risk of cancer are called carcinogens. Because more than one change is needed, many years may elapse between exposure to a carcinogen and the development of cancer. This is known as a latent period.

How Do Carcinogens Cause Cancer?

Carcinogens contribute to cancer by altering a cell's DNA, which is the set of instructions that tells the cell what to do. These changes in DNA are known as mutations. Mutations are actually very common, occurring up to a million times or more in the body each day. Most of these mutations are not due to carcinogens in our environment. Instead, they are due to the endogenous (internal) carcinogens that our bodies produce in the course of normal metabolism.

Other mutations are the result of errors in copying the DNA of our replicating cells. The cells in bodies are frequently dividing in order to replace old, worn out, or injured cells. Before each cell divides, it must create a new copy of its DNA. One way to think about this process is to imagine yourself repeatedly typing a page of text each time you need a new copy. Eventually, you will make some typographical errors, but most will be detected and corrected by your computer's spell checker program. Occasionally, your typo will produce a real word that is different from the original one, and your computer may not identify this. A few of these errors may seriously change the meaning of your message.

In much the same way, our cells contain DNA repair enzymes that detect most of the DNA mutations resulting from copying errors, carcinogens within our bodies, or environmental carcinogens. In most cases, these enzymes can correct the DNA errors, but if the errors cannot be repaired, they set a cell suicide program in motion that destroys the cell before it becomes cancerous.

Some mutations, however, may escape repair and get passed on to the next generation of cells. Some of these changes are harmless, but some might cause a cell to behave in a way it normally wouldn't. For example, a mutation of a gene in a particular part of DNA might cause a cell to grow more quickly than it normally would, or it might stop the cell from dying when it's supposed to. Carcinogens are capable of causing these kinds of harmful mutations.

It's important to keep in mind, though, that carcinogens do not cause cancer in every case, all the time. Agents classified as carcinogens may still have different levels of cancer-causing potential. And the degree of cancer risk posed by a carcinogen also depends on the concentration or intensity of the carcinogen, as well as the length of time that someone is exposed to it. Some substances or forms of radiation may only cause cancer at very high doses or after prolonged exposure. Lower levels may not have harmful effects. For example, Chapter 4 explains how ultraviolet (UV) radiation in sunlight can cause skin cancer, and discussed ways to lower your skin cancer risk. But, protecting yourself against skin cancer doesn't mean you have to live in complete darkness.

When concentrations are low and the duration of exposures is limited, the increase in risk is usually minor. Even when the risk of each low-dose exposure can be estimated accurately (which is not always the case), it remains difficult to predict the risk from the combination of many low-dose exposures we face each day. And low-dose exposures that pose only a small risk to each exposed person, but are widespread, can still have significant public health significance across an entire population. An example of this is secondhand tobacco smoke, which increases risk in large numbers of people who do not smoke but are exposed to the smoke other people produce.

How Are Carcinogens Classified?

Several monitoring and regulatory groups use similar systems to classify how much evidence exists that an agent is carcinogenic—in other words, will it cause cancer? The most widely used system comes from the International Agency for Research on Cancer (IARC), part of the World Health Organization (see Resources). It divides agents into general categories, ranging from certainty that a substance causes cancer in humans, to probable, possible, unknown, and probably not cancer causing, based on available scientific evidence.

Perhaps not surprisingly, most of the 750 or so agents listed by the IARC are possible/probable or of unknown risk. This is because there is not enough strong evidence either way that many substances definitely do or definitely do not cause cancer. About fifty are classified as carcinogens.

In the United States, the National Toxicology Program (NTP), formed from parts of several government agencies (including the National Institutes of Health, Centers for Disease Control and Prevention, and the Food and Drug Administration), puts out a *Report on Carcinogens* every few years, which classifies "known to be human carcinogens" or "reasonably anticipated to be human carcinogens." Examples of familiar substances known to cause cancer in humans include arsenic, asbestos, radon, tobacco smoke, and smokeless tobacco. Over 200 agents appear on this list. Refer to the NTP for a complete list (see Resources).

How Did We Make the Cancer Connection?

One of the earliest connections between a particular exposure and cancer was made in the early 1700s with what became known as "chimney sweepers' cancer." Percival Pott, in his book *Chirurgical Observations*, noted that chimney sweeps, usually small boys and adolescents who bathed very little, developed cancer of the scrotum more often than other workers. He associated the accumulation of soot with cancer, thereby linking occupation to cancer risk.

Similar to the chimney sweeps, young women employed in watch manufacturing facilities in the early 1900s were also noted to develop cancer from tasks they performed. Using brushes moistened with their tongues, these workers painted watch faces with radium to make them glow in the dark. Day after day, the young women repeatedly licked their tiny brushes and dipped them into the cancer-causing radium paint. Unknowingly, they ingested dangerous levels of radiation, and the number of workers who later developed tongue and jaw cancers was far higher than would have been expected in this population.

These were some of the first recognized examples of a relationship between exposures to high levels of substances and a significantly increased risk of cancer. This has since been shown in other settings where workers have been exposed to high doses of ionizing radiation (see pages 268–269) or to certain chemicals, as well as among atomic bomb survivors.

Often in the past, direct evidence of a cancer-causing agent has come from such instances of sustained or high-dose exposures. But unfortunately, the possible connection between an agent and cancer is not always so obvious. On the other hand, we now have better tools available to help us find these links when they exist.

The Process of Assessing Your Risk

Today, the potential hazards of an agent are determined through risk assessment. This process evaluates both the cancer-causing potential of a substance, as well as the levels of the substance in the environment. Risks are assessed to protect people against unsafe exposures and to set appropriate environmental standards. Although the process is effective, it is not perfect.

Risk assessment involves two basic steps: identifying what the hazard is, and then determining how (and how much) exposure to the hazard might cause cancer.

Identifying the Hazard

The first step is identifying the chemical or physical nature of a hazard and its cancer-producing potential. When a link between an agent and cancer is suspected, several types of scientific studies can be used to detect it. These include laboratory studies and epidemiological studies that evaluate the statistical associations between exposures and diseases in populations of humans. Because each type of study has its own strengths and weaknesses, the results from different types are often examined together to give a better overall picture of the risk an agent might pose. For more information on the types of studies, see pages 11–15.

Assessing Exposure

The second step in risk assessment measures levels of hazard in the environment (in the air, water, and food, for example) and the extent to which people are actually exposed (how much they eat of a particular food, use a particular water source, and so on). Knowledge of how the body absorbs chemicals or is exposed to radiation is essential for such dose measurements.

For most potential carcinogens, evidence of risk starts with high-dose experiments on animals or observations where high-dose exposures have occurred in humans. To set human safety standards, regulators must recalculate from animals to humans and from high-dose to low-dose conditions. Because both predictions involve a lot of uncertainty, cautious assumptions are used so that risk assessment will err on the side of safety. For cancer safety standards, increased risks of greater than one additional case per million persons over a lifetime is generally considered unacceptable.

Standing Watch—
Which Agencies Are Responsible for Maintaining and Enforcing Exposure Levels?

For substances determined to cause cancer, several government agencies are responsible for ensuring that levels of exposure are within safe limits. Safety standards developed by way of risk assessment are the basis for federal regulatory activities at the following government agencies, among others (see Resources).

- **Food and Drug Administration (FDA) (www.fda.gov):** The FDA has the authority to regulate not only the safety of food (labeling, additives, pesticide levels) and drugs, but also medical and radiation-emitting devices (such as cellular phones and microwaves), and even has limited authority over cosmetics.

- **Environmental Protection Agency (EPA) (www.epa.gov):** Established in 1970, the EPA is responsible for air, water, and food safety through the monitoring and control of environmental pollution.

- **Occupational Safety and Health Administration (OSHA) (www.osha.gov):** As part of the U.S. Department of Labor, OSHA is responsible for creating and enforcing workplace safety and health regulations, including those relating to potential carcinogen exposures.

Different Kinds of Carcinogens

The two major classes of carcinogens are certain chemicals and *some* types of radiation. As we discussed in the last chapter, some infectious diseases (especially viruses) can be considered to be carcinogens as well.

Living in a Hazardous World   **267**

Chemicals

Various chemicals (for example, benzene, benzidine, cadmium, soots, asbestos, vinyl chloride, and arsenic) show definite evidence of causing cancer in humans. Most of these are generally thought of in terms of workplace exposures. Other "chemical" carcinogens include medications, some of which are, ironically, used to treat certain cancers.

Other chemicals are considered probable human carcinogens (such as chloroform, formaldehyde, and polychlorinated biphenyls, or PCBs; see page 294) based on evidence from animal experiments.

Some environmental pollutants and chemicals in consumer products receive a lot of press coverage, but the actual evidence about their cancer-causing properties remains inconclusive.

Radiation

Radiation is the emission (sending out) of energy from any source. The light that comes from the sun is a source of radiation, as is the heat that is constantly coming off our bodies. When talking about radiation, however, most people think of specific kinds of radiation, such as radioactive materials or nuclear reactions. Only high frequency radiation (ionizing radiation and UV radiation) has been proven to cause genetic damage, which can lead to cancer. Most forms of radiation are nonionizing and have not been linked to cancer.

Types of ionizing radiation include x-rays, gamma rays, cosmic rays, and particles given off by radioactive materials such as alpha particles, beta rays, and protons. People may be exposed to three main sources of ionizing radiation.

- *Natural background radiation* comes from cosmic rays from outer space and radioactive elements normally present in the soil. This is the major contributor to worldwide radiation exposure.

- *Nonmedical synthetic radiation* occurs as a result of above-ground nuclear weapons testing that took place before 1962, as well as occupational and commercial sources.

- *Medical radiation* comes in the form of diagnostic x-rays and other tests, as well as from radiation therapy. Radiation therapy is currently used to treat some types of cancer and involves dosages many thousand times higher than those used in diagnostic x-rays.

- *Exposure to sunlight* (UV radiation) causes almost all cases of basal and squamous cell skin cancer and is a major cause of melanoma (see Chapter 4).

As is the case with chemicals, certain forms of radiation have not been clearly linked to cancer but still receive a large amount of attention. These are *nonionizing* forms of radiation, and because of their low frequencies, they don't have the energy to cause DNA damage. Forms of nonionizing radiation include microwaves, radio waves, and radar, as

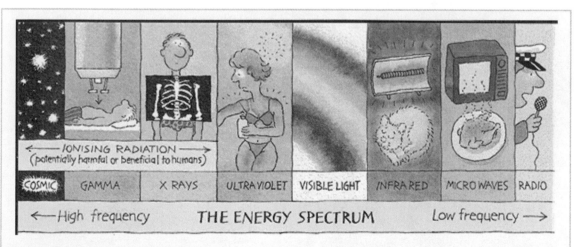

Reprinted from *Radiation and Life* web graphic by permission of Uranium Information Centre, Ltd., Melbourne, Australia. Available at: http://www.uic.com.au/ral.htm. Accessed February 25, 2002.

well as the electromagnetic radiation arising from power lines, cellular phones, and household appliances such as televisions. There is very little evidence that this type of radiation can cause cancer. While some studies have suggested associations with cancer, most of the now extensive research in this area does not. Furthermore, it has been difficult to come up with a possible mechanism by which this type of radiation could cause cancer. Research, and controversy, in this area continues.

Protect Yourself From Hazards in Your World

Some people wonder, "Is a cancer-causing product lurking in my home? Have I been exposed to something that may harm me or my family years from now?"

We take precautions every day to avoid substances that we *know* may trigger cancer. And we make reasonable assumptions about our risks when it comes to substances we *think* may cause cancer. But, many people don't have all the facts. The more you learn about the real, rather than imagined, risks related to developing cancer, the safer you will be. Here we'll examine the most commonly found cancer-causing products and discuss the actual risks as well as steps, if any, that are needed to protect yourself and your family.

The Places We Live

There are a lot of myths and misconceptions about things in your own home that may cause cancer. Most environmental risks are related to lifestyle, and you'll see that in most cases you have nothing to fear. In cases where there is a danger, we'll explain what steps you need to take to be safe

Radon

You can't see it. You can't smell or taste it. But radon is a problem. Major health organizations including the American Cancer Society agree that radon causes thousands of preventable lung cancer deaths every year.

Radon is a colorless, odorless gas that occurs naturally in soil, rocks, underground water, and air. It's produced by the natural breakdown (radioactive decay) of uranium in soil and rocks. The radon breaks down further into decay products that attach to particles in the air. Outdoor radon levels are minute. But when radon enters a building—or your home—its decay products can accumulate.

Uranium miners, who are exposed to high levels of radon, were first noted to have a higher than expected risk of lung cancer. Extensive studies have shown that radon causes lung cancer in nonsmokers. Smokers exposed to high levels of radon in their homes have even higher risks for lung cancer. When inhaled, radon decay products become trapped in the lungs where the ionizing radiation energy is believed to begin the gradual cancer-causing process.

Limited data on children suggest that they may be more susceptible to cancers caused by radiation. But until more definitive data becomes available, common sense tells us that if radon causes lung cancer in adults, children with their smaller lung volumes and higher breathing rates are just as much at risk or more.

Radon levels are highest in the Northeast and Midwest, but high radon levels have been found in every state and vary from area to area. Your home may have a high radon level, yet your neighbor's may be within acceptable limits. Radon is measured in picocuries per liter (pCi/L), and the EPA urges anyone whose level at home is above 4 pCi/L (an estimated 8 million American homes) to take action. By comparison, the average outdoor air radon level is about 0.4 pCi/L, but it can be higher in certain areas.

An airtight home with all cracks carefully sealed keeps warm air in during the winter, it also allows dangerous radon to accumulate year-round. However, radon can be found in any home whether it's new or old, insulated well or not, has a basement or a concrete slab. Until you test, you simply don't know.

What to Do to Protect Yourself

Both short-term and long-term tests are available and are relatively inexpensive (less than fifty dollars). The National Safety Council operates a Radon Hotline to answer questions and provide materials about radon, its health effects, and radon testing. If you're interested in obtaining more information, you can call the hotline at (800) 557-2366. Information about radon, and lists of contractors qualified to conduct radon testing and make home modifications to lower radon levels is available on the EPA web site at www.epa.gov/iaq/contacts.html.

- If you're buying a home, insist that it be tested before you buy. Be suspicious of cracked foundations or homes with crawl spaces under family rooms or bedrooms.

- If you're selling, test your home to assure potential buyers that your radon level is low. Each state has a radon information office. Call for information and a list of approved testing companies.

- If your radon test registers over 4 pCi/L, you can take action with simple solutions. Radon levels can be lowered. You may be able to install pipes and fans below concrete floors and foundations. Or a fan in your crawl space can provide necessary ventilation.

- Include radon-resistant techniques in your building plans for renovating, finishing your basement, or for new construction.

Personal Products

Personal care products are items such as cosmetics, hair and skin care items, fragrances, toothpastes, and deodorants. These types of products have been used for centuries. The FDA regulates them (loosely) under the Federal Food, Drug, and Cosmetic Act (FFDCA), but only after they are released to the marketplace. Neither cosmetic products nor cosmetic ingredients are reviewed or approved by the FDA before they are sold to the public.

The FFDCA does require that color additives used in cosmetics be tested for safety, although this does not apply to hair dyes. Regulations do restrict or prohibit the use of ingredients that are known to be toxic such as chloroform and mercury compounds.

In addition, the FDA requires that *all* ingredients be labeled in order of decreasing amounts used in the product. Although the FDA cannot require companies to test their cosmetic products for safety before marketing, if the safety of a cosmetic product has not been tested, the product's label must read: "WARNING: The safety of this product has not been determined." If the FDA wishes to remove a cosmetic product from the market, it must first prove in a court of law that the product may harm users, that it is improperly labeled, or otherwise violates the law.

Hair Dyes. Are hair dyes hazardous? Not even your hairdresser knows for sure. About one-third of adult American women, as well as a small but increasing number of men, use hair dyes. And with the aging of the population and an unwillingness to go gray without some protest, the numbers are likely to increase. Hair color may matter, but does it cause cancer?

Most of the concern regarding potential cancer risk revolves around the use of permanent and semi-permanent dyes, as opposed to temporary ones (those lasting only for a few washings). These products contain chemicals that have been found to cause cancer in laboratory animals. However, the animals in these studies were fed high levels of the dyes over a long period of time, so the relevance of this information to the use of hair dyes by humans is uncertain. Because dark brown and black dyes have higher concentrations of suspected carcinogens, these products are of greatest potential concern.

More than twenty studies across large populations have examined the association between exposure to permanent hair dyes and various cancers. The largest studies to date have found that death rates from all cancers combined appear to be about the same among women who do or do not use hair dyes. Some studies have found an association between hair dye use and bladder or blood cancers (such as leukemias), but others have not.

The IARC concluded in 1993 that hairdressers and barbers probably are exposed to work-related carcinogens, but that the evidence of increased cancer risk was limited. Insufficient evidence existed for that agency to evaluate the possible carcinogenic risks of personal use of hair color.

Most hair dyes don't have to go through premarket testing for safety that other cosmetic color additives do before hitting store shelves. That leaves you as a consumer on your own when deciding whether hair dyes are safe.

So what if you regularly dye your hair? Other than recommendations that apply to everyone when it comes to routine health screening and healthy lifestyle choice, no specific medical advice is needed for current or former hair-dye users. The bottom line is that most of the available evidence does not show hair dyes to be a significant cancer risk factor.

Talc. Talc (also known as talcum or hydrous magnesium silicate) is a white to grayish-white powder that may be contaminated with other minerals, such as asbestos, silica, or quartz. It is found in most body and baby powders, except those that are specifically labeled "talc-free" or "pure corn-starch," and is also used for medicinal and toiletry products, glove and shoe powders, fillers for pills, and soap and paper products. In some cases it may be contaminated with other minerals, such as asbestos, silica, or quartz.

How Should I Apply Hair Dye?

Because the conclusions among published studies are inconsistent, the FDA has provided some suggestions for people concerned about hair dyes as a cancer risk factor, or as a cause of eye or skin irritation.

- Don't leave the dye on your head any longer than necessary.

- Rinse your scalp thoroughly with water after use.

- Wear gloves when applying hair dye.

- Carefully follow the directions.

- Never mix different hair-dye products, because you can induce potentially harmful reactions.

- Be sure to do a patch test for allergic reactions before applying the dye to your hair.

- Never dye your eyebrows or eyelashes.

- Delay dyeing your hair until later in life when it starts to turn gray.

- Consider using henna (which is largely plant-derived) hair dyes that are lead acetate-based, or temporary hair coloring products.

The scientific evidence for the carcinogenicity of talc is based on two forms of talc exposure: inhalation exposure among workers and exposure among women who use genital powder.

Several studies have examined the connection between talc inhalation exposure and lung cancer. In many of the studies with positive results, there was evidence of asbestos contamination of the talc, so the substance responsible for the cancers may have been asbestos rather than the talc. Thus, the evidence for lung cancer is strongest for talc contaminated by asbestos. However, there is little available evidence to suggest that the grade of talc now used in consumer products increases the risk of developing lung cancer.

Several studies in the 1980s and 1990s suggested that the use of talc in genital hygiene could lead to the development of ovarian cancer. This link may be due to the presence of asbestos fibers in talc because the two substances are often found together in mineral deposits. Exposure may occur when a woman applies a talc-containing powder to her genital area, or possibly through sexual contact with a man who has applied this powder to himself. It may enter a woman's body through the vagina and pass through the uterus and fallopian tubes to reach the ovaries. However, the evidence for the risk of ovarian cancer is mixed. Published reviews of this association have called for caution in interpreting study results and the need for further research.

Neither the NTP nor the EPA has yet classified talc as carcinogenic. However, the IARC has determined that talc containing asbestos is known to be carcinogenic. For talc not containing asbestos, the IARC has determined that the evidence of carcinogenicity is inadequate (meaning there is not enough evidence to classify it as carcinogenic).

Nonetheless, if you use genital powders and are concerned about the evidence in this chapter, you may wish to use only cornstarch powders, or reduce or eliminate your use of powders. A recent review suggests that cornstarch is unlikely to increase cancer risk.

Antiperspirants. Did you receive the e-mail about antiperspirants causing breast cancer? It's not true, by the way, but many women were so concerned when their e-mail pen pals began circulating the alarming news, they forwarded the false message to their friends, and, well, you know how cyber-rumors spread.

The hazard, according to the e-mail, was that nicks from razors supposedly allow antiperspirants to be absorbed into the body, where they prevent the lymph nodes under the arms from removing cancer-causing toxins from the breasts. **There is no scientific evidence to support this claim.**

No population-based studies have reported an association between breast cancer risk and antiperspirant use. Furthermore, there is no evidence that the chemicals in antiperspirants are absorbed through the skin (regardless of whether or not the skin is shaved or has small razor nicks), nor is there any evidence that aluminum or any of the other chemicals in antiperspirants cause DNA damage that can lead to cancer.

Sweat glands, which are located in the skin, are not connected to lymph nodes. Lymph nodes help clear some potential cancer-causing toxins from the body, but they do not release these toxins through sweating. The fluid in lymph nodes enters the bloodstream, where toxins are eventually removed by the liver (and excreted in feces) or kidneys (and excreted in urine).

Some women wonder why they are advised not to use antiperspirants or deodorants on the day they are scheduled to receive a mammogram. Here's why: many of these products contain aluminum, which is a metal and can show up on a mammogram as tiny specks in the area. These specks can resemble microcalcifications, which are one of the things doctors look for as a possible sign of cancer. Avoiding the use of these products helps prevent any confusion when looking at the mammogram films.

Nonionizing Radiation

There are certain types of radiation that have not been linked with certainty to cancer, but still receive a large amount of attention. These are nonionizing forms of radiation, which include microwaves, radio waves, radar, and electromagnetic radiation (from power lines, cellular phones, and household appliances; see page 269). Because of their low frequencies, these forms of radiation don't have the energy to cause

DNA damage. There is very little evidence that this type of radiation can cause cancer.

Although some studies have suggested associations with cancer, most of the now extensive research in this area does not. Furthermore, it has been difficult to come up with a possible mechanism by which this type of radiation could cause cancer. Certainly research, and controversy, in this area continue.

Power Lines and Appliances. Electromagnetic radiation is a type of non-ionizing radiation produced by moving electric charges. It may be of natural origin (the sun) or human origin (electronic devices or power lines).

Electromagnetic fields have been the subject of much controversy. Recent extensive studies of electric utility workers showed a minimal increase in the risk of brain tumors and leukemia, but these increases were so small that they may have been due to chance. Results from studies on magnetic fields and childhood leukemia have been suggestive but inconsistent. While smaller studies have observed a link between cancer and activities such as the use of electric blankets and watching television, the most recent and largest study did not find a connection between electromagnetic fields and cancer.

In 1999, the National Institute of Environmental Health Sciences released results of an extensive six-year study. It stated that the evidence for a risk of cancer and other human disease from the electric and magnetic fields (EMF) around power lines is "weak" at best, but could not totally be discounted, and efforts to reduce exposures when possible should continue. The conflicting data concerning electromagnetic fields will undoubtedly continue to generate controversy. Clearly, the question of whether or not electromagnetic fields can cause cancer needs to be answered.

Cellular Phones. Recent media attention has focused on a possible link between cellular phone use and brain cancer. Cellular phones operate with radio frequencies (RF), a form of electromagnetic energy located on the electromagnetic spectrum between FM radio waves and the waves used in microwave ovens, radar, and satellite stations (see page 269). Cell phones do not emit ionizing radiation, the type that damages DNA.

Because widespread cellular phone use is little more than ten years old (remember that some cancers may take decades to develop), there has been limited opportunity to examine its long-term health effects. However, the lack of ionizing radiation and the low-energy level emitted from cell phones and absorbed by human tissues make it unlikely that these devices cause cancer. Moreover, several well-designed epidemiological studies find no consistent association between cell phone use and brain cancer. The FDA Center for Devices and Radiological Health has stated:

> If there is a risk from these products—and at this point we do not know that there is—it is probably very small. But if people are concerned about avoiding even potential risks, there are simple steps they can take. People who must conduct extended conversations in their cars every day could switch to a type of mobile phone that places more distance between their bodies and the source of the RF, since the exposure level drops off dramatically with distance. For example, they could switch to a mobile phone in which the antenna is located outside the vehicle; a hand-held phone with a built-in antenna connected to a different antenna mounted on the outside of the car or built into a separate package; or a headset with a remote antenna to a mobile phone carried at the waist. Again, the scientific data do not demonstrate that mobile phones are harmful. But if people are concerned about the radiofrequency energy from these products, taking the simple precautions outlined above can reduce any possible risk.

Cancer may not pose as great a risk as other potential health problems such as injuries in car accidents caused by the use of cell phones while driving.

Cleaning Products

By their very nature, many chemicals used in cleaning products have toxic properties, such as being poisonous or corrosive. Does this mean we should avoid using them to scrub our toilets or unclog our drains? Not at all! When used properly, most of them pose little health risk. What's important is not the potential of the substance to do harm, but the actual risk to *you* in how you use the product. Most household cleaners are reasonably safe and are not a significant cancer risk.

What to Do When You Have Questions About a Specific Product

You don't need an advanced degree in chemistry to determine whether a product you are using (or disposing of) may be dangerous. Although not always the case, a certain amount of information should be available on the product label. If not, it may take some investigation, but you can get assistance from the National Institute of Environmental Health Sciences (NIEHS) Office of Communications at (919) 541-3345 (www.niehs.nih.gov/external/faq/hsprod.htm). For specific information about possible carcinogenic properties, you may also want to visit the web site of the IARC (www.iarc.fr) or the NTP (ntp-server.niehs.nih.gov) to look for the ingredients on the complete lists of carcinogenic agents.

Household Pesticides

According to the EPA's Office of Pesticide Programs, a pesticide is any substance or mixture of substances intended to prevent, destroy, repell, or reduce any pest. Pests can be insects, mice, and other animals, unwanted plants (weeds), fungi, or microorganisms like bacteria and viruses. Though often misunderstood to refer only to insecticides, the term pesticide also applies to herbicides and fungicides.

About 75 percent of homes in the United States use at least one pesticide product indoors each year. In fact, most household exposure to pesticides occurs inside the home rather than outside due to airborne particles, chemicals tracked in from outdoors, and stored pesticide containers. (See pages 284–285 to learn about pesticides and food.)

But the health hazards of pesticides are primarily from direct contact with the chemicals at high doses. For example, farm workers who apply the chemicals and work in the fields after the pesticides have been applied, and people living near fields sprayed from the air are at a great risk.

The health effects associated with high-dose pesticide exposure include irritation to the eyes, nose, and throat, dizziness, muscle twitching and tingling sensations, and nausea. Repeated and long-term exposure can ultimately damage the central nervous system, liver, and kidneys, and, for some pesticides, cause an increased risk of cancer.

Yet other dangers still exist, and it pays to read product labels. Regardless of their potential to cause cancer, pesticides pose other health risks as well, involving the nervous and reproductive systems, and the liver. Other suspected health effects, based mostly on animal data, include reduced fertility, birth defects, and immune system dysfunction. To minimize any risk, consider the following guidelines for pesticide use.

- Read and follow the label directions for every product before use.

- Use a product specifically recommended for the job you want to do.

Pesticides and Breast Cancer

In recent years, some controversy has existed around the possible relationship between certain pesticides and cancers that are influenced by hormones, such as breast cancer. Dichloro-diphenyl-trichloroethane (DDT) and other organochlorine insecticides have been implicated because of their ability to mimic the effects of estrogen, a major female hormone. Although DDT and some of the organochlorine insecticides were banned from use in the United States in the 1970s, questions about their lingering effects remain.

Currently, research does not show a clear link between breast cancer risk and exposure to these environmental pollutants. Although a few studies have suggested certain pollutants increase breast cancer risk, the most recent analysis of available data, combining the results from several previous studies of women living in the northeastern United States, did not find such a link. Most experts believe that if such a connection exists, it accounts for a very small portion of breast cancer cases, but research in this area continues.

- Ventilate the area before and after application. Avoid inhaling the chemical.

- Use an alternative, nonchemical method if possible.

- Use the amount directed under the specific conditions mentioned. Avoid using more chemicals than necessary and never mix chemicals.

- Keep and store pesticides away from food and the kitchen area.

Herbicides and Lymphoma

Herbicides are chemicals that kill plants, weeds in particular. There are many chemical classes of herbicides, but it is the phenoxy herbicides (such as 2,4-dichlorophenoxyacetic acid, or 2,4-D, and 2,4,5-trichlorophenoxyacetic acid, or 2,4,5-T) that have been of greatest concern as a possible carcinogen.

Several studies have suggested an increased risk of non-Hodgkin's lymphoma (NHL) among farmers, and herbicides were one of the possible explanations considered. However, those studies are limited by absence of dose information, mixed chemical exposures, and exposures to infections and other possible causes of cancer. More recent epidemiologic studies have focused on herbicide industry workers. These have suggested a possible trend toward slightly increased risk of NHL in relation to phenoxy herbicide exposure, but the results have been inconsistent and the association, if present, appears to be weak. Animal evidence has not shown the phenoxy herbicides to be carcinogenic. Most expert agencies have found that no firm conclusions can be drawn.

- Keep pets and children away from stored pesticides and treated areas.

- Handle the container safely and maintain an adequate distance from the treated area.

- Dispose of chemical containers according to package directions.

- Wash thoroughly with soap and water after using pesticides and launder your clothes before wearing them again.

By their very nature, most pesticides create some risk of harm to humans, animals, or the environment because they are designed to kill living organisms. No pesticide is 100 percent safe, and care must be exercised in the use of any pesticide.

At the same time, pesticides are useful because of their ability to kill potential disease-causing organisms. The EPA (www.epa.gov/pesticides) is responsible for regulating pesticides for safety in the United States. They evaluate and register pesticides before they may be sold, distributed, or used. And safer, biologically based pesticides are becoming more popular.

The issue of health risk boils down to the question of the extent and application of any given pesticide. When used properly, most household pesticides pose no threat. As long as you follow the product instructions for applications, the threat to you and your family's health is minimal.

The Food We Eat

Food safety—specifically whether pesticides and irradiation are hazardous—has continued to be an issue of public concern in recent years. The majority of available scientific data, however, does not provide strong evidence for associations with cancer.

Pesticides on Food

We've discussed the problems in using pesticides around the house and for keeping bugs and fungi from destroying our yards and garden. Now we turn to the issue of pesticide residue that remains on the food we grow and eat.

Continued research is essential for maximum food safety, but pesticides play a valuable role in sustaining the food supply. In contrast to occupational and environmental health hazards, pesticide residues in the fruits and vegetables you buy or grow pose very little risk to human health. In fact, people who eat more fruits and vegetables, which may have pesticide residues on them, generally have lower cancer risks than people who eat few fruits and vegetables.

The American Cancer Society believes that the benefits of a balanced diet rich in fruits and vegetables far outweigh the largely theoretical risks posed by occasional, very low pesticide residue levels in foods.

What can you do if you are still concerned about pesticide residue on your fruits and vegetables? Washing fresh produce before eating it is a healthful habit. You can reduce and often eliminate residues present on food by following these simple tips provided by the FDA.

- Wash produce with large amounts of cold or warm tap water and scrub with a brush when appropriate. Do not use soap.

- Throw away the outer leaves of leafy vegetables such as lettuce and cabbage.

- Trim the fat from meat, and trim fat and skin from poultry and fish. Residues of some pesticides concentrate in animal fat.

Additional answers and suggestions can also be found on the EPA web site (www.epa.gov/pesticides/food). Information about specific pesticides and crops is also available.

Some people may also choose to buy produce grown without pesticides, commonly known as "organic."

Food Irradiation

Food irradiation, which has been in use for decades, is a way to prevent illness caused by bacteria such as *E. coli, Campylobacter, Salmonella,* and *Listeria,* and parasites in food, and perhaps even replace some pesticides currently being used.

Irradiation has been shown to be safe and effective, and it is now used in more than forty countries. In the United States, the FDA has approved the use of irradiation of meat and poultry and allows its use in some other foods, including fresh fruits and vegetables and spices.

In addition to reducing insects and parasites, irradiation of certain fruits and vegetables delays ripening, allowing foods to remain unspoiled much longer than would be possible otherwise. Irradiated strawberries, for example, stay unspoiled for up to three weeks. Untreated strawberries may last only three to five days.

The irradiation process exposes food to higher frequency radiation known as gamma rays or x-rays to kill the bacteria, but it does not make the food radioactive (just as an airport luggage scanner does not make luggage radioactive) or create harmful chemical compounds. It may cause a small loss of nutrients, but no more so than with other processing methods such as cooking, canning, or heat pasteurization.

Food is packed in containers and moved by conveyer belt into a shielded room. There the food is exposed briefly to a radiant-energy source—the amount of energy used depends on the food. Energy waves pass through the food and break molecular bonds in the DNA of bacteria, other pathogens, and insects. These organisms die or, unable to reproduce, their numbers are held down. Food is left virtually unchanged, but the number of harmful bacteria, parasites, and fungi is reduced and may be eliminated. There is no credible evidence that irradiated foods cause cancer or that irradiation significantly affects the antioxidant vitamins and other substances in certain foods that help prevent cancer.

The FDA requires that irradiated foods be labeled as such to distinguish them from nonirradiated foods. The Radura symbol along with a statement "treated with irradiation" or "treated by irradiation" on the label means the product was processed by irradiation.

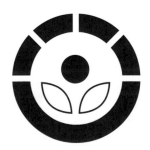

Artificial Sweeteners

Controversy has surrounded two approved sugar substitutes, saccharin and aspartame, for many years.

Saccharin. Discovered in 1879, saccharin is actually older than the FDA, and for many years was designated as a "generally recognized as safe" (GRAS) additive. When a Canadian study in the late 1970s showed that saccharin caused bladder cancer in rats, the FDA proposed to ban it. Because it was the only sugar substitute available at the time, a public outcry ensued, fueled in part by media reports that the test animals received the equivalent of hundreds of cans of diet soda a day. Congress responded by passing the Saccharin Study and Labeling Act, which placed a two-year moratorium on any ban of the sweetener while additional safety studies were conducted. Congress has since extended the moratorium several times, most recently renewing it until 2002. However, the law required that any foods containing saccharin must carry the now-familiar label:

Use of this product may be hazardous to your health. This product contains saccharin, which has been determined to cause cancer in laboratory animals.

The NTP removed saccharin from its roster of "reasonably anticipated carcinogens" in its most recent report in 2000. It has remained on the market and continues to generate demand as a tabletop sweetener, particularly in restaurants, where it is available in single-serving packets. It has continuing appeal because of its stability at high temperatures (unlike aspartame), which makes it an option for sweetening baked goods; its long shelf life; and because it is inexpensive to produce.

The bottom line? Studies have found high doses of saccharin cause or promote tumors of the bladder in laboratory rodents. However, a close look at the results of these rodent studies suggests they may not be relevant to humans. Saccharin causes deposits of irritating crystals in the bladder of male, but not female rats, and is associated with bladder cancer in male but not in female rats. Many researchers have concluded that irritation from crystals and from large crystal deposits, called calculi or stones, is the way saccharin increases bladder cancer risk in male rats. Due to differences in our metabolism, saccharin does not cause bladder crystals or stones in humans, leading many researchers to suspect that saccharin is unlikely to cause bladder cancer in humans. Large epidemiologic studies, however, have not reported increases in bladder cancers among people using saccharin, so if saccharin does increase cancer risk in humans, it does so only at unusually high doses.

Aspartame. Approved for use by the FDA in 1981, aspartame has been the subject of controversy as well. Rumors (many on the Internet) of aspartame causing health problems have abounded, linking it to everything from autoimmune diseases such as lupus and multiple sclerosis to brain cancer. However, there is very little, if any, evidence to back up any of these claims, other than the known risk to people with a rare genetic defect known as phenylketonuria.

Other Food Additives

So, you may be wondering, "What about Red No. 2?" Food dye is actually considered a food additive. In its most general sense, a food additive is any substance added to food. The FDA defines a food additive as a substance "which results or may reasonably be expected to result—directly or indirectly—in its becoming a component or otherwise affecting the characteristics of any food." This can include everything from spices or vitamins to preservatives or food coloring agents.

Additives are used in foods for five main reasons.

- To maintain the consistency of a food.

- To maintain or improve its nutritional value. (All products containing added nutrients must be appropriately labeled.)

- To reduce spoiling and extend shelf life.

- To control pH levels or provide leavening.

- To enhance flavor or color.

The Red Scare

In the early 1970s, data from Russian studies raised questions about Red No. 2's safety. Several subsequent studies showed no hazards. The FDA conducted its own tests, which were inconclusive. The consumer-oriented Health Research Group petitioned the FDA to ban the color, while congressional and public interest mounted.

The FDA turned the matter over to its Toxicology Advisory Committee, which evaluated numerous reports and decided there was no evidence of a hazard. The committee then asked the FDA to conduct follow-up analyses. Agency scientists evaluated biological data and concluded that "it appears that feeding FD&C Red No. 2 at a high dosage results in a statistically significant increase" in malignant tumors in female rats.

There still was no positive proof of either potential danger or safety in humans. The FDA ultimately decided to ban the color because it had not been shown to be safe. The agency based its decision in part on the presumption that the color might cause cancer. Though long gone from U.S. shelves, products tinted with Red No. 2 still can be found in Canada and Europe. Whether the color is gone forever in the United States remains to be seen. FDA and industry officials say it could stage a comeback.

Since 1958, all food additives (with the exception of GRAS additives in use prior to that time, such as sugar or salt) are required to have proof of safety at intended levels of use before the FDA allows them to be added to foods. Color additives in use before 1960, however, have had to undergo safety testing before being allowed continuous use. Of the 200 color additives in use at the time, 90 have since been listed as safe, and the remainder have been removed from use by the FDA or by industry.

Both of the congressional acts regulating food additives include a provision that prohibits the approval of an additive if it is found to cause cancer in humans or animals. This clause is often referred to as the Delaney Clause. Today, food and color additives are more strictly regulated than at any time in history. All additives are subject to ongoing safety reviews as scientific understanding and methods of testing continue to improve.

If you're interested in looking at what types of testing have been done on a particular food additive, the FDA maintains the "Everything Added to Food in the United States" (EAFUS) Database, which is available at http://www.cfsan.fda.gov/~dms/eafus.html.

"Natural" Carcinogens

Not all cancer-causing substances are manmade. Certainly several viruses such as HIV are known to cause cancer among humans (see Chapter 6). Some other infectious agents, including certain parasites (more common in Africa and Asia), and even bacteria, may also play a role in the development of cancer, although indirectly. More research is needed to better define these potential risks.

The most well-known "natural" carcinogen is aflatoxin, a chemical produced by a fungus (mold) that sometimes contaminates peanuts, wheat, soybeans, ground nuts, corn, and rice. Aflatoxin is a very potent cause of liver cancer, and contributes significantly to that disease in parts of Africa, where food spoilage caused by molds is common. In the United States, there is a comprehensive program that requires the USDA and

FDA to test certain foods to ensure that they do not contain dangerous amounts of aflatoxin. Peanuts and peanut products are among the most stringently tested. So, the risk of developing liver cancer from your peanut butter and jelly sandwich is remote!

Another group of "natural" carcinogens are those that, at high doses, cause cancer in laboratory animals, but have not been shown to be carcinogens to humans. Many chemicals naturally found in foods such as natural plant pesticides, are included in this category. Plants, including many edible ones, naturally produce pesticides to protect themselves against insects. Although some of these have been found to cause cancer in laboratory animals, epidemiologic studies have consistently found that a diet high in foods from these plant sources is associated with a higher, rather than lower, risk of cancer. Many substances found in nature can be as potent as manmade pollutants in causing cancer in animals. But the relevance of these substances to the safety of low levels of manmade chemicals is uncertain and highly controversial.

The Water We Drink
Arsenic

Arsenic, a naturally occurring element that is present in rocks and soil, can be a byproduct of some industrial processes, and it was once a component of many pesticides. It has the potential to seep into underground water sources. Arsenic is very poisonous when consumed in high doses. People who wish to poison (and kill) other people—in mystery novels and in real life—often choose arsenic. Although low levels of arsenic do not cause immediate effects, long-term exposure has been linked to bladder, lung, and possibly other cancers.

Arsenic levels tend to be highest in groundwater, which is tapped as a source of drinking water for about half of U.S. cities. Levels of arsenic tend to be high in small communities and in places with private wells. People who are concerned with how much arsenic is in their water can check the consumer confidence report mailed to them each year by their local water supplier.

The EPA is responsible for assuring the safety of drinking water. It does this by setting drinking water standards—regulations to control the level of contaminants in the water. After reviewing studies that look at possible health effects, the EPA sets a maximum level of a contaminant in drinking water at which no anticipated effect on health would occur, and which also allows for an adequate margin of safety.

Recently, even "safe" levels have been questioned. A report by the National Academy of Sciences released in 2001 claims that arsenic in drinking water may be much more harmful than previously thought. Even tiny amounts appear to be linked to increases in lung and bladder cancer. In fact, the EPA is reducing the amount of arsenic allowed in U.S. water supplies. This is a return to a tighter standard and will become fully effective in 2006.

Pesticides

Pesticides deserve mention once again because their use can potentially cause health problems through pollution of water. Chemical run-off from farm fields, yards, and golf courses treated with pesticides can contaminate streams and lakes, thus causing damage to natural food chains dependent on fish, shellfish, and other marine or fresh-water life.

In addition, contamination of groundwater from pesticides or other chemicals can affect drinking water and create potential health risks for humans. Such risks are now likely to be less than in past years because pesticides that persist in the environment (one of the most familiar is DDT) have been largely replaced by products that are quickly degraded. Thanks to water treatment processes, dangerous levels of suspected carcinogens in the water system are infrequent.

In Our Communities

When a specific type of cancer occurs more often than expected in a particular community, it is often called a "cancer cluster." Clusters can involve a few cases of a very rare type of cancer or a larger number of a more common type of cancer. At least one dozen "clusters" are reported in the press each year and cause widespread concern, typically in schools, workplaces, or other localized areas of communities.

Because of the nature of carcinogens and the way in which cancer develops, scientists suspect a group of cancers are more likely to be a true "cluster" if the cases involve the following.

- One type of cancer, rather than several different types

- A rare type of cancer, rather than common types

- A certain type of cancer in an age group not usually affected by that type of cancer

Suspected clusters of cancer should be reported to the local or state health department. The department then makes an initial assessment to determine if the cases are truly a cluster and should be studied further. Most state health departments report that fewer than 5 percent of cancer cluster investigations actually require thorough study. Sometimes local health officials will ask for assistance from the Centers for Disease Control and Prevention (CDC). If a situation is deemed an epidemic emergency, the CDC will send a team to investigate a reported cluster; however, this occurs rarely.

Two areas of particular concern to the public are nuclear power plants and toxic waste sites.

Ionizing radiation emissions from nuclear power plants are closely controlled and involve negligible levels of exposure for communities near the plants. Although reports about cancer clusters in such communities have raised public concern, large studies have shown that clusters do not occur more often near nuclear plants than they do by chance elsewhere in the population.

Toxic wastes in dumpsites can threaten human health through air, water, and soil pollution. Many toxic chemicals contained in such wastes can be carcinogenic at high doses, but most community exposures (and possible cancer clusters) appear to involve very low or negligible dose

What About PCBs?

Polychlorinated biphenyls (PCBs) are a group of over 200 related chemicals that were used by U.S. industries from the 1930s until they were banned in the late 1970s. Large amounts of PCBs are still present in the environment, and from breakdown of products. Very small amounts of PCBs are present in most food, water, and air. Most exposure of the general public occurs through the consumption of food or water from contaminated areas.

PCBs are known to increase the risk of cancer in experimental animals and are listed as a probable cause of cancer in humans by the IARC. In general, the levels of PCBs found in drinking water and the air are very low and insignificant. The concentrations found in food are also many thousand times below the concentrations that have been shown to cause cancer in experimental animals. Nevertheless, people should avoid consuming food from sources known to be heavily contaminated with PCBs, such as from areas where PCBs have been released into rivers, lakes, or onto soil.

If you are uncertain about PCB contamination in your area, it's best to check with local health authorities, such as the city, county, or state health department.

levels. Cleanup of existing dumpsites and close control of toxic materials in the future are essential to ensure healthy living conditions.

Increases in suspected cancer cases at one time and in one location often cause enormous distress to those involved. It is essential that these situations be confronted openly, promptly, and professionally. Although almost all investigations of clusters do not result in the recognition of a new or identified carcinogen, prompt efforts should be taken to confirm or refute the existence of a cluster and to hear and respond to the community's concerns.

In the Doctor's Office or a Hospital

You may find it surprising that some forms of medical therapy can actually lead to an increased risk of cancer in certain situations. Ironically, by far the majority of these are used to treat an already existing cancer. The medical community "fights fire with fire," so to speak, using powerful chemicals (or radiation) that can alter a cell's DNA, in the hopes of controlling a disease that might otherwise be fatal. Even though some of the treatments doctors use are technically carcinogens, the benefits arising from their use generally far outweigh the potential risks.

Chemotherapy

Chemotherapy is a drug treatment used to destroy cancer cells. Over one hundred drugs are currently used for chemotherapy—either alone or in combination. Many more are expected to become available. It is sometimes the first choice for treating many cancers. Chemotherapy is often used with surgery or radiation to treat cancer when the cancer has spread (metastasized), when it has come back, or when there is a strong chance that it could come back.

Chemotherapy differs from surgery or radiation in that it is almost always given as a systemic treatment. This means the medicines travel throughout the whole body or system rather than being confined or localized to one area such as the breast, lung, or colon. Because chemotherapy can reach cancer cells that may have spread to other parts of the body, it is often the most effective form of treatment for metastatic cancer.

Long-term side effects related to chemotherapy depend on the specific drugs received and whether you received other treatments such as radiation therapy. Longer-term effects can continue after the treatment is completed. Some of these effects can progress and become chronic, or new side effects may occur. Another cancer sometimes develops as a result of chemotherapy treatment. "Secondary" cancers can include Hodgkin's disease and non-Hodgkin's lymphoma, leukemias, and some solid tumors. Follow-up care after all treatment is completed is an essential component of cancer care for all cancer survivors.

Oncologists who prescribe chemotherapy drugs are aware that they increase the risk of secondary cancers. The risk for some chemotherapy drugs is greater than for others. For this reason and because of these drugs' other side effects, oncologists do not recommend chemotherapy unless they have good reason to believe it will help the patient and that the benefit will far outweigh the risk of a second cancer later on. They will attempt to use the least toxic chemotherapy drugs and the lowest doses that they expect to be effective for each patient.

Radiation Therapy

Radiation therapy uses high-energy ionizing radiation to destroy cancer cells in an effort to treat or control cancer. Radiation therapy's potential to also cause cancer was recognized many years ago. In fact, much of our knowledge about ionizing radiation has come from studying the survivors of the atomic bombs in Japan, from occupational exposure of workers, and from patients treated with radiation therapy for malignant and non-malignant disease.

While still a relatively rare occurrence, development of a second cancer is more common among those who receive radiation therapy than those who do not. Most cases of leukemia related to radiation exposure usually develop within a few years of exposure, peaking at five to nine years, then slowly declining. Most solid tumors do not occur until ten years after radiation exposure, and some cancers are diagnosed even fifteen or more years later. Radiation-related leukemia risk depends on a number of factors, such as the amount of radiation received, the percentage of bone marrow exposed, and whether the patient was also treated with chemotherapy.

Studies of radiation-related breast cancer have found the greatest risk in women who were irradiated as children and adolescents for other conditions. (The most common reason for chest radiation in adolescents is Hodgkin's disease, a type of lymphoma. The risk is highest for the youngest women.) Oncologists, who generally recommend especially vigilant lifetime screening for breast cancer, know the increased risk of breast cancer in these women. However, most studies have found no increased breast cancer risk among women who receive radiation at age thirty years and older.

X-rays and Mammography

Compared to radiation therapy, x-rays (including mammograms, which are x-rays of the breasts) use doses of radiation that are many times lower. Many people are concerned about their exposure to x-rays. As is the case with radiation therapy, studies in the past have shown that there appears to be some risk particularly in children who received multiple x-rays. The level of radiation in modern x-rays is much lower than that used even twenty-five years ago, and likely poses much less of a risk. Still, repeat exposures should be minimized whenever possible especially in children.

For women over forty years old, the dose of radiation received during modern mammograms does not significantly increase the risk for breast cancer. To put dose into perspective, a woman who receives radiation as a treatment for breast cancer receives several thousand rads (the units that measure radiation exposure). If a woman has yearly mammograms beginning at age forty and continuing until she is ninety years old, she will have received ten rads.

CT Scans

Computed tomography (CT) scans use larger doses of radiation than those found in conventional x-rays. Again, concern has been raised over the possibility of an increased cancer risk in children who receive multiple CT scans. Although study results have not been conclusive, some researchers are suggesting that children should receive lower doses of radiation during CT scans compared to those used for adults.

Another potential source of exposure are whole-body CT scans, which some people are now requesting as part of a regular health checkup (for lung cancer). Many groups, including the FDA, have expressed concern over this practice, because there is little evidence of its usefulness, and it exposes people to unnecessary doses of radiation. Controversy in this area will no doubt continue.

Other Imaging Tests

Nuclear medicine tests, such as positron emission tomography (PET) scans, inject radioactive chemicals into the body. The amount of radiation used is quite small and is not considered a cancer risk. Magnetic resonance imaging (MRI) scanners, which rely on magnets, and ultrasound tests, which use sound waves, do not use radiation at all.

Hormones

Hormones have been used to treat and prevent certain diseases for decades. Many cancers, including cancers of breast, cervix, uterus (endometrium), and ovaries, grow in response to hormones. And in the cases of diethylstilbestrol (DES), hormone replacement therapy

(HRT), oral contraceptives (OC), and tamoxifen, the use of hormones may increase a woman's risk of developing certain types of cancer. In contrast, these medications can also be used to prevent, or even treat, some cancers.

Tamoxifen has been approved by the FDA for treatment of breast cancer and for decreasing the risk of breast cancer in women who have an increased risk. At the same time, it is known that the very same hormone can increase a woman's risk of developing cancer of the uterus. The decision to take tamoxifen is a personal choice made by weighing the benefits against the risks—the same decisions we all make every day with any medication.

A thorough discussion of hormones is beyond the scope of this book. Any woman concerned about her cancer risk related to the use of hormones should discuss these concerns frankly and openly with her doctor.

In the Places We Work

Millions of U.S. workers are exposed to substances that have tested as carcinogens [cancer-causing agents] in animal studies. Less than 2 percent of chemicals in commerce have been tested for carcinogenicity [cancer-causing properties].
—National Institute for Occupational Safety and Health

Strong statements from a regulatory agency. But should you be worried? And if so, exactly what should you be worried about? The answer depends on where you work and what you do for a living.

Many of the chemicals used in manufacturing and other processes are potentially more dangerous (in a number of ways) than those found around the home. If you work in a high-risk occupation or worksite, you may be exposed to levels of cancer-causing substances much higher than you would with home hazards. An exhaustive list of all of the potential exposures is not possible here, but we'll touch on a few major ones.

For many years now, cancer risk has been associated with certain occupations and hazards. Substantial increases in risk have been shown in settings where workers have been exposed to high concentrations of ionizing radiation, certain chemicals, metals, and other substances that were later found to cause cancer. The cancers that arose in chimney sweeps and watch-dial painters are examples of how repeated and high-level exposure to a carcinogen can lead to cancer. Federal and local agencies have since been created to ensure safety and to enforce the regulations that are in place to protect employees.

The IARC now recognizes that many occupations and workplaces deal with substances that potentially can contribute to cancer. Certainly, others exist as well. Many will no doubt be identified in the future. These are some of the more prominent industries.

- Aluminum production

- Boot and shoe manufacture and repair

- Furniture and cabinet making

- Hematite mining (underground) with exposure to radon

- Iron and steel founding

- Nickel refining

- Painting (occupational exposure)

- Rubber industry

Examples of Specific Occupational Hazards

Asbestos. Asbestos is a group of naturally occurring fibrous minerals. It has been used to insulate factories, schools, homes, and ships, and to make automobile brake and clutch parts, roofing shingles, ceiling and floor tiles, cement, textiles, and hundreds of other products. Both the IARC and the NTP classify asbestos as a known human carcinogen.

People are exposed to asbestos mainly by inhaling of fibers in the air they breathe. Inhalation usually occurs during mining and processing of asbestos, during the production of asbestos-containing products, or during the installation of asbestos insulation. People with the heaviest exposure are those who worked in asbestos industries, such as ship-building and insulating.

Exposure may also occur when older asbestos-containing materials begin to break down. Although the risk has dropped dramatically in the United States, there is still a potential for exposure from asbestos that remains in place in older buildings, water pipes, and other settings.

Inhalation of asbestos fibers has been proven to cause lung cancer. The higher the exposure to asbestos, the higher the risk of lung cancer. There is synergy between cigarette smoking and asbestos exposure in causing the more common forms of lung cancer (small cell carcinoma and non-small cell carcinoma). In other words, asbestos workers who smoke face a much higher risk of developing lung cancer than asbestos workers who do not smoke.

Most cases of mesothelioma, a rare form of cancer that affects the thin membranes lining the abdomen and chest, result from asbestos exposure. The risk increases with the amount of asbestos exposure, but cases of mesothelioma have occurred even after low levels of exposure. Meso-theliomas have been observed not only among workers who are exposed, but also among their family members, such as in the case of Myrna Block, who was mentioned at the beginning of this chapter, as well as in people living in the neighborhoods surrounding asbestos factories and mines. The IARC has estimated that one third of the mesothelioma cases in the United States may be due to non-occupational exposures such as these. Unlike the usual type of lung cancer, mesothelioma risk is not increased among smokers.

How Can You Reduce Your Risk?

If there is a possibility of on-the-job exposure, say, in renovation of old buildings, you should use all protective equipment, work practices, and safety procedures designed for working around asbestos.

If you live in an older home, there may be asbestos-containing insulation or other materials. A knowledgeable expert can check your home to determine if there is any asbestos and if it poses any risk of exposure. You may then decide if you need to have the asbestos removed from your home. You should hire a qualified contractor to perform this job, to avoid contaminating your home further or causing any exposure to the workers. You should not attempt do remove asbestos-containing material yourself.

If you've already been exposed, it is important to assess the amount of your exposure. If you were exposed only very briefly, or only at very low levels, your risk of a resulting disease is minimal. However, it you were exposed at high levels, you may be at increased risk for developing diseases related to your exposure.

You can protect your health in several ways.

- If you are a smoker, it is essential that you stop smoking (see Chapter 5).

- Get regular health checkups from a doctor experienced with asbestos-related diseases. People with heavy asbestos exposure often have periodic chest x-rays and lung function tests.

- It may be advisable for you to receive vaccines against flu and pneumonia to prevent other respiratory illnesses that might weaken your lungs. Discuss this with your doctor.

- Get prompt medical attention for any respiratory illness.

Benzene. Benzene is a colorless, flammable liquid with a sweet odor. It is formed from natural processes, such as volcanoes and forest fires, as well as from human activities—it is even a component of cigarette smoke. Benzene is widely used in the United States and ranks among the top twenty chemicals produced. It is primarily used as a solvent, as a starting material for the synthesis of other chemicals, and as a component of gasoline. Both the IARC and the NTP classify benzene as a known human carcinogen.

The greatest risk for exposure to high doses of benzene occurs in the workplace, although it also exists in low levels in the environment and in some cleaning products. Workers in industries that make or use benzene, including the rubber industry, oil refineries, chemical plants, shoe manufacturers, and gasoline-related industries, may be exposed to high levels of this chemical.

The evidence linking benzene and cancer predominantly comes from studies of workers in the chemical, shoemaking, and oil refining industries who developed acute myeloid leukemia, a cancer of blood-forming cells in the bone marrow.

Steps have been taken to limit exposures to benzene both occupationally and environmentally. An EPA regulation limits concentrations of benzene in drinking water to five parts per billion, with an ultimate goal of zero parts per billion. The National Institute of Occupational Safety and Health (NIOSH) and the Occupational Safety and Health Administration (OSHA) have limited occupational exposures to benzene to 0.1 parts per million and also recommend personal protective equipment such as respirators (see Resources for agency information).

Other Occupational Hazards. Certain cancers have been linked to carpentry and furniture making and refinishing. Since the 1960s, higher rates of cancer in the nose, voice box (larynx), and lungs have been observed in people who work in the furniture manufacturing industry.

The IARC has since determined that exposure to hardwood dust is an increased risk for those types of cancer. Woodworkers (even in home workshops) should take protective measures, such as wearing masks and using suction or vacuum devices for equipment that generates sawdust, to reduce their risk of inhaling dust.

As mentioned earlier, workers exposed to high levels of pesticides, in industry or farming, may be at higher risk of certain cancers.

Chromium and chromium alloy production workers and chromium platers have demonstrated an increased risk for developing lung cancer. Chromium is a hard, steel-gray metallic element that occurs naturally in the environment. Chromium and its compounds are common in the stainless steel industry, in the production of brick, glass, and ceramics, and as a protective coating for automobiles and other equipment.

Another occupation that has raised some questions about cancer risk is painting. As a group, painters show an increased incidence of lung cancer, perhaps due in part to methylene chloride in paint strippers and the glycol ethers in paints.

Government Protection in the Workplace. Workers in a wide range of occupations, from health care to construction to bartending, are exposed daily to known and probable carcinogens such as metals, dusts, solvents, dyes, secondhand smoke, chemicals, and radioactive materials. Strong regulatory control and constant attention to safe occupational practices are required to minimize the workplace potential for exposure to high-dose carcinogens. Two government agencies are responsible for this.

NIOSH: This agency is responsible for conducting research and making recommendations to prevent work-related disease and injury. The NIOSH is part of the CDC. In addition to conducting research, NIOSH investigates potentially hazardous working conditions when requested by employers or employees.

OSHA: This agency is a part of the U.S. Department of Labor. It is responsible for generating workplace safety regulations, as well as for putting them into effect and disciplining employers who do not comply with them.

Although NIOSH and OSHA were both created by the Occupational Safety and Health Act of 1970, they are two distinct agencies with separate responsibilities. NIOSH is a research agency, while OSHA is responsible for creating and enforcing workplace safety and health regulations. NIOSH and OSHA often work together toward the common goal of protecting worker safety and health. Either of these agencies can be contacted if you have questions or concerns about hazards in your workplace, via the Internet (www.cdc.gov/niosh/homepage.html) or by consulting the government "blue" pages in your local telephone directory (see Resources).

Protect Yourself at Work. As an employee, you have a right to work in a safe environment. Occupational cancers are highly preventable when the risks are known and an effective regulatory system is in place. It's important for you to do what you can to help protect yourself. Part of your job is knowing what potentially dangerous substances you might come into contact with. Familiarize yourself with the Material Safety Data Sheets (MSDS) on file where you work. You are allowed access to them under an OSHA-enforced law. These sheets describe all of the chemicals you use in detail, including toxicity and safe handling information.

But while government agencies like OSHA attempt to protect employee work environments by creating and enforcing regulations, as a worker you have a responsibility to monitor your own work environment and report safety hazards. What's more, some employers may not update their data about chemicals, processes, and other cancerous substances on a regular basis. And, unfortunately, many substances have simply not been tested thoroughly.

The best advice: don't assume something is safe just because you are allowed to use it. Find out more information if you need to, and take advantage of all the safety measures available to you. These may include the following.

- Wear protective clothing, gloves, boots, and headgear.

- Make sure your work area has proper ventilation. If necessary, wear a properly fitted mask or respirator.

- Allow only properly protected employees in your work area.

- Focus on the task at hand to avoid spills or accidents. Advise your employer of hazardous or unsafe conditions and request that the situation be remedied as soon as possible.

- If you smoke, try to quit as soon as possible (see Chapter 5). Tobacco use combined with occupational exposures can greatly elevate your risk of cancer.

If you report a hazardous situation to your supervisor or union representative, corrective action must be taken within a reasonable amount of time. If this does not occur, you have the legal right to anonymously request an evaluation from either OSHA or NIOSH. For situations of immediate work-related danger, you can refuse to perform a task provided that your employer is advised of the hazard. In such a case, you should be willing to accept an alternate assignment.

Putting It All Together

Should we live in a bubble? Certainly not. Should we wring our hands and worry about hidden dangers and cancer-causing materials we don't even know about yet? Of course not.

Sometimes it is the perception of risk rather than the actual risk itself that seems to drive our fears or concerns. For example, members of the League of Women Voters and a group of college students were asked to prioritize their perceptions of the risk of death for thirty activities and technologies.

Both groups placed nuclear power first, ahead of smoking, ingestion of alcoholic beverages, and riding in motor vehicles. They perceived nuclear accidents and Chernobyl-type leaks as events to be concerned about. Yet professional risk experts ranked the real risks. At the top were smoking and motor vehicle accidents. Nuclear power fell way down the list at twentieth—in the same range as ingestion of food coloring and the use of home appliances.

Certainly Myrna Block didn't think a thing about laundering her husband's work clothes when he came home from his shift at the fiberglass plant. Since the 1960s, public health officials and the medical community have proven the dangers of asbestos and other worksite health hazards. Government regulations are now in place. Workers wear protective gear, and many plants require workers to shower and change clothes before leaving the facility. Even the very way hazardous, cancer-causing materials are handled has changed dramatically to save lives and reduce risks.

Unfortunately there are many things about cancer and what causes it that we are not yet able to prove. But we can, through population-based studies and laboratory experiments, get a reasonable idea of what's going on. For example, there's no question that smoking has killed many more people than industrial chemicals or radiation. But sometimes it's easier to believe that someone or something else is responsible. Sometimes we tend to be more concerned about things we can't control. But when it comes to your health, there's a lot you can control.

Not the Last Word

By far the majority of cancers seem to be caused by complex interactions of genetics and environmental factors. Although we still don't understand what causes a cell to go haywire and develop into cancer, we do know that lifestyle choices such as diet, exercise, and the use of alcohol or tobacco products account for, or at least contribute to, a very large percentage of cancer cases. Environmental factors—some we can closely control and others we can't—do play a role, directly or indirectly, in some of these cases. Continued research in this area, as well as efforts to protect people from unintended exposures, must continue.

CHAPTER 9

Your Action Plan:

Putting It All in Perspective

We can try to avoid making choices by doing nothing,
but even that is a decision.
—GARY COLLINS

If you have a sore throat, you see your doctor. A little backache means another trip to the medical clinic. When Johnny falls off his bike and bumps his head, you're off to the emergency room. But if you're feeling just fine, there's no reason to see the doctor, right?

Wrong. Doing nothing may not be the right choice. Doing something means forming a partnership with your doctor and scheduling regular screening examinations when you're well, just to make sure all systems are "go." But there are more compelling—and lifesaving—reasons to have regular screening exams for breast cancer, cervical cancer, and colorectal cancer. One of the best things you can do to protect your health is to follow recommended cancer screening guidelines. This simple step can improve your chances of survival by finding cancer early when it is highly curable. And that's the good news about cancer when it is detected early.

The Importance of Early Detection and Screening

Individuals should be informed about cancer screening. They need to know what leading organizations recommend, and they should talk with their doctors about establishing a plan so that they are appropriately screened for cancer at the right intervals.

—ROBERT A. SMITH, PH.D.,
Director of Cancer Screening
for the American Cancer Society

Check It Out!

The American Cancer Society (ACS) recommends that you schedule a cancer-related checkup with the doctor or other health care provider you have chosen as your partner in health care (see Chapter 1).

- If you are twenty to thirty-nine years old, have a cancer-related checkup every three years.

- If you are forty years and older, have a cancer-related checkup every year.

The checkup should include health counseling about tobacco use, sun exposure, diet and nutrition, risk factors, sexual practices, and environmental and occupational exposures—all the areas discussed in this book. Depending on your age and health, it might include examinations for cancers of the thyroid, testicles, ovaries, lymph nodes, and oral cavity, as well as for some nonmalignant diseases.

Screening is the search for disease in people who do not have symptoms of the disease, or who do not recognize that they have the disease. Although it usually does not prevent cancer from occurring, early detection through screening, followed by effective treatment, can extend your life, reduce the amount of treatment needed, and improve the quality of your life if you are diagnosed with cancer. In some cases, screening can actually prevent cancer by finding precancerous changes such as colon polyps or precancerous changes on the cervix. Treating these precancerous changes can prevent some cancers from ever occurring.

Regular screening can detect cancers of the breast, cervix, prostate, and colon/rectum at earlier stages, when treatment is more likely to result in a cure. If all Americans participated in regular cancer screenings, the ACS estimates that the relative five-year survival rates (number of people

Type of Cancer	Screening/Test Available
Breast	Mammography Clinical breast exam (CBE)
Cervical	Pap test Pelvic exam
Prostate	Digital rectal exam Prostate-specific antigen (PSA) blood test
Colorectal	Fecal occult blood test (FOBT) Flexible sigmoidoscopy Colonoscopy Double contrast barium enema (DCBE)
Skin	Self-examination, clinical examination*
Oral (mouth and tongue)	Clinical examination*
Testicular	Clinical examination*

*As part of a routine cancer-related checkup

The American Cancer Society Guidelines for the Early Detection of Breast Cancer

The following guidelines are for women who have no symptoms. They are designed to find breast cancer at the earliest stages when there is the best opportunity to treat it successfully.

- Women aged forty years and older should have a clinical breast examination (CBE) by a health professional and a screening mammogram every year. The CBE should be conducted close to, and preferably before, the scheduled mammogram so that if a mass is detected, the radiologist can look for it on the x-ray.

- Between the ages of twenty and thirty-nine years old, women should have a CBE by a health professional every three years.

- All women aged twenty years and older should perform breast self-examinations (BSE) every month. By doing the exam regularly, you get to know how your breasts normally feel and you can more readily detect any signs or symptoms.

If you notice a change in a breast, such as development of a lump or swelling, skin irritation or dimpling, nipple pain or retraction (turning inward), redness or scaliness of the nipple or breast skin, or a discharge

still alive *at least* five years after diagnosis) for these screening-accessible cancer sites would increase from about 80 percent to more than 95 percent.

These types of cancer account for about half of all new cancer cases. Some of the tests used to screen for their presence are relatively simple, and some you can do yourself.

other than breast milk, you should see your doctor as soon as possible for evaluation. However, remember that most of the time, these breast changes are not cancer.

Although there are some features of a mass that suggest whether it is likely to be benign or cancerous, a woman examining her own breasts should discuss any new lump with her doctor. The doctor can determine when additional tests are appropriate to rule out a cancer and when follow-up exams are the best strategy. If there is any suspicion of cancer, a biopsy will be done.

The use of mammography, clinical breast examination, and breast self-examination, according to the recommendations outlined above, offer you the best way to effective treatment and long survival if you have breast cancer. This combined approach is better than any one method alone. Without question, breast physical examination without mammography can miss the opportunity to detect many breast cancers that are too small for a woman or her doctor to feel but can be seen on mammograms.

On the other hand, mammography can miss some cancers that can be felt by a woman or her doctor. Monthly BSEs can find some cancers in women younger than forty years old that develop between their CBEs every three years. It can even find some cancers in women older than forty years old that become apparent between their annual mammograms and clinical exams.

The following information and guidelines are for the early detection of cancer in people without symptoms. Some people are at higher risk for certain cancers and may need to have tests more frequently. Talk with your doctor to find out how these guidelines relate to you.

Breast Cancer

Among American women, breast cancer is the most common form of cancer (excluding skin cancer), accounting for more than 30 percent of all cancers. Only lung cancer causes more cancer deaths among women. And contrary to popular belief, age is the single most important risk factor for breast cancer. Popular magazines often portray the disease as one that normally strikes women in their 30s and 40s, but the truth is that three-fourths of all breast cancers occur in women over the age of fifty years old. And a woman seventy years old is almost twice as likely to develop breast cancer in the next year as a woman aged fifty.

Women whose close female relatives—their mothers or sisters—have had the disease are at increased risk for breast cancer. This is especially true if the relative was diagnosed before menopause. But of the women who develop breast cancer, *more than 80 percent have no family history*. The take-home message here is that every woman is at risk for breast cancer, and her risk increases as she gets older.

Because we don't know yet how to prevent breast cancer entirely, the best protection is to detect it as early as possible and treat it promptly. Researchers are currently investigating the possible roles of heredity, environment, and lifestyle factors such as physical activity and obesity.

What Is Each Test?

Mammography. A mammogram is a low-dose x-ray picture of the breast taken with a special machine that uses only a small amount of radiation. Mammograms can find changes too small to be felt by even highly trained examiners. It is the single most effective method of early breast cancer detection because it can reveal cancer in its earliest stages, before symptoms develop.

Approximately 10 percent of women will require additional mammography. Only one or two mammograms out of every 1,000 lead to a diagnosis of cancer. Don't be alarmed if this happens to you. Only 8 to 10 percent of those women will need a biopsy, and 80 percent of those women will not have cancer.

Mammography is beneficial, and it is beneficial because it finds breast cancer early, when a woman has more treatment options.
—ROBERT A. SMITH, PH.D., Director of Cancer Screening
for the American Cancer Society

When you have a mammogram, you will be asked to undress above the waist, so wear pants or a skirt on the day of the procedure. A wrap will be provided by the facility for you to wear. A technologist will be present to

Does a Mammogram Hurt?

If mammography is done properly and at the appropriate time in the menstrual cycle, most women generally feel minimal discomfort or pain when their breast is pressed onto the x-ray plate. Of course, individuals may vary in their perception of the discomfort involved. A small percentage of women who have especially dense breasts do find that mammography can be painful. If you experience pain during the mammogram, tell the technologist. Because breasts are likely to be most tender just before or during menstruation, appointments should be scheduled for two weeks after menstruation.

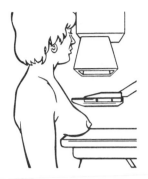

position your breasts for the mammogram. Most technologists are women. You and the technologist are the only ones present during the mammogram.

The specially trained technologist positions the breast between two plastic plates. Slight pressure will be applied for a few seconds to flatten and spread the breast tissue. Although this may be temporarily uncomfortable, it is necessary to get a good, clear picture. Two pictures are usually taken of each breast—a side view and a view from above. The entire procedure can usually be completed in less than fifteen minutes. A doctor who specializes in looking at x-rays, called a radiologist, will read the mammogram to see if there are any suspicious areas. All mammography facilities are now required to send the results within thirty days. You will be contacted within five working days if there is a problem with the mammogram.

If your doctor hasn't mentioned the need for a mammogram, ask about it yourself. Having a mammogram can provide peace of mind, because most women who are screened will not have breast cancer, and regular mammograms offer the best protection against having a breast cancer diagnosed late.

If you ask where you can get a mammogram, your doctor will probably be very helpful. You can also find out where mammograms are performed by contacting the ACS at 800-ACS-2345. The Food and Drug Administration maintains a list of certified mammography facilities as well (http://www.fda.gov/cdrh/mammography/certified.html). Mammogram costs, or a percentage of them, are covered by Medicare, Medicaid, and most private health plans. Low cost mammograms are available in most communities.

Clinical Breast Examination. A CBE is an examination of your breasts by a health professional, such as a doctor, nurse practitioner, nurse, or physician

Important Reasons to Get a Mammogram

- Breast cancer is the most common cancer (excluding skin cancer) among women.

- Finding breast cancer early can save your life.

- Early detection often means less extensive surgery.

- Having a mammogram once a year helps give you peace of mind.

- Getting a mammogram is easier than you think.

assistant. For this examination, you undress from the waist up. The health professional will first observe your breasts for changes in size or shape. Then, using the pads of the fingers, the examiner will gently palpate, or feel, your breasts. Special attention will be given to the shape and texture of the breasts, location of any lumps, and whether such lumps are attached to the skin or to deeper tissues. The area under both arms will also be examined.

During the CBE is a good time for the health professional to teach you how to examine your breasts. Ask your doctor or nurse to teach you and to watch your technique.

Breast Self-Examination. There are many good reasons for doing a BSE each month. One reason is that it is easy to do, and the more you do it, the better you will get at it. When you get to know how your breasts normally feel, you will quickly be able to recognize any change, and early detection is the key to successful treatment.

The best time for BSE is about a week after your period ends, when your breasts are not tender or swollen. If you are not having regular periods, do a BSE on the same day every month. Mark your calendar. Women who are pregnant, breast-feeding, or have breast implants also need to do regular breast self-examinations.

How to Do Your BSE

Lie down with a pillow under your right shoulder and place your right arm behind your head.

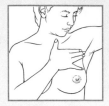

Use the finger pads of the three middle fingers on your left hand to feel for lumps in the right breast. (Your finger pads are the top third of each finger.)

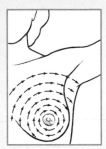

Press firmly enough to know how your breast feels. A firm ridge in the lower curve of each breast is normal. If you're not sure how hard to press, talk with your doctor or nurse. Or try to copy the way your health professional uses his or her finger pads during a breast exam. Learn what your breast feels like most of the time.

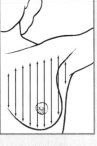

Move around the breast in a circular, up and down line, or wedge pattern. Be sure to do it the same way every time, check the entire breast area, and remember how your breast feels from month to month.

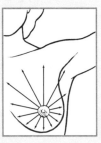

Repeat the exam on your left breast, using the finger pads of the right hand. (Put the pillow under your left shoulder.)

Repeat the examination of both breasts while standing, with one arm behind your head. The upright position makes it easier to check the upper and outer part of the breasts (toward your armpit). This is where about half of breast cancers are found. You may want to do the standing part of the BSE while you are in the shower. Some breast changes can be felt more easily when your skin is wet and soapy.

For added safety, you can check the appearance of your breasts for any dimpling of the skin, changes in the nipple, redness, or swelling while standing in front of a mirror right after your BSE each month. If you find any changes, see your doctor right away.

Breast cancer is not just a woman's disease. Although it is rare, men can, and do, develop breast cancer. Men should report any lumps in their breast and chest.

Most breast lumps are found by women themselves, but in fact, most lumps in the breast are not cancer. Be safe, be sure.

Cervical Cancer

Cervical cancer was once one of the most common causes of cancer death for American women. Today, it's not, thanks to a highly successful and easy-to-perform screening test. Amazingly, since the 1950s, the number of cervical cancer deaths in the United States declined by about 75 percent. The main reason for this change is the increased use of the Pap test—a screening procedure that permits diagnosis of precancerous and early cancerous cells before they have a chance to invade other areas. The death rate continues to decline at a rate of about 2 percent a year. When detected early, cervical cancer is one of the easiest cancers to treat successfully.

The most important risk factor for cervical cancer is infection by the human papillomavirus, or HPV (see Chapter 6). This virus can be passed from one person to another by sexual contact. More than 95 percent of cervical cancers are linked to HPV infection.

About the Uterus and Its Cervix

The cervix is the lower part of the uterus (womb) that connects the body of the uterus to the vagina (birth canal). The part of the cervix closest to the body of the uterus is called the endocervix. The part next to the vagina is the ectocervix.

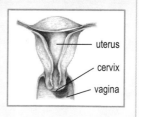

The American Cancer Society Guidelines for the Early Detection of Cervical Cancer

Getting screened for cervical cancer is currently the best thing a woman can do to detect any cervical changes that might have the potential to progress to cancer. Most women who develop the disease have not been getting Pap tests, either at all or on a regular basis.

—DEBBIE SASLOW, PH.D., Director of Breast and Cervical Cancer

for the American Cancer Society

The ACS recommends that all women begin yearly Pap tests (also called Pap smears) and a pelvic examination at age eighteen or when they become sexually active, whichever occurs earlier. If a woman has had three negative annual Pap tests in a row, this test may be done less often at the judgment of her doctor.

The vast majority of cervical cancers can be prevented. Because the most common form of cervical cancer starts with preventable and easily detectable precancerous changes, there are two ways to prevent this disease.

Reduce your risk—recommendations include delaying onset of sexual intercourse if you are young and being monogamous. Not smoking is another way to reduce the risk of cervical cancer and precancerous lesions.

Have a Pap test to detect precancerous changes—treatment of these disorders can stop cervical cancer before it is fully developed. Most invasive cervical cancers are found in women who have not had regular Pap tests.

What Is a Pap Test?

A Pap test is a simple procedure that can be performed by a doctor or trained health care professional as part of a pelvic exam. The Pap test is a way to check cells from the cervix (the lower part of the uterus or womb) and the vagina. This test can find precancerous changes or cancer

How to Get Ready For a Pap Test

Don't use tampons, douche, birth-control foams, jellies, or other vaginal creams for two to three days before the test. Do not have sexual intercourse for two days before the test. Try not to schedule your Pap test during your menstrual period. The best time is at least five days after your period stops.

How the Test Is Done

The Pap test can be done in a doctor's office, clinic, or hospital. Doctors and other specially trained health care professionals such as physician assistants, nurse midwives, and nurse practitioners may perform pelvic exams and take Pap test samples. The ACS does not recommend replacing the conventional methods of performing this test with the "at home" (self-administered) Pap test.

While you lie on an exam table, the health care professional inserts a speculum, a metal or plastic instrument that keeps the vagina open so that the cervix can be seen clearly. Next, a sample of cells and mucus is lightly scraped from the ectocervix (outer part of the cervix) using a small wooden or plastic spatula. A small brush or a cotton-tipped swab is then used to take a sample from the endocervix (inner part of the cervix). These samples can be smeared on glass slides right away. Or the spatula and brush can be rinsed in a preservative solution and sent to the lab, where cells are then attached to the glass slides using specialized equipment. In either case, specially trained laboratory technologists and doctors examine the samples under a microscope.

Taking the Pap test sample takes a few seconds. The entire procedure, including the speculum exam and pelvic exam, takes a few minutes. You typically feel some discomfort, cramping, or pressure, but the test should not be painful.

of the cervix or vagina. A Pap test will only rarely detect cancer of the ovaries or cancer of the upper part of the uterus (endometrial cancer). It can also find some infections of the cervix and vagina.

Some women believe they do not have to be examined by a health care professional once they have stopped having children, or have reached menopause. This is not correct. They should continue to follow the ACS guidelines. There is some disagreement among doctors as to whether women who have had a hysterectomy for a benign condition (such as uterine fibroids) need to continue having a Pap test. If a hysterectomy was done for cancer, more frequent Pap tests may be recommended initially. Another debate is whether women should continue Pap tests as long as they are in good health, or should stop at a certain age. The current ACS view is that all women should continue having Pap tests as long as they are in good health. However, if they have had three or more consecutive negative results, their doctor may recommend having the test less often, and the patient's age and history of hysterectomy may be a factor in their doctor's assessment. These issues, as well as others (such as the role of HPV testing) are currently being evaluated by an ACS advisory committee, which will update the cervical cancer screening recommendations in January of 2003. Check the ACS website (www.cancer.org) for updates.

While the Pap test has been more successful than any other screening test in preventing a cancer, it is not perfect. Because some abnormalities may be missed (even when samples are examined in the best laboratories), it is a good idea to have this test at least once a year, unless recommended otherwise (see page 320).

Endometrial (Body of the Uterus) Cancer

Endometrial cancer starts in the lining of the body (upper part) of the uterus. Although endometrial cancer and cervical cancer both start in the uterus, they are very different diseases, and the ACS has different recommendations for their early detection. Unlike cervical cancer, endometrial cancer is not related to HPV infection.

The American Cancer Society Guidelines for the Early Detection of Endometrial (Body of the Uterus) Cancer

The ACS opinion is that testing for endometrial cancer is not necessary for women who have no identified risk factors. Since early diagnosis usually results from symptoms such as abnormal uterine bleeding or discharge, the ACS recommends that doctors discuss the risks and symptoms of endometrial cancer with their patients at menopause, and should strongly encourage these women to report any unexpected bleeding or spotting.

It is especially important for doctors to discuss this information with women who are at increased risk because of the following:

- a history of unopposed (without progestin) estrogen therapy
- late menopause
- tamoxifen for treating breast cancer or reducing the risk of developing breast cancer
- never having had children
- difficulty becoming pregnant
- not ovulating due to hormone problems
- obesity, diabetes, or high blood pressure

Doctors should also tell women at increased risk about the potential benefits, risks, and limitations of testing for early endometrial cancer detection.

Hereditary nonpolyposis colon cancer, often abbreviated as HNPCC, is an inherited condition that greatly increases the risk of developing colon cancer and endometrial cancer. The ACS recommends annual endometrial cancer screening, starting at age thirty-five, for women known to have HNPCC, and those whose family history suggests they might have it. This recommendation is based on their high risk for developing endometrial cancer, even though there have not been enough studies to prove this will help them live longer. These women should also talk with their doctors about the benefits, risks, and limitations of testing.

Although endometrial cancer cells can sometimes be found by a Pap test, this test is not as reliable for endometrial cancer as it is for cervical cancer (see pages 320–322). Two screening tests for endometrial cancer, endometrial biopsy and vaginal ultrasound, are the subject of ongoing studies. (These tests are also used for women with symptoms.)

For an endometrial biopsy, a small sample of endometrial tissue is obtained by applying suction to a very thin flexible tube inserted into the uterus through the cervix. A transvaginal ultrasound or sonogram uses sound waves to create images of the uterus. A probe inserted into the vagina releases sound waves that echo off tissue of the pelvic organs. A computer translates these echo patterns into an image of the uterus.

Prostate Cancer

Prostate cancer is the second leading cause of cancer death in men in the United States, exceeded only by lung cancer. One man in six will be diagnosed with prostate cancer during his lifetime, but fortunately only one man in thirty will die of this disease. African-American men are more likely to have prostate cancer than white or Asian men are, as are those men with a family history of this cancer, especially those whose relatives were diagnosed at a young age. The risk of getting the disease increases with age and most men who get prostate cancer are sixty-five years or older.

About the Prostate

The prostate, found only in men, is a walnut-sized gland located in front of the rectum, at the outlet of the bladder. It contains gland cells that produce some of the seminal fluid, which protects and nourishes sperm cells in semen. Just behind the prostate gland are the seminal vesicles that produce most of the fluid

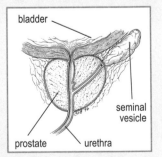

bladder

seminal vesicle

prostate   urethra

for semen. The prostate surrounds the first part of the urethra, the tube that carries urine and semen through the penis (see also page 338).

The American Cancer Society Guidelines for the Early Detection of Prostate Cancer

Whether or not all men should undergo testing for prostate cancer remains controversial for several reasons. Prostate cancer tends to occur in older men, and it generally grows very slowly. Even if it is left alone, many years can pass between when prostate cancer is diagnosed and when it actually starts causing problems. Men in their 70s and 80s with prostate cancer may actually be more likely to die of another cause. As the saying goes in the medical community, more men die *with* prostate cancer than *of* it.

Added to this is the fact that forms of treatment for prostate cancer, such as surgery and radiation therapy, can sometimes have serious side effects, such as impotence (inability to have an erection) or incontinence (inability to control urination).

Therefore, the decision about whether or not to undergo screening is often a difficult one. You should be sure you are aware of all of the facts before deciding one way or the other (see pages 342–343).

The ACS believes that health care professionals should *offer* you the prostate-specific antigen (PSA) blood test and digital rectal examination (DRE) yearly, once you become fifty years old. Factors to consider include your overall health and life expectancy. If you are African American or have a father or brother who developed prostate cancer at a young age, you are at higher risk and should begin testing at age forty-five. Your doctor should openly discuss with you the benefits and risks of testing at yearly checkups, so you can make an informed decision about whether or not to undergo testing. You should learn as much as you can about prostate cancer and the pros and cons of early detection and treatment of prostate cancer, so you can actively participate in the decision to have the tests.

The ACS believes that doctors should discuss testing for prostate cancer with men, and any policy that discourages or does not offer testing is not appropriate.

When prostate cancer is in its earliest stages, it usually causes no pain or other symptoms. As the cancer grows, it may cause slowing in the urinary stream, a need to urinate more often, or blood in the urine. These types of symptoms occur because the prostate gland is located just beneath the bladder. Although these symptoms also can be caused by noncancerous conditions, they need to be checked by a doctor.

What Is Each Test?

Be informed. Knowledge is the font of all human inspiration.
—MIKE WAYDA, cancer survivor

Prostate-Specific Antigen Blood Test. PSA is a substance made by the normal prostate gland. Although PSA is mostly found in semen, a small amount also makes its way into the blood. In the PSA screening test for prostate cancer, a small amount of blood is tested to see how much PSA it contains. If PSA levels rise above normal, there may be cancer in the prostate.

The PSA level can be affected by many factors that are not related to cancer. For example, it increases with noncancerous enlargement of the prostate (called benign prostatic hyperplasia, or BPH), something that many men have as they grow older, and with prostatitis, an inflammation of the prostate gland. The PSA will also normally go up slowly with age, even if there is no prostate abnormality. Ejaculation can cause a temporary increase in blood PSA levels, so some doctors will suggest that men abstain from ejaculation for two days before testing.

Most men have levels under 4 nanograms per milliliter (ng/mL) of blood. When prostate cancer develops, the PSA level usually goes above 4. If your level is above 4, but less than 10, you have about a twenty-five percent chance of having prostate cancer. If it goes above 10, your chance of having prostate cancer is over fifty percent and increases further as your PSA level increases. A biopsy (removal and microscopic examination of tissue) is needed to confirm if cancer is present.

Digital Rectal Exam. During this examination, a doctor inserts a gloved, lubricated finger into the rectum to feel for any irregular or abnormally firm area that might be a cancer. The prostate gland is located just in front of the rectum, and most cancers begin in the back part of the gland that can be reached by a rectal exam. While it is uncomfortable, the exam causes no pain and only takes a short time.

Although DRE is less effective than the PSA blood test in finding prostate cancer, it can sometimes find cancers in men with normal PSA levels. For this reason, the ACS guidelines recommend use of both the DRE and PSA blood test in men who decide to be screened for prostate cancer. However, men who would prefer not to have the DRE can still have the PSA test.

If Your Doctor Does the Exam Differently

The instructions your doctor gives you on how to prepare for a test and the way he or she performs a particular examination may differ slightly from what you read here and elsewhere.

To reassure yourself, discuss the examination with your doctor. You might bring a copy of the information you have read when you have your checkup and share it with him or her. Don't be hesitant to ask questions about how to prepare for a test. If you are not satisfied with the instructions you get or have questions that are not answered by the office or clinic staff, ask to speak to the doctor.

If you think that a part of the examination has not been done or has been performed differently from what you expected, ask why. Usually there is a logical explanation that will set your mind at ease. If you are still not satisfied, consider having the test or examination repeated elsewhere.

Colon and Rectal Cancer

Knowing and not doing are equal to not knowing at all.

—UNKNOWN

Colon and rectal cancers (also called colorectal cancer) develop in the digestive system, which is also called the gastrointestinal, or GI, system. Colon cancer and rectal cancer have many features in common; sometimes they are referred to together as colorectal cancer.

Among men and women, colorectal cancer is the third most common cancer diagnosed in Americans, excluding skin cancers. The death rate from colorectal cancer has been going down for the past twenty years. This could probably be because there are fewer cases (some cases were likely prevented by removal of precancerous polyps), more of the cases are found at earlier, more treatable stages, and the treatments themselves have improved.

Researchers have identified several factors that increase a person's risk of developing colorectal cancer.

- Aging—risk increases with increasing age.

- A diet that consists mainly of foods from animal sources

- Intestinal polyps

- Chronic inflammatory bowel disease (ulcerative colitis or Crohn's disease)

- A personal history of colorectal cancer

- A family history of colorectal cancer or certain inherited syndromes, such as familial adenomatous polyposis (FAP) or hereditary nonpolyposis colon cancer (HNPCC)

- Obesity

- Lack of physical activity

- Smoking

Even though the exact cause of most colorectal cancer is not known, it is possible to prevent many colon cancers. Following screening guidelines can lower the number of cases of the disease by detecting and removing polyps that could become cancerous. Also, screening can lower the death rate from colorectal cancer by finding disease early when it is most treatable. People can also lower their risk of developing colorectal cancer by managing the lifestyle risk factors that are under their control, such as diet and physical activity. Because some colorectal cancers can't be prevented, finding them early is the best way to improve the chance of successful treatment and reduce the number of deaths caused by this disease.

About the Colon and Rectum

The five-foot-long large intestine has five sections. It begins at the ascending colon, where waste passes from the small intestine into the colon. This ascends upward on the right side of the abdomen and connects to the transverse colon, which goes across the body to the left side and connects to the descending colon, which continues downward on the left side. This becomes the sigmoid colon, which joins the final six inches or so of the large intestine called the rectum. The anus is the opening where waste matter passes from the rectum out of the body.

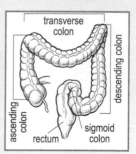

The American Cancer Society Guidelines for the Early Detection of Colorectal Cancer

The goal of screening for colorectal cancer is to find polyps and cancers before they cause symptoms, and to detect colorectal cancer early. These tests offer the best opportunity to detect colorectal cancer at an early stage when successful treatment is likely and to prevent some colorectal cancers by detection and removal of polyps. Several tests can be used to screen for colorectal cancer, so someone with an average risk can choose from various options. Ask your doctor which tests are available where you live and which option is best for you.

Beginning at age fifty, men and women at average risk should follow one of the five screening options below.

- Fecal occult blood test (FOBT) every year*

- Flexible sigmoidoscopy every five years+

- Fecal occult blood test every year plus flexible sigmoidoscopy every five years* +

  (Of the three options above, yearly FOBT and flexible sigmoidoscopy every five years is preferable.)

- Double-contrast barium enema every five years

- Colonoscopy every ten years+

* For FOBT, the take-home multiple sample method should be used.
+ A digital rectal examination is not recommended as a stand-alone exam, but it should be done before insertion of a sigmoidoscope or colonoscope.

All positive test results should be followed up with colonoscopy.

People with certain risk factors should begin screening earlier or have screening more often. Based on your individual situation and any risk factors you may have, such as a family history of colorectal cancer, your doctor can suggest which screening option is best for you as well as any modifications in the schedule based on your individual risk. Each test has different levels of accuracy, risks, and costs, so discuss these with your doctor and make an informed decision.

What Is Each Test?

One or more of the following tests may be used to screen for colorectal cancer based on your risk of colorectal cancer. These tests as well as others are also used when people have symptoms of colorectal cancer and other digestive diseases.

Fecal Occult Blood Test. The FOBT is used to find occult, or hidden, blood in feces. Blood vessels at the surface of colorectal polyps or adenomas or cancers are often fragile and easily damaged by the passage of feces. The damaged vessels usually release only a small amount of blood into the feces. You cannot see the blood. Only rarely is there enough bleeding to change the color of the stool (usually to a darker brown or black). The FOBT detects blood even if it can't be seen.

If this test result is positive (blood is detected), then additional testing is needed to see if there is a tumor, polyp, or other cause of bleeding such as hemorrhoids or diverticulitis. Even foods or drugs can affect the test, so you should follow these instructions carefully.

- Do not take nonsteroidal anti-inflammatory drugs (NSAIDs) such as ibuprofen (Advil), naproxen (Aleve), or aspirin (more than one adult aspirin per day) for seven days before the test (they can cause bleeding).

- Avoid taking vitamin C in excess of 250 milligrams from either supplements or citrus fruits and juices for three days before testing (it affects the chemicals in the test).

- Do not eat red meat for three days before testing (substances in the meat may cause the test to be positive).

Some other foods such as turnips and horseradish, as well as other medications, including colchicine, steroids, blood thinners, and iron supplements can also interfere with FOBT results. Ask your doctor if there are other foods or medications that you should avoid before testing.

People having this test will receive a test kit with instructions that explain how to take a stool or feces sample at home (usually three specimens). The kit is then returned to the doctor's office or a medical laboratory for testing. A one-time test of a stool sample that your doctor took from a digital rectal exam is not an adequate substitute, and is not recommended.

Flexible Sigmoidoscopy. A sigmoidoscope is a slender, flexible, hollow, lighted tube about the thickness of a finger. It is inserted through your rectum into the lower part of your colon. Not only can your doctor look through this to find any abnormality, the sigmoidoscope can be connected to a video camera and video display monitor for a better view. This test may be somewhat uncomfortable, but it should not be painful. Because the scope is only sixty centimeters long (around two feet), the doctor is able to see less than half of your colon. However, if the doctor sees polyps in that part of the colon, he or she may recommend a colonoscopy. Before the sigmoidoscopy, you will need an enema to clean out your lower colon.

Double-Contrast Barium Enema. This procedure is also called a barium enema with air contrast or a DCBE. Barium sulfate, a chalky substance, is used to partially fill and open up the colon. The barium sulfate is given through a small tube placed in your anus. When the colon is about half-full of barium, you will be turned on the x-ray table so the barium spreads throughout the colon. Then air will be pumped into your colon through the same tube to make it expand. This produces the best pictures of the lining of your colon. You will need to cleanse your bowel the night before with laxatives and may need to have an enema the morning of the exam.

Colonoscopy. A colonoscope is a longer and more complex version of a sigmoidoscope. It is inserted through the rectum up into the colon and allows your doctor to see the lining of your entire colon. The colonoscope is also connected to a video camera and video display monitor so the doctor can closely examine the inside of the colon.

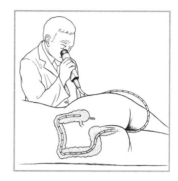

If you have a colonoscopy, you will need a liquid diet, laxatives, and an enema to clean your colon so there will not be any stool to block the view. Colonoscopy usually does not cause pain because you will be given medication through a vein to make you feel relaxed and sleepy during the procedure. Colonoscopy may be done in a hospital outpatient department, in a clinic, or in a doctor's office, and usually takes fifteen to thirty minutes, although it may take longer if polyp removal is necessary.

If a small polyp is found, your doctor may remove it. Polyps, even those that are not cancerous, could eventually become cancerous. For this reason, they are usually removed. This is done by passing a wire loop through the colonoscope to cut the polyp from the wall of the colon with an electrical current. The polyp can then be sent to a lab to be checked under a microscope to see if it has any areas that have changed into cancer.

If your doctor sees a large polyp or tumor or anything else abnormal, a biopsy will be done. To do this, a small piece of tissue is taken out through the colonoscope. Examination of the tissue can help determine if it is a cancer, a benign (noncancerous) growth, or the result of inflammation.

Digital Rectal Examination. As described earlier, the doctor inserts a gloved finger into the rectum to feel for anything not normal. This simple test, which is not painful, can detect masses in the anal canal or lower rectum. It is not a very sensitive test for detecting colorectal cancer due to its limited reach. While a DRE is often included as part of a routine physical examination, it is not recommended as a stand-alone test for finding colorectal cancer. DRE should be done before the doctor inserts the sigmoidoscope or colonoscope.

Skin Cancer

Cancer of the skin is the most common of all cancers. In fact, it's about as common as all other forms of cancer *combined*. Both melanoma and other forms of skin cancer are serious diseases. Although melanoma is much less common than basal cell and squamous cell cancers, all three types of skin cancer are almost always curable in their early stages. But melanoma is much more likely than basal or squamous cell cancer to spread (metastasize) to other parts of the body. For more information regarding cancer of the skin and how to prevent skin cancers, refer to Chapter 4.

Changes in the skin can be found early. You can play an important role in finding skin cancer early, when it is curable.

The American Cancer Society Recommendations for the Early Detection of Skin Cancer

A routine cancer-related checkup should include a skin examination by a health care professional qualified to diagnose skin cancer (see page 310, "Check It Out!").

It's also important to check your own skin, preferably once a month. You should know the patterns of moles, blemishes, freckles, and other marks on your skin, so that you'll notice any changes in existing ones, or any new ones that develop. Chapter 4 has a description of how to perform a skin self-examination.

Oral Cancer

Doctors can't say for sure what causes each case of cancer in the mouth, tongue, and throat. But we do know what many of the risk factors are and how some of these risk factors cause cells to become cancerous. We know that tobacco and alcohol can damage cells in the lining of the mouth and throat, and that cells in this layer must grow more rapidly to repair this damage. This, in turn, leads to an increased risk of cancer.

Most oral cancers can be prevented by avoiding risk factors, such as tobacco and alcohol. The best way to avoid these cancers is never to start smoking or using smokeless tobacco. For more information on quitting tobacco products, see Chapter 5. Limit your intake of alcoholic beverages, if you drink at all. Quitting tobacco and alcohol significantly lowers your risk of developing these cancers, even after many years of abuse.

The American Cancer Society Recommendations for the Early Detection of Oral Cancer

The ACS recommends that a health care professional examine the mouth and throat as part of a routine checkup (see page 310, "Check It Out!"). In addition, regular dental checkups that include an examination of the entire mouth by a dentist are important in the early detection of mouth and throat cancers and precancerous conditions. Many doctors and dentists also recommend oral self-examination.

Many oral cancers can be found early. Some early cancers have symptoms that cause patients to seek medical or dental attention. Unfortunately, others may not cause symptoms until they reach an advanced stage or may cause symptoms that appear to be due to a disease other than cancer, such as a toothache.

Cancers of the Mouth and Throat: What to Look For

Many doctors and dentists recommend that you take an active role in the early detection of mouth and throat cancer by doing monthly self-examinations. This means looking in a mirror to check for any of these signs and symptoms.

- A sore in the mouth that does not heal (most common symptom)

- Pain in the mouth that doesn't go away (also very common)

- A persistent lump or thickening in the cheek

- A persistent white or red patch on the gums, tongue, tonsil, or lining of the mouth

- A sore throat or a feeling that something is caught in the throat that doesn't go away

- Difficulty chewing or swallowing

- Difficulty moving your jaw or tongue

- Numbness of your tongue or other area of your mouth

- Swelling of your jaw that causes dentures to fit poorly or become uncomfortable

- Loosening of your teeth or pain around your teeth or jaw

- Voice changes

- A lump or mass in your neck

- Weight loss

Many of these signs and symptoms may be caused by other cancers or by less serious, harmless problems. It is important to see a medical doctor or dentist if any of these conditions lasts more than two weeks. Remember, the sooner you receive a correct diagnosis, the sooner you can start treatment and the more effective your treatment will be.

Testicular Cancer

Although testicular cancer is rare (fewer than 8,000 cases per year are diagnosed in the United States), it is still the most common cancer found in men between the ages of fifteen and thirty-five. The exact cause of

---

 The American Cancer Society Recommendations for the Early Detection of Testicular Cancer

Doctors agree that examination of a man's testicles is an important part of a general physical examination. The ACS includes the examination in its recommendations for routine checkups (see page 310, "Check It Out!").

The issue of regular testicular self-examination is more controversial. The ACS believes it is important for men to be aware of testicular cancer and remind them that any testicular mass should be evaluated by a doctor without delay. (Some doctors feel that the most common reason for a delay in treatment is a delay in seeking medical attention after discovering a mass.) Other doctors feel that not noticing masses promptly is also an important factor in delaying treatment, and they recommend monthly testicular self-examination by all men after puberty.

The ACS does not feel that there is any medical evidence to suggest that, for men with average testicular cancer risk, monthly examination is any more effective than simple awareness and prompt medical evaluation. However, each man should choose whether or not to perform this examination, so instructions for testicular examination are included in this section. Men with certain risk factors (cryptorchidism, previous testicular tumor, family history) who have an increased risk of developing testicular cancer, should seriously consider monthly examinations, and the ACS suggests they discuss this issue with a doctor.

most cases is not known. The most important known risk factor for testicular cancer is a history of one or both testicle(s) not moving into the scrotum properly before school age, a condition known as cryptorchidism, or undescended testicle(s). Other known risk factors, such as being white and having a family history of the disease, are unavoidable because they are present at birth. But most men who develop testicular cancer have no known risk factors. For these reasons, it is not currently possible to prevent most cases of this disease.

Quite often, cases of testicular cancer can be found at an early stage. In some cases, early testicular cancers cause symptoms that lead men to seek medical attention. Unfortunately, however, some testicle cancers may not cause symptoms until they reach an advanced stage, and others may cause symptoms that appear to be due to a condition other than cancer. In about 90 percent of cases, men have a painless or an uncomfortable lump on a testicle, or they may notice testicular enlargement or swelling. Men with testicular cancer often report a sensation of heaviness or aching in the lower abdomen or scrotum.

About the Testicles

Each of the two testicles is somewhat smaller than a golf ball. Both are contained within a sac of skin called the scrotum, which hangs below either side of the penis. The testicles manufacture the male hormones, the most abundant of which is testosterone. They also produce sperm, the male reproductive cells. Sperm cells are carried from the testicle by the vas deferens to the seminal vesicles, where they are mixed with fluid produced by the prostate gland (see also page 324).

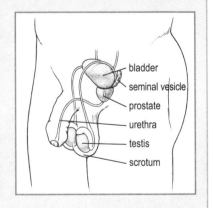

bladder
seminal vesicle
prostate
urethra
testis
scrotum

What Is a Testicular Self-Exam?

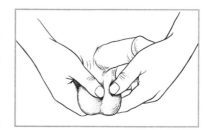

Testicular Self-Exam. If you plan to examine your testicles, the best time to do so is during or after a bath or shower, when the skin of the scrotum is relaxed. Stand in front of a mirror and hold the penis out of the way. Examine each testicle separately. Hold the testicle between the thumbs and fingers with both hands and roll it gently between the fingers. Look and feel for any hard lumps or nodules (smooth rounded masses) or any change in the size, shape, or consistency of the testes. Contact your doctor if you detect any troublesome signs. Be aware that the testicles contain blood vessels, supporting tissues, and tubes that conduct sperm and that some men may confuse these with a cancer. If you have any doubts, ask your doctor.

If you find that one of your testicles is much larger or firmer than the other, or you find a lump, whether painful or not, don't panic. The problem is usually not cancer, but you'll need to see your doctor to make sure. Ignoring any changes in your testicles or not seeing a doctor right away could make whatever problem you may have more difficult to treat successfully.

Luckily, even if it is testicular cancer, in most cases, it can be cured. Most men still have the ability for normal sexual activity, but fertility may be affected. Sperm banking may be recommended.

Ongoing Debates About Early Detection

In the introduction to this book, we mentioned how the ACS uses the results from numerous scientific studies of various types as the basis for conclusions on what causes cancer, how to prevent cancer, and how to find it early. But we didn't mention that there are some issues that remain unresolved or incompletely resolved, because there is not enough scientific information or because studies find contradictory results. Sometimes individual experts or health organizations have different interpretations of these studies, and reach different conclusions and recommendations.

On most screening issues, the differences among major medical organizations are relatively small. The ACS early detection recommendations described in this book are very similar to those of the National Cancer Institute, the National Comprehensive Cancer Network, the American College of Physicians, the American Association of Family Physicians, the American College of Obstetricians and Gynecologists, the American Urological Association, the American Gastroenterological Association, the U.S. Preventive Services Task Force, and others. This is probably because these organizations all use a similar approach in evaluating all of the available scientific evidence.

Most of the controversy you read about in newspapers and hear on TV news is in response to individual studies. For most medical organizations, any one study will probably not have a large impact on early detection policy since policy is typically based on numerous studies conducted over many years. However, by their very nature, news organizations often focus on the latest controversy, rather than on long-term consensus, and favor headlines such as "Latest Study Questions Value of Mammography" over "Major Medical Organizations Still Agree About Value of Mammography, As They Have For Many Years."

The following is our advice for coping with conflicting reports on screening tests or cancer prevention.

- Don't be overly influenced by reports of individual studies in newspapers or on TV news programs. Leading medical organizations don't have their confidence shaken by a single study, and you shouldn't either.

- Check out recommendations of major public health organizations and medical specialty organizations.

- Ask your doctor which recommendations he or she follows and why.

- Ask your doctor to explain the issues in terms you can understand.

- Ask how these issues could affect your health.

To help get you started in understanding the most significant debates in cancer screening, we have included these very brief summaries.

Mammography

Most breast cancers found by mammography are less advanced than those felt by a women or her doctor. Most experts agree that women who regularly have good quality mammograms and who have access to high-quality oncology care are less likely to die of breast cancer than are women who do not have mammograms. Simply put, the accumulation of scientific evidence has shown that when breast cancer is detected when it is small, women have more treatment options, and a better chance of successful treatment. Most of the current debate covered in recent news articles is over whether having mammograms will measurably increase a woman's overall life expectancy.

Why haven't researchers resolved this issue yet? One problem is that it is no longer ethical to conduct a randomized study that invites some women to have mammograms, but does not extend an invitation to others. Most of the available data is from studies done years ago, when x-ray equipment was less sophisticated, when screening was done differently, and when today's high-quality treatment for breast cancer was not widely available. By current research standards, none of the studies were perfectly designed (few studies are), so researchers make statistical adjustments and assumptions in analyzing the data.

Depending on how you adjust and interpret the data, and which studies you believe to be most reliable, most researchers conclude that mammography is of substantial value. Only a small group feels the evidence is not sufficient to reach that conclusion, and an even smaller group feels that it is worthless in saving lives. On top of this, some researchers question the balance of the value of a saved life against the cost, anxiety, and discomfort of false-positives (biopsies are done because of suspicious findings on a mammogram in women who ultimately are shown to not have cancer so biopsy results turn out benign).

Doctors and scientists at ACS, and all major U.S. medical and public health organizations that have issued statements about breast cancer screening agree that the value of mammography is clear. Moreover, in a recent study of U.S. women, a majority demonstrated an awareness and tolerance of false positive results as an acceptable tradeoff for saving lives from breast cancer.

PSA Testing for Prostate Cancer

As with mammography, few doctors would disagree with the fact that PSA testing finds prostate cancers long before they are advanced enough to cause symptoms. The big debate is about whether early detection and prompt treatment helps men live longer.

Because prostate cancer often occurs in older men and tends to grow slowly, many seventy-five- or eighty-year-old men with prostate cancer eventually die of other, unrelated causes, before their prostate cancer caused any symptoms that had a significant impact on their quality of life. For these men, there would be have been no value to early detection and treatment. In fact, side effects of treatment, which might have included impotence and incontinence, would have had a negative impact on their quality of life.

Consider, on the other hand, a healthy fifty-year-old man with prostate cancer. Even if his cancer might not start to cause symptoms for five years or might not kill him for ten years, we would expect it to have a very negative impact on the length and quality of his life. And we would expect early diagnosis and treatment to be of substantial benefit to most men in this situation.

Although doctors have learned quite a bit about how to predict which men are likely to benefit from PSA testing, much more remains to be learned, and thus uncertainty still exists. The current ACS view (and that of the majority of medical organizations) is that each man, with his doctor's help, should decide whether testing is right for him based on his state of general health and his attitudes about the common side effects of prostate cancer treatment. For men at increased risk (African-American men and those with a family history of prostate cancer at a young age), ACS believes that the benefits clearly outweigh the risks, and testing is recommended.

Several studies are being done that will help determine whether or not PSA testing reduces the risk of dying from prostate cancer and how much screening adds to the life expectancy of a typical man. Preliminary results from some of these studies are already available, and the results are compelling. However, for the time being, the ACS and most other organizations recommend *a process of informed decision making* about testing for prostate cancer by giving men the pros and cons.

HPV Testing for Cervical Cancer Screening

Several recent studies have evaluated HPV testing as a replacement for the Pap test. The current view of ACS (and most medical organizations) is that HPV results may help decide which women with slightly abnormal Pap test results need further evaluation and which can be safely followed by a repeat Pap test. But, HPV testing is not currently recommended as a substitute for the Pap test.

CT Scans for Lung Cancer Screening

Recently, a new x-ray technique called low-dose spiral, or helical CT scanning has been successful in detecting early lung cancers in smokers and former smokers. Studies are in progress to determine if routine use of this procedure will actually save lives. Until those studies are complete, the ACS recommends that doctors tell their patients at higher lung cancer risk about the benefits and limitations of current screening methods, and about follow-up tests and treatments that might be used if screening suggests lung cancer might be present. People who choose to be screened for lung cancer by CT scanning should find a facility that uses state-of-the-art methods and is associated with a multi-specialty group of doctors that can provide appropriate follow-up tests and treatment.

Your Action Plan

Experts at the ACS recommend that you participate fully in your health care. That means coming to your checkup (see page 310, "Check It Out!") prepared and well informed. You should know your risk factors and your personal medical history. Use the worksheets on pages 346–347 to assess your risk, to follow preventive behaviors, to make healthy lifestyle choices, and to guide you in scheduling regular screening tests. Know which tests you should have. If your doctor does not recommend a particular test, ask him or her to explain why it's not needed (the test may not be recommended because it isn't appropriate).

Screening Tests Save Lives

"It's highly unlikely that physicians are going to refuse to order or perform screening tests for their patients if directly asked," says Durado Brooks, M.D., M.P.H., director of Prostate and Colorectal Cancers for the American Cancer Society. "Physicians know these tests save lives, and want their patients to have them. In many cases, they're just not asked because there is so little promotion of the tests," he adds. Dr. Brooks advises that you educate yourself about screening recommendations and then talk with your doctor about having the tests that are appropriate for you.

"That's probably the most assured way for the patient to get the screening done," says Brooks. "And it's their due—it's something that could save their lives by finding cancers early, or abnormalities that could become cancer."

Some risk factors may place you at higher risk than others, and some behaviors may lower your risk more than others. The information in this book can help you live longer and live healthier—despite a family history or previous poor lifestyle choices. You *can* take control of your health because no one else will.

Worksheets for Doctor Visits

Before you go to the doctor, make sure you know what questions to ask and what to expect. The Cancer Prevention and Early Detection Worksheets will help. Use them to learn more about the most common cancers that can affect you, what puts you at risk, how you can lower this risk, and ways that you can make sure that if you do develop cancer, it is found early when it is most easily treated. The final column on the worksheet allows room for you to write down your own plan of action to combat cancer.

Cancer Prevention and Early Detection Worksheets for Women

Screening for Cancer in General

The American Cancer Society recommends that all women get a cancer-related checkup every three years between the ages of twenty and forty, and every year thereafter. This checkup should include health counseling and, depending on the woman's age, might include examinations for cancers of the skin, thyroid, mouth, lymph nodes, and ovaries, as well as for some diseases other than cancer.

It's important to realize that some factors may place you at higher risk than others, and some behaviors may lower your risk more than others. Many cancers develop without any of these risk factors present. There is not enough room here to go into more detail—this is intended only as a general guide. For a more thorough explanation of cancer risk factors, visit us at www.cancer.org, or call us any time, day or night, at 800-ACS-2345.

And if you have any risk factors or haven't had your early detection tests, please take these worksheets and discuss this with your doctor.

Lung Cancer

Risk Factors	Preventive Behaviors

Risk Factors

- Do you smoke tobacco? _____

- Do you work around asbestos? _____

- Have you been exposed to radon? _____

- Have you been exposed to uranium? _____

- Have you been exposed to arsenic? _____

- Have you been exposed to vinyl chloride? _____

- Do you smoke marijuana? _____

- Are you regularly exposed to secondhand smoke? _____

Preventive Behaviors

- Quitting smoking.

- Encouraging those you live with or work with to quit.

- If you smoke, let your doctor know if you develop any of the following symptoms (some may have causes other than cancer):

  - A cough that does not go away
  - Chest pain, often aggravated by deep breathing
  - Hoarseness
  - Weight loss and loss of appetite
  - Bloody or rust-colored sputum (spit or phlegm)
  - Shortness of breath
  - Fever without a known reason
  - Recurring infections such as bronchitis and pneumonia
  - New onset of wheezing

Special tests for certain cancers are recommended as outlined under "Screening Tests."

Screening Tests	Your Action Plan
None have been found to be effective. Usually found on x-ray, but there are often no symptoms.	Steps to Lower Your Risk:

- Talk to your doctor about possible screening if you have any of the risk factors listed.

Screening:

_____

_____

_____

_____

_____

_____

Colorectal Cancer

Risk Factors

- Do you have a family history of colon or rectal cancer? _____

- Do you have a colorectal cancer syndrome in your family (such as familial adenomatous polyposis (FAP) or hereditary nonpolyposis colon cancer (HNPCC))? _____

- Do you have a personal history of colorectal cancer? _____

- Do you have a personal history of intestinal polyps? _____

- Do you have a personal history of chronic inflammatory bowel disease (Crohn's disease or ulcerative colitis)?

  _____

- Are you over fifty years of age? _____

- Do you consume a diet mostly from animal sources? _____

- Are you physically inactive? _____

- Are you overweight? _____

- Do you use tobacco? _____

Preventive Behaviors

- Following screening guidelines to remove adenomatous polyps before they become cancer.

- Getting at least thirty minutes of physical activity on most days.

- Achieving and maintaining a healthy weight.

- Eating plenty of fruits, vegetables, and whole grain foods and limiting intake of high-fat foods.

- Quitting smoking.

Screening Tests	Your Action Plan
Beginning at age fifty, you should follow one of the five screening options below:	Steps to Lower Your Risk:

* Fecal occult blood test (FOBT) every year
* Flexible sigmoidoscopy every five years
* Fecal occult blood test every year plus flexible sigmoidoscopy every five years

(Of the three options above, yearly FOBT combined with flexible sigmoidoscopy every five years is preferable.)

* Double-contrast barium enema every five years
* Colonoscopy every ten years

Talk to your doctor about beginning screening earlier and/or more often if you have any of the following risk factors:

Screening:

* Strong family history of colorectal cancer or polyps (cancer or polyps in a first-degree relative younger than sixty or in two first-degree relatives of any age). Note: a first degree-relative is defined as a parent, sibling, or child.
* A known family history of colorectal cancer syndromes.
* A personal history of colorectal cancer or adenomatous polyps.
* A personal history of chronic inflammatory bowel disease.

Skin Cancer

Risk Factors

- Do you sunbathe? _____
- Do you use tanning booths? _____
- Do you have fair skin with blonde or red hair? _____
- Do you sunburn easily or have many freckles? _____
- Did you have severe sunburns as a child? _____
- Do you have many or unusually shaped moles? _____
- Do you live in a southern climate or at a high altitude? _____
- Do you spend a lot of time outdoors (for work or recreation)? _____
- Have you ever received radiation treatments? _____
- Do you have a family history of skin cancer? _____
- Do you have a weakened immune system due to an organ transplant or due to another condition? _____
- Were you born with xeroderma pigmentosum, basal cell nevus syndrome, or dysplastic nevus syndrome? _____
- Have you been exposed to any of the following chemicals? _____
  - Arsenic
  - Coal tar
  - Paraffin
  - Radium

Preventive Behaviors

- Staying out of the sun, especially between 10 AM and 4 PM.
- Wearing a broad-brimmed hat, a shirt, and sunglasses when out in the sun.
- Using a sunscreen with an SPF of 15 or higher, and reapplying it often.
- Not using tanning beds or sunlamps.
- Protecting young children from excess sun exposure.
- Checking your skin regularly for abnormal or changing areas, especially moles, and having them examined by your doctor.

Screening Tests	Your Action Plan
Cancer-Related Checkup (including skin exam):	Steps to Lower Your Risk:
• Over twenty: every three years	_____
• Over forty: every year	_____
Self exam (monthly):	_____
• Become familiar with any moles, freckles or other abnormalities on your skin. Use a mirror or have a family member or close friend look at areas you can't see (ears, scalp, lower back).	_____
• Check for changes once a month. Show any suspicious or changing areas to your doctor.	_____
	Screening:
	_____
	_____
	_____
	_____

Cervical Cancer

Risk Factors

- Were you (are you) sexually active before age seventeen?_____

- Have you had multiple sex partners or a partner who has had multiple partners? _____

- Have you had unprotected sex? _____

- Do you have a history of a sexually transmitted disease (especially HPV with genital warts), or HIV? _____

- Do you smoke? _____

- Do you eat a diet low in fruits and vegetables? _____

- Did your mother take diethylstilbestrol (DES) during her pregnancy? _____

- Are you over age fifty? _____

Preventive Behaviors

- Abstaining from or practicing safer sex using barrier protection each time you have intercourse.

- Quitting smoking.

- Eating a diet rich in fruits and vegetables.

- Watching for and reporting signs and symptoms (although all of these can have other causes):

  – Abnormal uterine bleeding or spotting
  – Abnormal vaginal discharge
  – Pain during intercourse

Screening Tests

- Yearly pelvic exam with Pap test to begin at age eighteen or when sexually active, whichever is earlier.

- After three or more consecutive satisfactory normal yearly examinations, the Pap test may be performed less frequently at the discretion of your doctor.

Your Action Plan

Steps to Lower Your Risk:

_____

_____

_____

_____

_____

Screening:

_____

_____

_____

_____

Breast Cancer

Risk Factors

- Are you over age fifty? _____

- Do you have a personal history of breast cancer? _____

- Do you have a family history of breast cancer (especially mother, sister, or daughter)? _____

- Did you have your first child after age thirty (or have no children)? _____

- Did you have chest radiation as a child or young woman as treatment for another cancer? _____

- Did you begin menstruating before age twelve, or go through menopause after age fifty? _____

- Have you been on hormone replacement therapy for more than five years? _____

- Do you drink one or more alcoholic beverages a day? _____

- Are you physically inactive? _____

- If you are postmenopausal, have you gained weight, especially around your waist? _____

Preventive Behaviors

- Following recommended guidelines for early detection of breast cancer.

- Talking with your doctor about the risks and benefits of hormone replacement therapy for your risk of cancer and other diseases (like heart disease and osteoporosis).

- Getting at least thirty minutes of physical activity on most days.

- Achieving and maintaining a healthy weight.

- Eating plenty of fruits, vegetables, and whole grain foods and limiting intake of high-fat foods.

- Decreasing your alcohol intake.

Women at high risk:

- Considering taking tamoxifen or enrolling in a chemoprevention study.

- Talking with your doctor about more frequent tests for early detection.

Screening Tests	Your Action Plan
Ages twenty to thirty-nine:	Steps to Lower Your Risk:
• Breast self-examination each month	
• Clinical breast examination by health care professional every three years	
Age forty and over:	
• Yearly mammogram	
• Yearly clinical breast examination by a health care professional, near the time of the mammogram	
• Breast self-exam every month	
	Screening:

Endometrial Cancer

Risk Factors

- Are you over age forty? _____

- Did you begin menstruating before age twelve, or go through menopause after age fifty? _____

- Do you have a history of infertility or never giving birth? _____

- Are you obese (very overweight)? _____

- Do you eat a diet high in animal fat? _____

- Do you have a history of diabetes? _____

- Have you taken tamoxifen or long-term estrogen replacement therapy *without progesterone* (if you still have your uterus)? _____

- Do you have a history of breast or ovarian cancer? _____

- Have you had radiation therapy to your pelvis? _____

- Do you have a family history of hereditary nonpolyposis colorectal cancer (HNPCC), or are you at risk for this cancer? _____

Preventive Behaviors

- Watching for and reporting any abnormal uterine spotting or bleeding.

- Using oral contraceptives for many years.

- Talking with your doctor about the risks and benefits of hormone replacement therapy for your risk of cancer and other diseases (like heart disease and osteoporosis).

- If taking hormone replacement therapy with your uterus still intact, taking estrogen *with progesterone*.

Screening Tests	Your Action Plan
Average Risk	Steps to Lower Your Risk:
• Talk with your doctor, especially at the time of menopause, about the risks and symptoms of endometrial cancer.	_____
	_____
• Report any vaginal bleeding or spotting to your doctor	_____
• Yearly pelvic exam	
	_____
Increased Risk (includes women with any of the first nine risk factors in the left column)	_____
• Discuss endometrial cancer early detection testing with your doctor.	_____
HNPCC	Screening:
• If you have or are at risk for HNPCC, consider yearly testing with endometrial biopsy beginning at age thirty-five.	_____
	_____
	_____
	_____

Ovarian Cancer

Risk Factors

- Have you already gone through menopause? _____

- Did you begin menstruating before age twelve, or go through menopause after age fifty? _____

- Did you have your first child after age thirty (or have no children)? _____

- Do you have a family history of ovarian cancer? _____

- Do you have a personal history of breast cancer? _____

- Have you been on hormone replacement therapy for more than five years? _____

Preventive Behaviors

- Using oral contraceptives for several years.

- Watching for and reporting signs and symptoms (although all of these can have other causes):

  – Abdominal swelling
  – Vaginal bleeding
  – Back and/or leg pain
  – Chronic stomach pain

- Talking with your doctor about the risks and benefits of hormone replacement therapy and your risks of cancer and other diseases, like heart disease and osteoporosis.

- Talking with your doctor about having your ovaries removed, if you are at high risk. (This surgery causes sudden menopause.)

Screening Tests

There are currently no effective and proven tests for early detection of ovarian cancer.

- As part of your regular health maintenance, you should undergo a periodic and thorough pelvic examination as directed by your doctor.

Your Action Plan

Steps to Lower Your Risk:

_____

_____

_____

_____

_____

Screening:

_____

_____

_____

_____

_____

Cancer Prevention and Early Detection Worksheets for Men

Screening for Cancer in General

The American Cancer Society recommends that all men get a cancer-related checkup every three years between the ages of twenty and forty, and every year thereafter. This checkup should include health counseling and, depending on the man's age, might include examinations for cancers of the skin, thyroid, mouth, lymph nodes, and testes, as well as for some diseases other than cancer.

Prostate Cancer

Risk Factors	Preventive Behaviors
• Are you over age fifty? _____	• Eating a diet low in fat and high in vegetables, fruits, and grains.
• Are you African American? _____	• Getting at least thirty minutes of physical activity on most days.
• Do you eat a diet high in fat? _____	• Achieving and maintaining a healthy weight.
• Are you overweight? _____	
• Are you inactive? _____	
• Do you have a family history of prostate cancer? _____	

It's important to realize that some factors may place you at higher risk than others, and some behaviors may lower your risk more than others. Many cancers develop without any of these risk factors present. There is not enough room here to go into more detail—this is intended only as a general guide. For a more thorough explanation of cancer risk factors, visit us at www.cancer.org, or call us any time, day or night, at 800-ACS-2345. And if you have any risk factors or haven't had your early detection tests, please take these worksheets and discuss this with your doctor.

Special tests for certain cancers are recommended as outlined under "Screening Tests."

Screening Tests	Your Action Plan
• Consider a yearly PSA blood test and digital rectal exam starting at age fifty, or at age forty-five if you are at high risk (African American, or have a father or brother diagnosed with prostate cancer at a young age).	Steps to Lower Your Risk: _____ _____
• Talk to your doctor about the pros and cons of prostate cancer screening.	Screening: _____ _____

Lung Cancer

Risk Factors

- Do you smoke tobacco? _____

- Do you work around asbestos? _____

- Have you been exposed to radon?
  _____

- Have you been exposed to uranium?
  _____

- Have you been exposed to arsenic?
  _____

- Have you been exposed to vinyl
  chloride? _____

- Do you smoke marijuana? _____

- Are you regularly exposed to
  secondhand smoke? _____

Preventive Behaviors

- Quitting smoking.

- Encouraging those you live with or
  work with to quit.

- If you smoke, let your doctor know if you
  develop any of the following symptoms
  (some may have causes other than cancer):

  - A cough that does not go away
  - Chest pain, often aggravated by
    deep breathing
  - Hoarseness
  - Weight loss and loss of appetite
  - Bloody or rust-colored sputum
    (spit or phlegm)
  - Shortness of breath
  - Fever without a known reason
  - Recurring infections such as bronchitis
    and pneumonia
  - New onset of wheezing

Screening Tests

None have been found to be effective. Usually found on x-ray, but there are often no symptoms.

- Talk to your doctor about possible screening if you have any of the risk factors listed.

Your Action Plan

Steps to Lower Your Risk:

_____

_____

_____

_____

_____

_____

Screening:

_____

_____

_____

_____

Colorectal Cancer

Risk Factors

- Do you have a family history of colon or rectal cancer? _____

- Do you have a colorectal cancer syndrome in your family (such as familial adenomatous polyposis (FAP) or hereditary nonpolyposis colon cancer (HNPCC))? _____

- Do you have a personal history of colorectal cancer? _____

- Do you have a personal history of intestinal polyps? _____

- Do you have a personal history of chronic inflammatory bowel disease (Crohn's disease or ulcerative colitis)? _____

- Are you over fifty years of age? _____

- Do you consume a diet mostly from animal sources? _____

- Are you physically inactive? _____

- Are you overweight? _____

- Do you use tobacco? _____

Preventive Behaviors

- Following screening guidelines to remove adenomatous polyps before they become cancer.

- Getting at least thirty minutes of physical activity on most days.

- Achieving and maintaining a healthy weight.

- Eating plenty of fruits, vegetables, and whole grain foods and limiting intake of high-fat foods.

- Quitting smoking.

Screening Tests

Beginning at age fifty, you should follow one of the five screening options below:

- Yearly fecal occult blood test (FOBT)
- Flexible sigmoidoscopy every five years
- Yearly fecal occult blood test plus flexible sigmoidoscopy every five years

(Of the three options above, yearly FOBT combined with flexible sigmoidoscopy every five years is preferable.)

- Double-contrast barium enema every five years
- Colonoscopy every ten years

Talk to your doctor about beginning screening earlier and/or more often if you have any of the following risk factors:

- Strong family history of colorectal cancer or polyps (cancer or polyps in a first-degree relative younger than sixty or in two first-degree relatives of any age). Note: a first degree-relative is defined as a parent, sibling, or child.
- A known family history of colorectal cancer syndromes.
- A personal history of colorectal cancer or adenomatous polyps.
- A personal history of chronic inflammatory bowel disease.

Your Action Plan

Steps to Lower Your Risk:

_____

_____

_____

_____

_____

Screening:

_____

_____

_____

_____

Skin Cancer

Risk Factors

- Do you sunbathe? _____
- Do you use tanning booths? _____
- Do you have fair skin with blonde or red hair? _____
- Do you sunburn easily or have many freckles? _____
- Did you have severe sunburns as a child? _____
- Do you have many or unusually shaped moles? _____
- Do you live in a southern climate or at a high altitude? _____
- Do you spend a lot of time outdoors (for work or recreation)? _____
- Have you ever received radiation treatments? _____
- Do you have a family history of skin cancer? _____
- Do you have a weakened immune system due to an organ transplant or due to another condition? _____
- Were you born with xeroderma pigmentosum, basal cell nevus syndrome, or dysplastic nevus syndrome? _____
- Have you been exposed to any of the following chemicals? _____
  - Arsenic
  - Coal tar
  - Paraffin
  - Radium

Preventive Behaviors

- Staying out of the sun, especially between 10 AM and 4 PM.

- Wearing a broad-brimmed hat, a shirt, and sunglasses when out in the sun.

- Using a sunscreen with an SPF of 15 or higher, and reapplying it often.

- Not using tanning beds or sunlamps.

- Protecting young children from excess sun exposure.

- Checking your skin regularly for abnormal or changing areas, especially moles, and having them examined by your doctor.

Screening Tests	Your Action Plan
Cancer-Related Checkup (including skin exam):	Steps to Lower Your Risk:
• Over twenty: every three years	_____
• Over forty: every year	_____
Self exam (monthly):	_____
• Become familiar with any moles, freckles or other abnormalities on your skin. Use a mirror or have a family member or close friend look at areas you can't see (ears, scalp, lower back).	_____
	_____
• Check for changes once a month. Show any suspicious or changing areas to your doctor.	_____
	Screening:
	_____
	_____
	_____
	_____
	_____

Resources

American Cancer Society

The American Cancer Society (ACS) provides educational materials and information on cancer, offers a variety of patient programs, and directs people to services in their community. To find your local office, contact us at 800-ACS-2345 or visit our web site (*http://www.cancer.org*).

National Home Office

1599 Clifton Road NE
Atlanta, GA 30329-4251
Toll-Free: 800-ACS-2345 (800-227-2345)
Web site: *http://www.cancer.org*

Other Organizations

The following listings represent organizations that operate on a national level and provide some type of service or resource to consumers. This list is organized by chapter and designed to give you a starting point for seeking information, support, and needed resources. If you have a question that cannot be answered by one of the sources listed here, many of these organizations provide referrals, and your questions may be directed to other organizations or individuals.

Most of the organizations listed here can be contacted via phone, fax, or e-mail, and some through their web site. Many of the web sites provide much of the same information that is available by postal mail. Some organizations are solely web-based and will require Internet access. Keep in mind that new web sites appear daily while old ones expand, move, or disappear entirely. Some of the web sites or content outlined below may change. Often, a simple Internet search will point you to the new web site for a given organization. The ACS web site (*http://www.cancer.org*) provides links to other sources of cancer information and more.

The ACS does not endorse the agencies, organizations, corporations, and publications represented in this resource guide. This guide is provided for assistance in obtaining information only.

General Health Information

Consumer Information Center

Pueblo, CO 81009
Toll-free: 888-878-3256
Fax: 719-948-9724
Web site: *http://www.pueblo.gsa.gov*
The Consumer Information Center distributes consumer publications on topics related to children, food and nutrition, health, exercise, and weight control.

Health Information on the Internet

There is a vast amount of information about nutrition, physical activity, and many other topics on the Internet. This information can be very valuable to those making decisions about their health. However, since any group or individual can publish on the Internet, it is important to consider the credentials and reputation of the organization providing information. Always discuss health information you find on the Internet with your doctor. Internet information should not be a substitute for medical advice.

Discovery Health

Discovery Communications, Inc.
7700 Wisconsin Avenue
Bethesda, MD 20814-3579
Phone: 301-986-0444
E-mail: comments@discoveryhealth.com
Web site: *http://www.discoveryhealth.com*
Discoveryhealth.com provides users with health information that is comprehensive, accurate, and nonbiased. The site has original features, tools, and updated articles.

FamilyDoctor.org

Attn: Special Projects Department
American Academy of Family Physicians
11400 Tomahawk Creek Parkway
Leawood, KS 66211-2672
E-mail: email@familydoctor.org
Web site: *http://www.familydoctor.org*
As a consumer-oriented site, Familydoctor.org provides information about health topics, drug information, self-care, and herbal remedies. The site also has a directory of family physicians by state. Content is written and reviewed by physicians and patient education professionals at the American Academy of Family Physicians.

Health.gov

Web site: *http://www.health.gov*
Health.gov is a portal to the web sites of a number of multi-agency health initiatives and activities of the U.S. Department of Health and Human Services and other Federal departments and agencies. The web site also has a link to healthfinder.gov, a guide to reliable consumer health information from the Federal Government.

HealthScout

Web site: *http://www.healthscout.com*
Healthscout is a general health web site that provides health care news and medical information. It also provides connections to other health resources.

Mayo Clinic Consumer Health on the Internet

Web site: *http://www.mayoclinic.com*
This web site contains a database searchable by keyword and topic. It also offers a question-and-answer link to a doctor at the Mayo Clinic, as well as links to reference articles and cancer organizations.

Medscape

Web site: *http://www.medscape.com*
Although a no-cost registration is required to view some of the content, this web site offers a great deal of information on prescription drugs and medical articles. There are also links to several organizations, cancer centers, database and education web sites, journals, and government sites. The web site is searchable by key word.

MedWatch

U.S. Food and Drug Administration (FDA)
MedWatch Office
5600 Fishers Lane, HFD-200
Rockville, MD 20857
Phone: 301-827-7240
Toll-free: 800-332-1088 to report an adverse event, medical error, or medical product quality problem or 888-INFO-FDA (888-463-6332) for information on an FDA-regulated product
Fax: 301-827-7241
Web site: *http://www.fda.gov/medwatch*
Through MedWatch, the FDA maintains an adverse event and product-reporting program. The organization accepts reports of problems with food, drugs, or devices from the general public. The web site includes medical product safety alerts and an e-mail feedback form, as well as searchable FDA safety databases and FDA medical bulletins.

Quackwatch

Web site: *http://www.quackwatch.com*
Quackwatch, Inc. is a nonprofit corporation whose purpose is to combat health-related frauds, myths, fads, and fallacies. The Quackwatch web site is a comprehensive source of information regarding fraudulent claims. *Information is offered in German, Spanish, French, and Portuguese as well as in English.*

WebMD

Web site: *http://www.webmd.com*
WebMD is a consumer-focused health-care information web site. Users can access health news, articles, research reports, condition-specific centers and support communities, interactive tools and programs, as well as on-line health and lifestyle product catalogues and ordering services.

Health Organizations (Chapter 1)
Agency for Healthcare Research and Quality (AHRQ)

Office of Health Care Information, Executive Office Center
2101 E. Jefferson Street, Suite 501
Rockville, MD 20852
Phone: 301-594-1360
Web site: *http://www.ahrq.gov*

The AHRQ, an office within the U.S. Department of Health and Human Services, provides consumers with science-based, easily understandable information that will help them make informed decisions about their own personal health care. They offer a number of clinical practice guidelines on common health problems in consumer versions for the public.

AMC Cancer Research Center and Foundation

Cancer Information and Counseling Line
1600 Pierce Street
Denver, CO 80214
Phone: 303-239-3422
Toll-free: 800-525-3777
Fax: 303-233-1863
E-mail: cicl@amc.org
Web site: *http://www.amc.org*
The AMC Cancer Research Center and Foundation is a nonprofit research institute dedicated to the prevention of cancer and other chronic diseases. The Center offers the Cancer Information and Counseling Line (CICL), a toll-free line staffed by professionals with degrees in counseling or related health areas. The web site contains general information on nutrition, exercise, sun safety, and smoking, as well as links to cancer-related resources.

American Board of Medical Specialties (ABMS)

1007 Church Street, Suite 404
Evanston, IL 60201-5913
Phone Verification: 866-ASK-ABMS
(866-275-2267)

Phone: 847-491-9091
Fax: 847-328-3596
Web site: *http://www.abms.org*
The ABMS is the umbrella organization for the twenty-four approved medical specialty boards in the United States. This organization provides information about specialization and certification in medicine. Their web site includes the Doctor Verification Service. Some libraries may carry the *Official ABMS Directory of Board Certified Medical Specialists,* which lists those doctors who have had additional training and who have passed special qualifying tests.

American Medical Association (AMA)

515 North State Street
Chicago, IL 60610
Phone: 312-464-5000
Web site: *http://www.ama-assn.org*
The AMA develops and promotes standards in medical practice, research, and education. Under the Doctor Finder section, the web site contains databases on doctors and hospitals, which can be searched by name, location, or medical specialty.

Centers for Disease Control and Prevention (CDC)

Public Inquiries/MASO
MS/F07
1600 Clifton Road NE
Atlanta, GA 30333
Phone: 404-639-3534
Toll-free: 800-311-3435

Web site: *http://www.cdc.gov*
The CDC is an agency of the U.S. Department of Health and Human Services. Their mission is to promote health and quality of life by preventing and controlling disease, injury, and disability. Their web site contains a searchable map of centers, information about health topics, downloadable publications, and links to related sources.

National Center for Chronic Disease Prevention and Health Promotion
4770 Buford Highway NE
MS/K64
Atlanta, GA 30341
Toll-free: 888-842-6355
Fax: 770-488-4760
E-mail: ccdinfo@cdc.gov
Web site: *http://www.cdc.gov/nccdphp*
This division of the CDC provides information, sponsors programs, identifies risk behaviors, and performs surveillance in the area of chronic disease prevention.

DIVISION OF CANCER PREVENTION AND CONTROL (DCPC)
E-mail: cancerinfo@cdc.gov
Web site: *http://www.cdc.gov/cancer*
DCPC conducts, supports, and promotes efforts to prevent cancer and to increase early detection of cancer. DCPC works with partners in the government, private, and nonprofit sectors to develop, implement, and promote effective cancer prevention and control practices nationwide.

National Council Against Health Fraud
P.O. Box 141
Fort Lee, NJ 07024
Phone: 201-723-2955
E-mail: ncahf@worldnet.att.net
Web site: *http://www.ncahf.org*
This agency focuses on health misinformation, fraud, and quackery. It can refer people to lawyers and help those who have had negative experiences to share their story.

National Institutes of Health (NIH)
9000 Rockville Pike
Bethesda, MD 20892
Phone: 301-496-4000
E-mail (please submit questions and requests via e-mail): nihinfo@od.nih.gov
Web site: *http://www.nih.gov*
The NIH is an agency of the Public Health Services, which in turn is part of the U.S. Department of Health and Human Services. The NIH mission is to uncover new knowledge that will lead to better health for everyone. NIH conducts research in its own laboratories, supports the research of nonfederal scientists, helps in the training of research investigators, and fosters communication of medical information.

National Cancer Institute (NCI)
(See page 391 – Early Detection and Screening Resources, Chapter 9)

National Center for Complementary and Alternative Medicine (NCCAM)

NCCAM Clearinghouse
P.O. Box 8218
Silver Spring, MD 20907-8218
Phone: 301-231-7537, ext. 5 (for calling from outside the U.S.)
Toll-free: 888-644-6226
Fax: 301-495-4957
Web site: *http://nccam.nih.gov*
This center provides information on complementary and alternative methods being promoted to treat different diseases.

National Institute on Aging

Building 31, Room 5C27
31 Center Drive, MSC 2292
Bethesda, MD 20892-2292
Phone: 301-496-1752
Toll-free: 800-222-2225 (information center)
E-mail: webmaster@nia.nih.gov
Web site: *http://www.nih.gov/nia*
The NIA, one of the National Institutes of Health, leads a broad scientific effort to understand the nature of aging and to extend the healthy, active years of life. The NIA's mission is to improve the health and well-being of older Americans through research and public information.

National Institutes of Health Consensus Program

P.O. Box 2577
Kensington, MD 20891
Toll-free: 800-644-2667
E-mail: consensus@od.nih.gov
Web site: *http://consensus.nih.gov*

This program updates practicing doctors and the public with current responsible information on the pros and cons of various medical technologies.

U.S. National Library of Medicine

8600 Rockville Pike
Bethesda, MD 20894
Web site: *http://www.nlm.nih.gov*
This is an extensive on-line library that provides a search engine for health, medical, scientific literature, and research, as well as links to other government resources.

INTERNET GRATEFUL MED

Web site: *http://igm.nlm.nih.gov*
Provides access to millions of literature references and abstracts in Medline and other databases, with links to on-line journals. The site is searchable by key words.

NLM GATEWAY

Web site: *http://gateway.nlm.nih.gov/gw/Cmd*
Offers links to searchable databases and allows users to search simultaneously in multiple retrieval systems.

PUBMED

Web site:
http://www.ncbi.nlm.nih.gov/PubMed
Provides access to millions of literature references and abstracts in Medline and other databases, with links to on-line journals. The site is searchable by keyword.

National Safety Council (NSC)

1121 Spring Lake Drive
Itasca, IL 60143-3201
Phone: 630-285-1121
Fax: 630-285-1315
E-mail: webmaster@nsc.org
Web site: *http://www.nsc.org*
The NSC is a membership organization dedicated to protecting life and promoting health. The Fact Sheet Library, available on the NSC web site, provides over eighty handy resource guides offering statistics, tips, and suggestions for improving safety.

National Women's Health Information Center (NWHIC)

8550 Arlington Boulevard, Suite 300
Fairfax, VA 22031
Phone: 703-560-6618
Toll-free: 800-994-WOMAN
(800-994-9662)
Fax: 703-560-6598
Web site: *http://www.4woman.gov*
The NWHIC is a federally funded women's health information and referral service. NWHIC is staffed by information specialists who clarify information needs, identify appropriate federal and private sector referral organizations, and order selected materials for callers.

World Health Organization (WHO)

Regional Office for the Americas/Pan American Health Organization
525 23rd Street NW
Washington, DC 20037

Phone: 202-974-3000 (Main); 202-974-3457 (Office of Public Information)
Fax: 202-974-3663
E-mail: info@who.ch
Web site: *http://www.who.org*
Founded in 1948, the WHO leads the world alliance for Health for All. A specialized agency of the United Nations, WHO promotes technical cooperation for health among nations, carries out programs to control and eradicate disease, and strives to improve the quality of human life.

Food and Nutrition Resources (Chapter 2)

American Dietetic Association (ADA)

216 West Jackson Boulevard, Suite 800
Chicago, IL 60606-6995
Phone: 312-899-0040
Web site: *http://www.eatright.org*
The ADA is the world's largest organization of food and nutrition professionals. The ADA serves the public by promoting nutrition, health, and well-being. The web site contains information on diet and nutrition and a registered dietitian locator service.

National Center for Nutrition and Dietetics (NCND) Information Line

Phone: 800-366-1655
Web site: *http://www.eatright.org/ncnd.html*
NCND's Consumer Nutrition Information Line offers the public direct access to objective, credible food and nutrition information from registered dietitians.

Recorded messages (in English and Spanish) with practical nutrition information, monthly Nutrition Fact Sheets, and referrals to registered dietitians are available twenty-four hours a day.

American Institute for Cancer Research (AICR)

1759 R Street NW
Washington, DC 20009
Phone: 202-328-7744
Toll-free: 800-843-8114
E-mail: aicrweb@aicr.org
Web site: *http://www.aicr.org*
This organization focuses on the relationship between diet and nutrition and cancer prevention and treatment. The AICR creates public health education programs, funds research, and provides information to the public and health care professionals.

International Food Information Council (IFIC) Foundation

1100 Connecticut Avenue NW, Suite 430
Washington, DC 20036
Phone: 202-296-6540
Fax: 202-296-6547
E-mail: foodinfo@ific.org
Web site: *http://ific.org*
As the educational arm of the IFIC, the IFIC Foundation communicates science-based information on food safety and nutrition to health and nutrition professionals, educators, journalists, and others for distribution to consumers. The IFIC has established partnerships with a wide range of professional organizations and academic institutions to develop science-based information for the public.

United States Department of Agriculture (USDA)

Fourteenth and Independence Avenue SW
Washington, DC 20250-9410
Phone: 202-720-2791
Web site: *http://www.usda.gov*
The USDA strives to enhance the quality of life for the American people by supporting production of agriculture. The USDA is also responsible for the food supply, managing agricultural products, forest, and rangeland, and community development.

USDA Food and Nutrition Information Center (FNIC)

National Agricultural Library, Room 304
10301 Baltimore Avenue
Beltsville, MD 20705-2351
Phone: 301-504-5719; 301-504-5414 (for inquiries to dietitians and nutritionists)
Fax: 301-504-6409
E-mail: fnic@nal.usda.gov
Web site: *http://www.nal.usda.gov/fnic*
The USDA's FNIC is an information center for the National Agricultural Library. FNIC materials and services include dietitians and nutritionists available to answer inquiries, publications on food and nutrition, and resource lists and bibliographies. The FNIC web site includes information on dietary supplements, food safety, dietary guidelines, food composition facts (including fast food), a list of available publications, and information on frequently asked topics.

U.S. Food and Drug Administration (FDA)

5600 Fishers Lane
Rockville, MD 20857-0001
Phone: 888-INFO-FDA (888-463-6332)
Fax: 301-443-9767
Web site: *http://www.fda.gov*
The FDA is a public health agency charged with protecting American by enforcing the Federal Food, Drug, and Cosmetic Act and other laws, promoting health by helping safe and effective products reach the market in a timely way, and monitoring products for continued safety after they are in use. The FDA regulates food, cosmetics, medicines, medical devices, and radiation-emitting consumer products, as well as feed and drugs for pets and farm animals.

Center for Food Safety and Applied Nutrition (CFSAN) Outreach and Information Center

200 C Street SW
Washington, DC 20204
Toll-free: 888-SAFEFOOD (888-723-3366); TYY: 800-877-8339
Web site: *http://www.cfsan.fda.gov*
The goal of the Outreach and Information Center is to enhance CFSAN's ability to provide and respond to the public's desire/demand for more useful, timely, and accurate information regarding its regulated products. In addition to providing food safety information, the Outreach and Information Center will provide assistance with other CFSAN issues, including nutrition, dietary supplements, food labeling, cosmetics, food additives, and food biotechnology.

Physical Activity Resources (Chapter 3)

American Alliance for Health, Physical Education, Recreation, and Dance (AAHPERD)

1900 Association Drive
Reston, VA 20191-1598
Phone: 800-213-7193
Fax: 703-476-9527
Web site: *http://www.aahperd.org*
The AAHPERD is the largest organization of professionals involved in physical education, leisure, fitness, dance, health promotion, and education and all specialties related to achieving a healthy lifestyle. AAHPERD is an alliance of other associations with a comprehensive and coordinated array of resources, support, and programs to help practitioners improve their skills and further the health and well-being of Americans. The other organizations can be reached through the AAHPERD web site.

American College of Sports Medicine (ACSM)

401 W. Michigan Street
Indianapolis, IN 46202-3233
Phone: 317-637-9200
Fax: 317-634-7817
E-mail: publications@acsm.org (for publication materials)
Web site: *http://www.acsm.org*
The ACSM promotes and integrates scientific research, education, and practical

applications of sports medicine and exercise science to maintain and enhance physical performance, fitness, health, and quality of life.

American Council on Exercise (ACE)

5820 Oberlin Drive, Suite 102
San Diego, CA 92121-3787
Phone: 858-535-8227
Toll-free: 800-825-3636
Fax: 858-535-1778
Web site: *http://www.acefitness.org*
The ACE is a nonprofit organization committed to promoting active, healthy lifestyles and their positive effects on the mind, body, and spirit. ACE sets certification and education standards for fitness instructors and provides ongoing public education about the importance of exercise.

American Health Foundation (AHF)

Publications
1 Dana Road
Valhalla, NY 10595
E-mail: health@ahf.org
Web site: *http://www.ahf.org*
The AHF is the only National Cancer Institute-designated cancer center devoted to cancer prevention. The AHF is a national resource for innovative approaches to nutritional and environmental health promotion programs. Its staff works with leaders throughout the country to promote healthy lifestyle behaviors.

American Heart Association (AHA)

7272 Greenville Avenue
Dallas, TX 75231
Phone: 214-373-6300
Toll-free: 800-AHA-USA1 (800-242-8721) —Customer heart and stroke information; 888-MY-HEART (888-694-278) — Women's health information
Web site: *http://www.americanheart.org*
The AHA is a nonprofit, voluntary health organization with a mission to reduce disability and death from cardio-vascular diseases and stroke. The AHA web site includes information about heart disease, stroke, and prevention, as well as an AHA Chapter locator.

National Association for Health and Fitness (NAHF): The Network of State and Governor's Councils

401 West Michigan Street
Indianapolis, IN 46202-3233
Phone: 317-955-0957
Fax: 317-634-7817
E-mail: info@physicalfitness.org
Web site: *http://www.physicalfitness.org*
The NAHF is a nonprofit organization that exists to improve the quality of life for individuals in the U.S. through the promotion of physical fitness, sports, and healthy lifestyles and by fostering and supporting State Governor's Councils on Physical Fitness and Sports in every state and U.S. territory.

National Center for Chronic Disease Prevention and Health Promotion

Division of Nutrition and Physical Activity (DNPA)
4770 Buford Highway NE, MS/K24
Atlanta, GA 30341-3717
Phone: 770-488-5820
Fax: 770-488-5473
E-mail: ccdinfo@cdc.gov
Web site: *http://www.cdc.gov/nccdphp/dnpa*
As part of the CDC and the National Center for Chronic Disease Prevention and Health Promotion, the DNPA provides science-based activities for children and adults that address the role of nutrition and physical activity in health promotion and the prevention and control of chronic diseases. The scope of DNPA programs includes epidemiology, applied research, public health policy, surveillance, community interventions, evaluation, and communications.

National Heart, Lung, and Blood Institute (NHLBI)

NHLBI Information Center
P.O. Box 30105
Bethesda, MD 20824-0105
Phone: 301-592-8573
Toll-free: 800-575-9355 (for recorded information about high blood pressure and cholesterol; cannot leave a message other than name and mailing address to where materials can be sent)
Fax: 301-592-8563
E-mail: NHLBIinfo@rover.nhlbi.nih.gov
Web site: *http://www.nhlbi.nih.gov*

The NHLBI is a branch of the National Institutes of Health. The NHLBI web site provides information to the public, health care professionals, and the media about heart and vascular, lung, and blood diseases, as well as sleep disorders.

National Institute of Diabetes & Digestive & Kidney Diseases (NIDDKD)

Weight-control Information Network (WIN)
1 WIN Way
Bethesda, MD 20892-3665
Phone: 202-828-1025; 877-946-4627
Fax: 202-828-1028
E-mail: win@info.niddk.nih.gov
Web site:
http://www.niddk.nih.gov/health/nutrit/nutrit.htm
The WIN is a national service of the NIDDKD of the National Institutes of Health. WIN was established in 1994 to raise awareness and provide up-to-date, science-based information on obesity, physical activity, weight control, and related nutritional issues to health professionals, people who are overweight or obese, the media, Congress, and the general public.

President's Council on Physical Fitness and Sports (PCPFS)

Department W
200 Independence Avenue SW
Room 738-H
Washington, DC 20201-0004
Phone: 202-690-9000
Fax: 202-690-5211

E-mail: pcpfs@osophs.dhhs.gov
Web site: *http://www.fitness.gov*
The PCPFS serves to promote, encourage and motivate Americans of all ages to become physically active and participate in sports. Assisted by elements of the U.S. Public Health Service, the PCPFS advises the President and the Secretary of Health and Human Services on how to encourage more Americans to be physically fit and active.

Shape Up America!

6707 Democracy Boulevard, Suite 306
Bethesda, MD 20817
E-mail: suainfo@shapeup.org
Web site: *http://www.shapeup.org*
Shape Up America! is a high-profile national initiative founded by former U.S. Surgeon General C. Everett Koop to promote healthy weight and increased physical activity in America. The web site provides credible, science-based health messages in a distinctive way so that people will understand the importance of healthy weight and increased physical activity.

YMCA of the USA

Association Advancement
101 North Wacker Drive
Chicago, IL 60606
Phone: 312-977-0031
Web site: *http://www.ymca.net*
The YMCA of the USA is the national resource office for the nation's YMCAs. Located in Chicago, with satellite offices across the country, the YMCA of the USA exists to serve YMCAs. Each

YMCA is an independent organization, autonomous and separate from the YMCA of the USA. In the U.S., the more than 2,400 YMCAs offer sporting and recreational programs, summer camps, childcare, art classes, and community development for all groups of people. Users can find their local YMCA using the web address above.

Sun and Skin Cancer Resources (Chapter 4)

American Academy of Dermatology (AAD)

930 North Meacham Road
P.O. Box 4014
Schaumburg, IL 60168-4014
Phone: 847-330-0230
Toll-free: 888-462-DERM (888-462-3376)—to locate a dermatologist
Fax: 847-330-0050
Web site: *http://www.aad.org*
The AAD is a professional organization that is dedicated to achieving the highest quality of dermatologic care for everyone. On their web site, the Patient Information section provides the general public with links to foundations and patient support groups, news updates related to dermatologic conditions, patient education, and skin cancer updates.

The National Coalition for Skin Cancer Prevention in Health, Physical Education, Recreation, and Youth Sports

American Association for Health Education

1900 Association Drive
Reston, VA 20191
Phone: 703-476-3427
Fax: 703-476-6638
E-mail: aahe@aahperd.org
Web site: *http://www.sunsafety.org*
This organization was created by the
American Alliance for Health, Physical
Education, Recreation and Dance through
a cooperative agreement with Centers for
Disease Control and Prevention to increase
the awareness of skin cancer prevention.
The Coalition strives to be the driving force
behind skin cancer prevention education
strategies for children.

The National Skin Cancer Prevention Education Program

Centers for Disease Control and
Prevention (CDC)
National Center for Chronic Disease
Prevention and Health Promotion
Division of Cancer Prevention and Control
4770 Buford Highway NE
MS/K64
Atlanta, GA 30341
Toll-free: 888-842-6355
Fax: 770-488-4760
E-mail: cancerinfo@cdc.gov
Web site: *http://www.cdc.gov/cancer/nscpep*
The National Skin Cancer Prevention
Education Program is the CDC's skin
cancer prevention and education program.
It is designed to reduce illness and death
in order to achieve the *Healthy People 2010*
skin cancer prevention goals of increasing
to at least 75% the proportion of adults
who regularly use at least one protective

measure, limit sun exposure, and use
sunscreen.

The National Weather Service (NWS)

National Oceanic and Atmospheric
Administration (NOAA)
1325 East-West Highway
Silver Spring, MD 20910
E-mail: w-nws.webmaster@noaa.gov
Web site: *http://www.nws.noaa.gov*
The NWS provides weather, hydrologic,
and climate forecasts and warnings for
the U.S., its territories, adjacent waters,
and ocean areas for the protection of life
and property and the enhancement of the
national economy. NWS data and products
include current weather and UV Index
information, climate archives, statistical
tables, and links to other sites.

Skin Cancer Foundation

245 5th Avenue, Suite 1403
New York, NY 10016
Phone: 212-725-5176
Toll-free: 800-754-6490 (for information
packet only)
Fax: 212-725-5751
E-mail: info@skincancer.org
Web site: *http://www.skincancer.org*
The Skin Cancer Foundation is a nonprofit national and international organization concerned with skin cancer. It
conducts public and medical education
programs and provides support for medical training and research. Access the web
site for information about skin cancer
including melanoma, basal cell, and

squamous cell, pictures and descriptions of skin cancers, as well as information about sun safety and self-examination.

The SunWise School Program

1200 Pennsylvania Avenue (6205J)
Washington, DC 20460
Phone: 202-564-2289
Fax: 202-565-2096
Web site: *http://www.epa.gov/sunwise*
To help raise awareness about the effects of overexposure to the sun's harmful ultraviolet (UV) rays and ways to reduce risk, the U.S. Environmental Protection Agency (EPA) created the national SunWise School Program. SunWise is an environmental and health education program designed to teach students (grades K-8) and their caregivers how to protect themselves from overexposure to the sun.

Smoking Information and Quit Smoking Resources (Chapter 5)

American Lung Association (ALA)

1740 Broadway
New York, NY 10019
Phone: 212-315-8700
Toll-free: 800-LUNG-USA (800-586-4872)
Fax: 212-265-5642
Web site: *http://www.lungusa.org*
The mission of the ALA is to prevent lung disease and promote lung health. ALA fights lung disease in all its forms, with special emphasis on asthma, tobacco control, and environmental health.

Nicotine Anonymous-World Services

419 Main Street, PMB #370
Huntington Beach, CA 92648
Phone: 415-750-0328
E-mail: info@nicotine-anonymous.org
Web site: *http://www.nicotine-anonymous.org*
Nicotine Anonymous is an anonymous support group, based on a twelve-step fellowship, of people who want to live free of nicotine addiction. The Nicotine Anonymous web site provides nicotine cessation and support literature in five languages, answers to frequently asked questions about nicotine addiction, and a worldwide list of meetings.

The Office on Smoking and Health (OSH)

Centers for Disease Control and Prevention (CDC)
National Center for Chronic Disease Prevention and Health Promotion
4770 Buford Highway NE
MS/K50
Atlanta, GA 30341-3724
Phone: 770-488-5705
Toll-free: 800-CDC-1311 (800-232-1311) for prepared voice/fax information only
E-mail: tobaccoinfo@cdc.gov
Web site: *http://www.cdc.gov/tobacco*
This CDC office is a division within the National Center for Chronic Disease Prevention and Health Promotion. OSH is responsible for leading and coordinating strategic efforts aimed at preventing tobacco use among youth, promoting tobacco cessation, and protecting nonsmokers

from environmental tobacco smoke (ETS). The web site offers public education and information on smoking and how to stop.

The Office of the Surgeon General
5600 Fishers Lane, Room 18-66
Rockville, MD 20857
Toll-free: 800-789-2547 for information, reports, and fact sheets
Web site: *http://www.surgeongeneral.gov*
The Office of the Surgeon General is part of the Office of Public Health and Science. It is also a part of the larger U.S. Department of Health and Human Services. Reports of the Surgeon General and other publications are available via the web site.

Resources for STDs and Infectious Agents (Chapter 6)

American Social Health Association (ASHA)
P.O. Box 13827
Research Triangle Park, NC 27709
Phone: 919-361-8400
Toll-free: CDC National HIV/AIDS Hotline 800-342-2437; CDC National STD Hotline 800-227-8922
Fax: 919-361-8425
E-mail: hiv-stdnet@ashastd.org for general STD and HIV/AIDS questions; hpvnet@ashastd.org for questions about HPV and cervical cancer; and herpesnet@ashastd.org for herpes questions
Web site: *http://www.ashastd.org*
The ASHA is a nonprofit organization dedicated to stopping sexually transmitted diseases. ASHA is the managing agency for several hotlines that are funded and supported by the Centers for Disease Control and Prevention.

HIV InSite
4150 Clement Street, Building 16
VAMC 111V – University of California
San Francisco
Fax: 415-379-5547
E-mail: info@hivinsite.ucsf.edu
Web site: *http://hivinsite.ucsf.edu/InSite.jsp*
HIV InSite is a web site developed by the University of California San Francisco, in collaboration with three other leading health science institutions. The site aims to be a source for comprehensive, in-depth HIV/AIDS information and knowledge. The HIV InSite Knowledge Base is a complete textbook with extensive references and related links organized by topic.

HIV/AIDS Treatment Information Services (ATIS)
P.O. Box 6303
Rockville, MD 20849-6303
Phone: 301-519-0459
Toll-free: 800-HIV-0440 (800-448-0040)
Fax: 301-519-6616
E-mail: Atis@hivatis.org
Web site: *http://www.hivatis.org*
ATIS is a service of the Department of Health and Human Services. Information specialists answer questions about HIV treatment options using a network of federal, national, and community-based information resources. The web site provides information about federally approved

medications and therapies, AIDS-related conditions, public education materials, clinical trial updates, and a glossary.

National Center for Infectious Diseases (NCID)

Office of Health Communication
Centers for Disease Control and
Prevention (CDC)
MS/C14
1600 Clifton Road
Atlanta, GA 30333
Web site: *http://www.cdc.gov/ncidod*
The mission of the NCID is to prevent illness, disability, and death caused by infectious diseases in the U.S. and around the world. By working in partnership with other public health officials on a local, national, and international level, the Center conducts surveillance, epidemic investigations, epidemiologic and laboratory research, training, and public education programs to develop, evaluate, and promote prevention and control strategies for infectious diseases.

CDC National Prevention Information Network (CDC NPIN)

P.O. Box 6003
Rockville, MD 20849-6003
Phone: 301-562-1098
Toll-free: 800-458-5231
Fax: 888-282-7681; 301-562-1050
Web site: *http://www.cdcnpin.org*
The CDC NPIN is a reference, referral, and distribution service for information on HIV/AIDS, sexually transmitted diseases (STDs), and tuberculosis (TB).

CDC NPIN provides publications on HIV/AIDS, STDs, and TB by mail or fax and referrals to HIV/AIDS organizations, local services, and treatment centers. The CDC NPIN web site includes publications on HIV/AIDS, STDs, and TB, other related organizations, local services, and conference dates.

Stress and Mental Health Resources (Chapter 7)

American Psychological Association (APA)

750 First Street NE
Washington, DC 20002-4242
Phone: 202-336-5510
Toll-free: 800-374-2721
E-mail: public.affairs@apa.org
Web site: *http://www.apa.org*
The APA is a nonprofit corporation working toward the advancement of psychology as a science, a profession, and a means of promoting human welfare. The APA has a Division on Health Psychology that addresses a range of health issues. The APA provides a hotline to obtain literature and discuss psychological conditions referrals to state psychological associations to locate a psychologist in a specific area. The APA web site provides information about psychological issues.

Center for Mental Health Services (CMHS)

5600 Fishers Lane, Room 17-99
Rockville, MD 20857
Created by Congress, the CMHS leads Federal efforts to treat mental illnesses

by promoting mental health and by preventing the development or worsening of mental illness when possible. CMHS is a component of the Substance Abuse and Mental Health Services Administration, a division of the U.S. Department of Health and Human Services.

Knowledge Exchange Network (KEN)
P.O. Box 42490
Washington, DC 20015
Toll-free: 800-789-2647
Fax: 301-984-8796
E-mail: ken@mentalhealth.org
Web site: *http://www.mentalhealth.org*
The KEN, a service of CMHS, is a national clearinghouse for free information about mental health, including publications, references, and referrals to local and national resources and organizations. KEN provides a publications list, articles, booklets, fact sheets, and videos about various mental health issues, information about community resources, and more. The web site provides the same information on-line.

National Institute of Mental Health (NIMH)
NIMH Public Inquiries
6001 Executive Boulevard, RM 8184, MSC 9663
Bethesda, MD 20892-9663
Phone: 301-443-4513 (information specialists available)
Toll-free for automated system for ordering free materials: 800-421-4211 for depres

sion; 800-647-2642 for panic disorders; 888-826-9438 for anxiety disorders
Fax: 301-443-4279
E-mail: nimhinfo@nih.gov
Web site: *http://www.nimh.nih.gov*
The NIMH is a branch of the National Institutes of Health. Its goal is to alleviate suffering due to depressive illnesses. NIMH services include answering questions about depression and other mental disorders and providing printed materials. The NIMH web site includes a section with information about the symptoms, diagnosis, and treatment of mental illnesses. Included are brochures and information sheets, reports, press releases, fact sheets, and other educational materials.

National Mental Health Association (NMHA)
1021 Prince Street
Alexandria, VA 22314-2971
Phone: 703-684-7722
Toll-free: 800-969-NMHA (800-969-6642) for Mental Health Information Center
Fax: 703-684-5968
E-mail: infoctr@nmha.org
Web site: *http://www.nmha.org*
The NMHA is the country's oldest and largest nonprofit organization addressing all aspects of mental health and mental illness. The organization is dedicated to promoting mental health, preventing mental disorders, and achieving victory over mental illness through advocacy, education, research, and service.

American Public Health Association (APHA)

800 I Street NW
Washington, DC 20001-3710
Phone: 202-777-APHA (202-777-2742)
Fax: 202-772-2534
E-mail: comments@apha.org
Web site: *http://www.apha.org*
The APHA is a nonprofit membership organization of public health professionals that seeks to protect and promote personal and environmental health. The web site provides information on APHA, membership, and public health news and information.

CHEMTREC®

1300 Wilson Boulevard
Arlington, VA 22209
Phone: 703-741-5500 (Customer Service)
Toll-free: 800-262-8200
Fax: 703-741-6037
E-mail: chemtrec@americanchemistry.com
Web site: *http://www.chemtrec.org*
CHEMTREC (Chemical Transportation Emergency Center) was established in 1971 by the chemical industry as a public service hotline for fire fighters, law enforcement, and other emergency responders to obtain information and assistance for emergency incidents involving chemicals and hazardous materials. The twenty-four-hour Call Center maintains a Manufacturers Safety Data Sheet (MSDS) database.

Consumer Federation of America (CFA)

1424 16th Street NW, Suite 604
Washington, DC 20036
Phone: 202-387-6121
Fax: 202-265-7989
E-mail: cfa@consumerfed.org
Web site: *http://www.consumerfed.org*
Established in 1968, CFA is an advocacy, education, and membership organization. It gathers facts, analyzes issues, and distributes information to the public, legislators, and regulators. Specific areas of interest include finances, utilities, product safety, transportation, health care, and food safety.

The Radon Fix-it Program

Toll-free: 800-644-6999
Web site: *http://www.radonfixit.org*
The Radon Fix-it Line is supported by the CFA Foundation, a nonprofit organization established to complement the CFA's activities. The toll-free phone line provides information that will allow consumers to take the necessary steps toward fixing radon problems in their homes.

Cosmetic, Toiletry, and Fragrance Association (CTFA)

1101 17th Street NW, Suite 300
Washington DC 20036-4702
Phone: 202-331-1770
Fax: 202-331-1969
Web site: *www.ctfa.org*
As a U.S. trade association for the personal care products industry, CTFA works to protect the freedom of the industry to

compete in a fair and responsible market-place. The web site provides safety and general interest information about personal care products under the Consumer Information link.

Environmental Health Center

1025 Connecticut Avenue NW, Suite 1200
Washington, DC 20036
Phone: 202-293-2270
Fax: 202-293-0032
E-mail: ehc@nsc.org
Web site: *http://www.nsc.org/ehc.htm*
As a division of the National Safety Council (see page 375), the Environmental Health Center is a leading provider of credible and timely information and community-based programs on environmental and public health issues.

Radon Hotline

Toll-free: 800-557-2366 to speak to an information specialist; 800-767-7236 to request a brochure about radon
E-mail: airqual@nsc.org
Web site: *http://www.nsc.org/ehc/radon.htm*
The National Safety Council in conjunction with the Environmental Health Center has established a Radon Hotline to answer questions and provide materials about radon, its health effects, and radon testing.

Environmental Protection Agency (EPA)

Ariel Rios Building
1200 Pennsylvania Avenue NW
Washington, DC 20460-2403
Phone: 202-260-2090

E-mail: public-access@epa.gov
Web site: *http://www.epa.gov*
The mission of the EPA is to protect human health and to safeguard the natural environment. The EPA provides information and materials on many topics, including radon, hazardous waste, air and water pollution, environmental tobacco smoke (ETS), pesticides, drinking water, and programs and activities of the EPA. A full listing of information topics, publications, and hotlines is available on the web site.

Envirofacts Data Warehouse and Applications

Web site: *http://www.epa.gov/enviro*
Envirofacts contains chemical data from several different program system data-bases. The Envirofacts Master Chemical Integrator (EMCI) identifies the chemicals in these systems. Using this integrator, you can learn details about a chemical substance, such as chemical names, discharge limits, and reported releases without knowing how the chemical is identified in the various program office systems throughout the Envirofacts database.

International Agency for Research on Cancer (IARC)/ Centre International de Recherche sur le Cancer (CIRC)

150 Cours Albert-Thomas
F-69372 Lyon Cedex 08
France
Phone: (0) 4-72-73-84-85 (country code 33)
Fax: (0) 4-72-73-85-75 (country code 33)
Web site: *http://www.iarc.fr*

The IARC is part of the World Health Organization (WHO). The organization is involved in both epidemiological and laboratory cancer research. The IARC disseminates scientific information, including statistics, through publications, meetings, courses, and fellowships. The IARC web site contains three databases with information on the occurrence of cancer worldwide and carcinogenic risks to humans, a list of publications, links to related cancer sites, and a web-based e-mail form for other inquiries.

National Institute for Occupational Safety and Health (NIOSH)

Centers for Disease Control and Prevention (CDC)
4676 Columbia Parkway
Cincinnati, OH 45226-1998
Phone: 513-533-8573
Toll-free: 800-35-NIOSH (800-356-4674)
Fax: 513-533-8573; toll-free fax-on-demand: 888-232-3299
E-mail: pubstaft@cdc.gov
Web site: *http://www.cdc.gov/niosh*
NIOSH is the division of the CDC responsible for conducting research and making recommendations for the prevention of work-related illnesses and injuries. NIOSH also investigates potentially hazardous working conditions as requested by employers or employees. NIOSH information specialists and the NIOSH web site provide information on many work safety topics including lung diseases, cancer, asbestos and other chemical haz-ards, indoor air quality, electromagnetic fields, and personal protective equipment.

National Institute of Environmental Health Sciences (NIEHS)

111 Alexander Drive
P.O. Box 12233
Research Triangle Park, NC 27709
Phone: 919-541-3345 (Office of Communications)
Fax: 919-541-2242
E-mail: webcenter@niehs.nih.gov
Web site: *http://www.niehs.nih.gov*
The mission of the NIEHS, a part of the National Institutes of Health and the U.S. Department of Health and Human Services, is to reduce the burden of human illness and dysfunction from environmental causes by understanding each of these elements and how they interrelate. NIEHS provides environmental health information via its web site.

Electric and Magnetic Fields Research and Public Information Dissemination (EMF RAPID)

Web site: *http://www.niehs.nih.gov/emfrapid*
NIEHS and the Department of Energy (DOE) coordinate the EMF RAPID program and web site. This program has the goal of determining if electric and magnetic fields associated with the generation, transmission, and use of electrical energy pose a risk to human health. The EMF RAPID web site provides information on electromagnetic fields and links to other EMF information sources.

National Pesticides Telecommunication Network (NPTN)

Oregon State University
333 Weniger
Corvallis, OR 97331-6502
Toll-free: 800-858-7378 (National Pesticides Telecommunication Network)
Fax: 541-737-0761
E-mail: nptn@ace.orst.edu
Web site: *http://www.ace.orst.edu/info/nptn*
The NPTN is a cooperative service of Oregon State University and the EPA that provides information about a wide variety of pesticide-related subjects, including pesticide products, recognition and management of pesticide poisoning, toxicology, and environmental chemistry. NPTN provides assistance in interpreting and understanding toxicology and environmental chemistry information about pesticides, pesticide label information, referrals to other agencies for information about pesticide incident investigation, emergency human and animal treatment, safety practices, clean-up and disposal, and laboratory analyses and general information on the regulation of pesticides in the United States.

National Toxicology Program (NTP)

National Institutes of Health
National Institute of Environmental Health Sciences
P.O. Box 12233
Research Triangle Park, NC 27709-2233

E-mail: ntpwm@niehs.nih.gov
Web site: *http://ntp-server.niehs.nih.gov*
The NTP's mission is to evaluate agents of public health concern by developing and applying tools of modern toxicology and molecular biology. The NTP's *Report on Carcinogens* identifies substances and mixtures or exposure circumstances that are *"known"* or are *"reasonably anticipated"* to cause cancer and to which a significant number of Americans are exposed. The *Report on Carcinogens* is published every two years and is available on the NTP web site.

Occupational Safety and Health Administration (OSHA)

U.S. Department of Labor
200 Constitution Ave NW
Washington, DC 20210
Phone: 202-693-1999 (Public Affairs Office)
Toll free: 800-321-OSHA (800-321-6742) for workplace safety and health-related questions
Web site: *http://www.osha.gov*
OSHA is responsible for creating and enforcing workplace safety and health regulations. Look on the OSHA web site for information about lists of known and suspected carcinogens, hazardous information bulletins, information on reproductive hazards, links to other Department of Labor web sites, an e-mail feedback form, and regulations and compliance links.

U.S. Food and Drug Administration (FDA)

(See page 377 – Food and Nutrition Resources, Chapter 2)

National Center for Toxicological Research (NCTR)

3900 NCTR Road
Jefferson, AR 72079
Phone: 870-543-7130
Web site: *http://www.fda.gov/nctr*
The mission of the NCTR is to conduct scientific research that supports and anticipates the FDA's future regulatory needs, such as identifying the biological mechanisms that make a substance toxic and developing methods to improve assessment of human exposure, susceptibility, and risk.

Early Detection and Screening Resources (Chapter 9)

American Board of Medical Specialties (ABMS)

(See page 371 – Health Organizations, Chapter 1)

Center for Devices and Radiological Health

U.S. Food and Drug Administration (FDA)
CDRH/FDA Consumer Staff
1350 Piccard Drive
HFZ-210
Rockville, MD 20850
Phone: 301-827-3990 (press 5)
Toll-free: 888-463-6332
Fax: 301-443-9535

Web site: *http://www.fda.gov/cdrh*
The Center for Devices and Radiological Health protects public health by providing reasonable assurance of the safety and effectiveness of medical devices and eliminating unnecessary human exposure to radiation emitted from electronic products.

FDA's Mammography Program

Toll-free: 800-838-7715 (Mammography Facility Hotline)
Fax: 410-290-6351
E-mail: MQSAhotline@SSSI.net
Web: *http://www.fda.gov/cdrh/mammography/fda_certified_mammography_faci.html*
Charged by Congress to develop and implement the Mammography Quality Standards Act, the FDA created the Division of Mammography Quality and Radiation Programs (DMQRP). The web site can be searched by state or zip code to find FDA-certified mammography centers in your area.

National Alliance of Breast Cancer Organizations (NABCO)

9 East Thirty-seventh Street, 10th floor
New York, NY 10016
Toll-Free: 888-80-NABCO (888-806-2226)
Phone (emergencies only): 212-889-0606
Fax: 212-689-1213
E-mail: nabcoinfo@aol.com
Web site: *http://www.nabco.org*
This nonprofit organization includes a network of more than 400 organizations. The NABCO web site includes information about breast cancer and breast health, a directory of nationwide events,

a resource list, a list of local support groups, and a directory of clinical trials. The site also allows women to register for a mammography e-mail reminder.

National Cancer Institute (NCI)

NCI Public Inquiries Office
Building 31, Room 10A31
31 Center Drive, MSC 2580
Bethesda, MD 20892-2580
Phone: 301-435-3848
Toll-free: 800-4-CANCER (800-422-6237) for Cancer Information Service
Fax: CancerFax: 800-624-2511 or 301-402-5874, which contains PDQ (Physician Data Query) full-text summaries on cancer treatment, screening, prevention, genetics, and supportive care; fact sheets on current cancer topics; and topic searches from the CANCERLIT database
E-mail: webmaster@cancer.gov
Web site: *http://www.nci.nih.gov*
The NCI leads the nation's fight against cancer by supporting and conducting groundbreaking research in cancer biology, causation, prevention, detection, treatment, and survivorship. Through CancerNet, it provides materials for health professionals, patients, and the public, including information from PDQ (Physician Data Query) about cancer treatment, screening, prevention, supportive care, and clinical trials and from CANCERLIT, a bibliographic database.

Division of Cancer Prevention

Web site: *http://cancer.gov/prevention*

The Division of Cancer Prevention is the primary unit of the NCI devoted to cancer prevention research.

Screen for Life: National Colorectal Cancer Action Campaign

Centers for Disease Control and Prevention (CDC)
Cancer Prevention and Control
4770 Buford Highway NE
MS/K64
Atlanta, GA 30341
Toll-free: 888-842-6355
Fax: 770-488-4760
E-mail: cancerinfo@cdc.gov
Screen for Life is a program implemented by the CDC, the Centers for Medicare and Medicaid Services, and the National Cancer Institute. It serves to inform men and women aged fifty years and older about the importance of having regular colorectal cancer screening tests. The web site contains information about colorectal cancer facts, educational materials, and other resources.

The Susan G. Komen Breast Cancer Foundation

5005 LBJ Freeway, Suite 250
Dallas, TX 75244
Toll-free (Breast Care Helpline): 800-IM-AWARE (800-462-9273)
Phone: 972-855-1600
Fax: 972-855-1605
E-mail: helpline@komen.org
Web site: *http://www.komen.org*
This organization promotes research,

education, screening, and treatment. The web site contains the latest news and information regarding breast health, drug therapies, treatment options, educational events and meetings, survivor stories, and other breast cancer–related information.

US TOO! International, Inc.

5003 Fairview Avenue
Downers Grove, IL 60515
Toll-free: 800-80-US-TOO (800-808-7866)
Phone: 630-795-1002
Fax: 630-795-1602
E-mail: ustoo@ustoo.com
Web site: *http://www.ustoo.com*
This independent group provides prostate cancer survivors and their families with emotional and educational support.

Y-ME National Breast Cancer Organization

212 West Van Buren, Suite 500
Chicago, IL 60607
Toll-free hotline: 800-221-2141; toll-free (Spanish): 800-986-9505
Phone: 312-986-8338
Fax: 312-294-8597
Web site: *http://www.y-me.org*
Web site (Spanish version): *http://www.y-me.org/spanish.htm*
This organization focuses on providing information and support to people with breast cancer and their families. Y-ME provides a national hotline, public meetings and seminars, workshops for professionals, referral services, support groups, a newsletter, a resource library, a teen program, and advocacy information.

Glossary

ABCD rule: a guide to the warning signs for *melanoma* skin cancer, where **A** is for asymmetry, **B** is for border, **C** is for color, and **D** is for diameter.

abstinence: the act of not participating in an indulgence, such as food, alcohol, drugs, or sexual intercourse.

acquired immunodeficiency syndrome: see *AIDS*.

actinic keratosis: also known as solar keratosis, a *precancerous*, slow-growing skin condition caused by overexposure to the sun. It is possible, but not common, for actinic keratoses to turn into *squamous cell* cancer.

acute: having a sudden onset over a short time; intense and severe as related to a condition or disease.

aerobic: physical activity that involves increased and sustained cardiovascular levels (respiration and heart rate).

aflatoxin: a chemical produced by a fungus (mold) that sometimes contaminates peanuts, wheat, soybeans, ground nuts, corn, and rice. Aflatoxin is a very potent cause of liver *cancer*.

AIDS: the acronym for acquired immunodeficiency syndrome; an immune disorder caused by infection with the *retrovirus HIV*. AIDS develops over time, as the immune system becomes weaker, resulting in a suppressed response to other infections and *cancers*. See also *HIV* and *retrovirus*.

alternative therapy: an unproven therapy used *instead of* standard (proven) therapy. Some alternative therapies have dangerous or even life-threatening side effects. With others, the main danger is that the patient may lose the opportunity to benefit from proven treatment. See also *complementary therapy* and *integrative therapy*.

animal study: a study that uses animals (a more complex subject than *cells* or simple organisms), which can be researched in a well-controlled environment.

anthropometry: the science (a branch of anthropology) of measuring the human body with regard to height, weight, and component size, including skin-to-skin thickness using an instrument called a caliper(s).

antibody: a *protein* produced by *immune system* cells and released into the blood in response to infection. Antibodies defend against foreign agents such as bacteria, which contain substances called antigens. Each antibody works against a specific *antigen*.

antigen: a substance that causes the body's immune system to react. This reaction often involves production of antibodies. For example, the immune system's response to antigens that are part of bacteria and *viruses* helps people resist infections.

arsenic: a naturally occurring element that is present in rocks and soil, a by-product of some industrial processes, and, at one time, a component of many *pesticides*. Often present in low levels in drinking water, arsenic is very *toxic* when consumed in high doses. Long-term exposure increases the risk of certain cancers.

artificial sweetener: also called a sugar substitute, it is a chemical equivalent of sugar such as aspartame (NutraSweet, Equal) or saccharin (Sweet'N Low).

asbestos: a group of naturally occurring fibrous minerals used as insulation and to make commercial textiles. It causes scarring of the lungs and can eventually lead to asbestos-related cancers.

B cell: a type of lymphocyte (white blood cell important to immune response) that helps protect the body against bacteria by producing *antibodies*. Also called B lymphocyte.

basal cell carcinoma: the most common *nonmelanoma skin cancer*, which arises in the *basal layer*. It usually develops on sun-exposed areas, especially the head and neck. Basal cell cancer is slow growing and is not likely to spread to distant parts of the body.

basal layer: the lowest part of the *epidermis* formed by basal cells. These cells continually divide to form new *keratinocytes*.

beedies: see *bidis*.

behavioral therapy: a type of psychotherapy that helps a person to change the way he or she responds to certain circumstances, such as reacting calmly to a stressful situation.

benign: not *cancer*, not *malignant*.

benign prostatic hyperplasia (BPH): noncancerous enlargement of the *prostate* that may cause problems with urination, such as trouble starting and stopping the flow.

benzene: a colorless, flammable liquid with a sweet odor that is formed from both natural and man-made sources, including cigarette smoke. It is considered a human *carcinogen*.

bidis: flavored cigarettes imported from India; also called beedies.

biopsy: the removal of a sample of tissue to see whether *cancer cells* are present. There are several kinds of biopsy procedures. In some, a very thin needle is used to draw fluid and cells from a lump. In a core biopsy, a larger needle is used to remove more tissue.

body mass index (BMI): an index of *obesity* that uses weight and height to determine levels of body fatness for adults aged twenty and older. The formula to calculate BMI is mass in kilograms (kg) divided by the square of height in meters (m^2).

botanicals: a group of *dietary supplements* that includes herbal remedies, skin care products, and oils, teas, or capsules that are plant-derived, either in whole or in part.

breast self-exam (BSE): a method of checking one's own breasts for lumps or suspicious changes. BSE is recommended for all women over age twenty, to be done once a month, usually at a time other than the days before, during, or immediately after her menstrual period.

Burkitt's lymphoma: a deadly type of *non-Hodgkin's lymphoma* that occurs in the lymphoid tissue. This type of *cancer* usually affects children in central Africa, where chronic infections with malaria and Epstein-Barr virus (EBV) are important *risk factors* for this disease. It was named after Denis Parsons Burkitt, a British surgeon.

cancer: a group of diseases that cause *cells* in the body to change and grow out of control. Most types of cancer cells form a lump or mass called a *tumor*, which can invade and destroy healthy tissue. Cells from the tumor can break away, travel, and spread to other parts of the body, where they can continue to grow. This spreading process is called *metastasis*. When cancer spreads, it is still named after the part of the body where it started. For example, if breast cancer spreads to the lungs, it is still breast cancer, not lung cancer. Some cancers, such as blood cancers, do not form a tumor. Not all tumors are cancer.

cancer cluster: the occurrence of a specific type of *cancer* more often than expected in a particular community. Most true cancer clusters involve a single or rare type of cancer or a certain type of cancer in an age group not usually affected by that type of cancer.

carbohydrate: an essential *nutrient* and main source of energy in the form of sugar and starches for the human body. Carbohydrates are found in foods such as pasta, grains, breads and cereals, fruits and vegetables, and simple sugars such as honey and table sugar.

carcinogen: any agent—chemical, physical, or biological—that causes *cancer*. Carcinogens are capable of causing harmful *mutations* in the DNA of a person's cells, which can lead to cancer.

carcinogenesis: the process that changes normal *cells* into *cancer*.

carcinoma: a type of *malignant tumor* that tends to arise from *epithelial* (surface) cells on the outside or inside of the body, such as the skin or colon. At least 80 percent of all cancers are carcinomas.

cell: the basic unit of which all living things are made. Cells replace themselves by splitting and forming new cells. In *cancer*, the processes that control the formation of new cells and the death of old cells are disrupted.

cervical cancer: a *cancer* that begins in the lining of the cervix (the neck of the uterus). Cervical cancers do not form suddenly. The change from normal cervical tissue to precancer to cancer is gradual.

cervical intraepithelial neoplasia (CIN): abnormal growth of the cervical *cells* that represents a potentially *precancerous* change in the cervix.

chemotherapy: treatment with drugs to destroy cancer cells. Chemotherapy is often used with surgery or radiation to treat cancer when it has spread, when it has come back (recurred), or when there is a strong chance that it could recur.

cholesterol: a naturally produced compound present in all animal tissues. It is responsible for maintaining cell membranes, as well as aiding in the digestion of fats. High levels of cholesterol in the blood are associated with an increased risk of heart disease. See also *dietary cholesterol*.

chronic: of long duration; usually relating to disease that progresses slowly.

cigar: a roll of tobacco wrapped in a tobacco leaf or in any substance containing tobacco that is smoked. Cigar smoking increases the smoker's risk of lung cancer to nearly three times higher than that of nonsmokers.

cigarillo: a small *cigar*, usually about the size of a cigarette.

cirrhosis: chronic liver disease in which the normal tissue becomes scarred, affecting liver function. There are a number of potential causes, including alcohol abuse, nutritional deficiencies, hemochromatosis (a hereditary disease in which too much iron is absorbed into the liver), and infection with any of the hepatitis viruses.

clinical breast examination (CBE): an examination of the breasts done by a health professional such as a doctor or nurse.

clinical nurse specialist: a registered nurse with a master's or other advanced degree who specializes in the direct care of patients in specific areas, such as oncology or mental health nursing (Psych CNS).

cofactor: a substance that works in combination with something else to bring about a certain effect.

cognitive therapy: a type of psychotherapy that helps a person to change attitudes or patterns of thinking.

collagen: a fibrous *protein* found in the *dermis* of the skin that gives it resilience and strength.

colon: the part of the large intestine (large bowel) that extends from the end of the small intestine (small bowel) down to the rectum.

colonoscopy: an examination in which a colonoscope (a long, flexible, hollow, lighted tube about the thickness of a finger) is inserted through the rectum up into the colon. It allows a doctor to see the lining of the entire colon. The colonoscope is connected to a video camera and video display monitor so that the doctor can closely examine the inside of the colon.

colposcopy: an examination of the vagina and cervix using a colposcope, which is an instrument with magnifying lenses similar to binoculars. The colposcope magnifies the walls of the vagina and the surface of the cervix in order to verify abnormal growth or an abnormal *Pap test* result.

complementary therapy: supportive methods or therapies used *in addition to* standard (conventional or mainstream) treatments. Complementary methods are not intended to cure disease; rather, they are provided to help control symptoms and improve quality of life. Some methods, such as massage therapy, yoga, and meditation, which are now called complementary, have been previously referred to as "supportive care." See also *alternative therapy* and *integrative therapy*.

computed tomography: an imaging test in which many x-rays are taken from different angles of a part of the body. A computer combines the images to produce cross-sectional pictures of soft tissues, especially internal organs. It is often referred to as a "CT" or "CAT" scan.

congenital: present at birth. This can refer either to something inherited (from parents' genes) or to something caused by environmental factors.

congenital melanocytic nevus: also called a congenital mole or birthmark; a mole present at birth.

contagious: able to be spread from one to another easily, either by direct or indirect contact; communicable or transmissible.

CT scan: see *computed tomography*.

dermatologist: a doctor who specializes in skin diseases.

dermis: the middle, thicker layer of the skin, located below the *epidermis*. It contains hair follicles, nerve endings, sweat glands, and blood and *lymph* vessels held in place by a *protein* called *collagen*.

diagnosis: identifying a disease by its signs or symptoms and by using imaging procedures and laboratory findings. The earlier a diagnosis of cancer is made, the better the chance for long-term survival.

dietary cholesterol: *cholesterol* consumed as part of the human diet. All animal food products contain cholesterol. Plant foods contain no cholesterol. Because the body produces enough of its own cholesterol, limiting the amount of dietary cholesterol is important for reducing the risk of heart disease. See also *cholesterol*.

dietary fat: *fat* consumed as a part of the human diet. Foods from animal sources are the major contributors of dietary fat. There are several types of dietary fats, some of which appear to increase the risk of certain diseases more than others. See also *fat*.

dietary supplements: also called nutritional supplements, products that include *vitamins*, *minerals*, herbs, amino acids, and *botanicals* that are not already approved by the FDA as drugs.

dietitian: a health care professional who applies the science of nutrition in a variety of settings. Dietitians and nutritionists help prevent and treat illnesses by promoting healthy eating habits, scientifically evaluating people's diets, and suggesting ways to improve them. A registered dietitian (R.D.) has at least a bachelor's degree and has passed a national competency exam. The term nutritionist is also used, but no educational requirements are associated with this title. See also *nutritionist*.

digital rectal examination (DRE): an exam in which the doctor inserts a gloved finger into the rectum to feel for anything abnormal. Some *tumors* of the rectum and *prostate* gland can be felt during a DRE.

DNA: abbreviation for deoxyribonucleic acid; genetic material in each *cell* that contains information on growth, division, and function.

doctor of osteopathy (D.O.): this health care professional attends an osteopathic medical school, which focuses on a more holistic (whole person) approach to medicine.

double-contrast barium enema (DCBE): an imaging test sometimes used to screen for colorectal cancer. Also called barium enema with air contrast, it involves the use of barium sulfate, a chalky substance, to partially fill and open up the colon. When the colon is about half full of barium, air is inserted to cause the colon to expand. This allows x-ray films to show abnormalities of the colon.

dysplasia: abnormal development of tissue.

dysplastic nevus: also known as an atypical mole, it increases a person's risk of *melanoma*. Dysplastic nevi usually look more irregular than normal moles and may appear anywhere on the body. They often run in families (known as dysplastic nevus syndrome).

early detection: finding cancer at an early stage, before it has grown large or spread to other sites. Many forms of cancer can reach an advanced stage without causing symptoms, which is why early detection is so important.

environment: the combination of circumstances, physical conditions, and outside influences surrounding an individual.

environmental tobacco smoke: see *secondhand smoke*.

epidemiology: the study of diseases in populations by collecting and analyzing statistical data. In the field of cancer, epidemiologists look at how many people have cancer, who gets specific types of cancer, and what factors (such as exposures, job hazards, family patterns, and personal habits, such as smoking and diet) play a part in the development of cancer.

epidermis: the top layer of the skin that serves as the body's outer protection from injury, infection, and dehydration.

epithelium: the outer layer of cells that covers many of the internal and external surfaces of the body, such as the skin and the lining of the intestines.

Epstein-Barr virus (EBV): a herpesvirus that causes infectious mononucleosis ("the kissing disease") and is also sometimes associated with certain types of *cancer*. It is estimated that nearly 90 percent of the U.S. population has been exposed to EBV.

exposure assessment: the determination of the levels of a hazard in the environment (such as in air, water, and food) and the extent to which people are actually exposed.

fat: an essential *nutrient* that helps the body absorb certain *vitamins*, stores energy, and helps maintain hair and skin. When stored in fat cells, it helps protect vital organs as well. See also *dietary fat*.

fatty acids: the building blocks of *fats*.

fecal occult blood test (FOBT): a test for "hidden" blood in the stool. The presence of such blood could be a sign of *cancer*.

first-degree relative: a parent, sibling, or child.

flexible sigmoidoscopy: an examination in which a slender, flexible, hollow, lighted tube (called a sigmoidoscope) about the thickness of a finger is inserted through the rectum up into the colon. It allows a doctor to look at the lining of the rectum and part of the colon for *cancer* or *polyps*. The sigmoidoscope is connected to a video camera and video display monitor so that the doctor can view, and even videotape, any abnormal findings.

gene: a segment of *DNA* that contains information on hereditary characteristics such as hair color, eye color, and height, as well as susceptibility to certain diseases.

general practitioner (G.P.): a doctor with a basic level of training; also referred to as a generalist.

genetic: determined by genes; inherited, as opposed to having an environmental cause.

hepatitis: the general condition of inflammation or swelling of the liver caused by certain toxins, drugs, or alcohol abuse or caused by infection with certain *viruses*, bacteria, parasites, or fungi. Hepatitis B virus (HBV) and hepatitis C virus (HCV) can cause chronic hepatitis, a risk factor for liver cancer.

herbal remedies: *dietary supplements* derived from the leafy parts of plants.

hereditary: inherited; capable of being transmitted genetically from a parent to a child.

HHV-8: an acronym for human herpes virus type 8, which is also known as *Kaposi's sarcoma-associated herpes virus (KSHV)*. It is a member of the herpes family of *viruses*.

HIV: an acronym for human immunodeficiency virus; a *retrovirus* that can be transmitted by injection into the bloodstream (using contaminated needles); by vaginal or anal intercourse; through blood products or organ or tissue transplant; or from mother to child during pregnancy, birth, or breast-feeding. The *virus* infects and destroys the *T cells* of the immune system, which, over time, may result in the development of acquired immunodeficiency syndrome, or *AIDS*. See also *AIDS* and *retrovirus*.

hormone: a chemical substance released into the body by the endocrine glands, such as the thyroid and adrenal glands, or by organs such as the ovaries. Hormones travel through the bloodstream and set in motion various body functions. Testosterone and estrogen are examples of male and female hormones.

hormone replacement therapy (HRT): the use of estrogen and progesterone from an outside source after the body has stopped making it because of natural or induced *menopause*. This type of hormone therapy is often given to relieve symptoms of menopause and may offer protection against heart disease and thinning of the bones *(osteoporosis)* in women after menopause.

HTLV-1: an acronym for human T-cell leukemia/lymphoma virus type 1, a *retrovirus* that causes adult T-cell leukemia/*lymphoma*. It can be transmitted by sexual intercourse; via a contaminated needle; from mother to child during pregnancy, birth, or breast-feeding; or by transfusion of blood products. See also *retrovirus*.

human herpes virus type 8: see *HHV-8*.

human immunodeficiency virus: see *HIV*.

human papillomavirus (HPV): any number of *papillomaviruses* that cause warts or *papillomas*, which are *benign* (noncancerous) *tumors*. These warts can appear on the skin, mouth, larynx (voice box), anus, or genital organs. HPV infection is a *risk factor* for some types of *cancers*, particularly cervical cancer.

human T-cell leukemia/lymphoma virus type 1: see *HTLV-1*.

hydrogenation: the process of adding hydrogen to a compound, particularly in the case of converting an unsaturated *fat* or *fatty acid* to a solid. An example is vegetable oil converted to margarine. Hydrogenation produces trans fats, which can increase the risk of heart disease when eaten in large amounts.

immune system: the complex system by which the body resists infection by microbes such as bacteria or viruses and rejects transplanted tissues or organs. The immune system may also help the body fight some cancers.

incidence: the number of new cases of a disease that occur in a population each year.

infectious disease: a disease caused by an organism, such as bacteria, a *virus*, or fungi, invading the body where it grows and spreads.

informed consent: the process of explaining a course of treatment, along with the risks, benefits, and possible alternatives; the legal document signifying that a patient understands this information and agrees to treatment.

inherited: transmitted genetically from parent to child.

integrative therapy: the combined use of evidence-based proven therapies (conventional or standard treatments) and *complementary therapies*.

invasive cancer: *cancer* that has spread beyond the layer of *cells* where it first developed to tissues or organs nearby.

in vitro study: a study that uses bacteria or animal *cells* grown in laboratory dishes or test tubes. In the case of possible *carcinogens*, researchers add suspected carcinogens and then examine the *DNA* of the cells for *mutations*.

involuntary smoking: breathing in the smoke from others or from burning cigarettes, especially by a nonsmoker; also called passive smoking.

Kaposi's sarcoma (KS): a *cancer* that develops in connective tissue such as cartilage, bone, fat, muscle, blood vessels, or fibrous tissues (related to tendons or ligaments). This disease typically causes *tumors* to develop in the tissues below the skin surface or in the mucous membranes of the mouth, nose, or anus. Once considered rare, KS *incidence* has increased along with the number of *HIV* infections; it is now considered an "*AIDS*-defining condition."

Kaposi's sarcoma-associated herpes virus (KSHV): see *HHV-8*.

keratin: the main *protein* that makes up the structure of the hair, nails, and other hard tissues. It is produced by skin cells called *keratinocytes*. Keratin also contributes to the skin's ability to protect the rest of the body.

keratinocytes: *squamous cells* that are the main type of *cell* of the *epidermis* of the skin.

kreteks: another name for clove cigarettes, a type of tobacco product imported from Indonesia.

latent period: the time between exposure to a *carcinogen* and the development of *cancer (carcinogenesis)*.

leukemia: cancer of the blood or blood-forming organs. People with leukemia often have a noticeable increase in white blood cells (leukocytes).

lipids: a group of organic compounds that includes *fats*, oils, *cholesterol*, and triglycerides. Lipids do not dissolve in water. Along with *carbohydrates* and *proteins*, lipids are part of the basic composition of *cells*.

lipoproteins: *proteins* that are combined with at least one *lipid* component; the main transport for lipids (such as cholesterol) through the blood.

lymphatic system: the tissues and organs (including *lymph nodes*, spleen, thymus, and bone marrow) that produce and store *lymphocytes* (*cells* that fight infection) and the channels that carry the lymph fluid. The entire lymphatic system is an important part of the body's immune system. Invasive *cancers* sometimes penetrate the lymphatic vessels (channels) and spread (metastasize) to lymph nodes.

> *lymph:* clear fluid that flows through the lymphatic vessels and contains *cells* known as *lymphocytes*. These cells are important in fighting infections and may also have a role in fighting *cancer*.

> *lymph nodes:* also called lymph glands, small bean-shaped collections of immune system tissue found along lymphatic vessels. They remove *cell* waste and fluids from *lymph*.

> *lymphocyte:* a type of white blood *cell* that helps the body fight infection. Lymphocytes are the main cell type found in lymphoid tissue, of which there are two main types: *B cells* (B lymphocytes) and *T cells* (T lymphocytes).

lymphoma: a *cancer* of the *lymphatic system*. Lymphoma involves *lymphocytes*. The two main types of lymphoma are Hodgkin's disease and *non-Hodgkin's lymphoma*.

magnetic resonance imaging (MRI): a method of taking internal pictures of the soft tissues (such as internal organs) using a powerful magnet to transmit radio waves through the body; the images appear on a computer screen as well as on film.

mainstream smoke: the part of *secondhand smoke* that is exhaled by a smoker (as opposed to *sidestream smoke*).

malignant: cancerous.

mammogram: a low-dose x-ray of the breast using a special type of machine used only for this purpose. A mammogram can show a developing breast *tumor* before it is large enough to be felt by a woman or even by a highly skilled health care professional. Screening mammography is used to help find breast cancer early in women without any symptoms. Diagnostic mammography helps the doctor learn more about breast masses or the cause of other breast symptoms.

maximum contaminant level goal (MCLG): a designation set by the EPA of the maximum level of a contaminant in drinking water at which no anticipated effect on health would occur.

melanin: a pigment produced by skin cells called *melanocytes* that helps protect the body from the harmful rays of the sun.

melanocyte: an epidermal *cell* that produces the skin's coloring *(melanin)*.

melanoma: a cancerous (malignant) tumor that begins in the cells that produce the skin coloring (melanocytes). Melanoma is almost always curable in its early stages. Melanoma is much less common than *basal cell* and *squamous cell* skin cancers but is more likely to spread to other parts of the body.

menarche: a woman's first menstrual period. Early menarche (before age twelve) is a risk factor for breast cancer, possibly because the earlier a woman's periods begin, the longer her exposure to estrogen.

menopause: the time in a woman's life when monthly cycles of menstruation cease forever and the level of hormones produced by the ovaries decreases. Menopause usually occurs in the late forties or early fifties, but it can also be brought about by surgical removal of both ovaries (oophorectomy) or by some forms of *chemotherapy* that destroy ovarian function.

metastasis: the spread of *cancer cells* to distant areas of the body by way of the lymph system or bloodstream.

minerals: elements found in nature that are also essential *nutrients*, such as potassium, sodium, calcium, and iron; also considered a *dietary supplement* because it can be reproduced synthetically.

mole: see *nevus*.

mutation: a change in the structure of *DNA*, the set of genetic instructions each *cell* follows. In some instances this may lead to the development of cancer.

nasopharyngeal cancer: *cancer* that develops in the *nasopharynx*. Epstein-Barr virus (EBV) infection is a strong risk factor for nasopharyngeal cancer in some parts of the world.

nasopharynx: an area in the back of the nose and upper throat that lies just below the base of the skull and just above the soft palate.

neoplasia: the process of *tumor* formation. Intraepithelial neoplasia simply refers to abnormal growth of *cells* within the body. Depending on the organ involved, intraepithelial neoplasia may be given more specific names, such as cervical intraepithelial neoplasia (CIN), vulvar intraepithelial neoplasia (VIN), or vaginal intraepithelial neoplasia (VAIN).

neoplasm: an abnormal growth *(tumor)* that starts from a single altered *cell*; a neoplasm may be *benign* or *malignant*. *Cancer* is a malignant neoplasm.

neurotransmitter: a chemical in the brain that transmits nerve signals across a synapse.

nevus: a *benign* (noncancerous) *tumor* that occurs as a result of a *melanocyte* multiplying rapidly; the clinical term for a mole.

nicotine: the colorless chemical found in tobacco that is responsible for its addictive properties.

nicotine patch: see *transdermal nicotine system*.

nicotine replacement therapy: methods, such as the nicotine patch, gum, nasal spray, and prescription medications, that provide nicotine without the other harmful components of tobacco. These therapies treat the very difficult withdrawal symptoms and cravings. Also known as nicotine substitutes.

nicotine substitutes: see *nicotine replacement therapy*.

non-Hodgkin's lymphoma: *cancer* that starts in *lymphoid tissue* (also called *lymphatic* tissue). B-cell *lymphomas*, which are often associated with Epstein-Barr virus infection, are much more common than T-cell lymphomas.

nonmelanoma skin cancer: the more common, but less deadly, form of skin cancer, including *basal cell carcinoma* and *squamous cell carcinoma*.

nucleus: the center of a cell where the DNA is found and where it begins to reproduce.

nurse practitioner (N.P.): a *registered nurse* (R.N.) with a master's or other advanced degree who is trained in primary care and other specialties, like oncology (cancer care) and acute care, and shares many tasks with doctors, such as taking patient histories, conducting physical exams, and prescribing medications within their scope of practice.

nutrients: compounds that are found in food, such as *carbohydrates, proteins,* or *fats (lipids),* and are essential to life.

nutritional supplements: see *dietary supplements.*

nutritionist: an expert in the area of food and diet. Nutritionists and dietitians help prevent and treat illnesses by promoting healthy eating habits, scientifically evaluating people's diets, and suggesting ways to improve them. See also *dietitian.*

obesity: an increase above healthy weight (usually by more than 20 percent) that reduces life expectancy; clinically, obesity is a *body mass index (BMI)* of 30 kg/m^2 or greater.

oncogenes: *genes* that promote cell growth and multiplication. These genes are normally present in all cells; however, oncogenes may undergo *mutations* (changes) that activate them, causing *cells* to grow too quickly and form *tumors.*

opportunistic infections: infections with organisms that do not normally cause problems in healthy individuals. These infections usually occur in people with suppressed *immune systems.*

oral contraceptives: pills, usually containing estrogen and/or progesterone (female hormones), used to prevent pregnancy; also known as birth control pills.

osteoporosis: thinning of bone tissue, resulting in less bone mass and weaker bones, which can cause pain, deformity (especially of the spine), and broken bones. This condition is common among postmenopausal women but may be prevented by *hormone replacement therapy.*

overweight: body weight above normal for one's age, height, and build; a *body mass index (BMI)* between 25 to 29.9 kg/m^2.

palpation: using the hands to examine. For example, a palpable mass in the breast is one that can be felt.

papilloma: a *benign* epithelial *tumor,* such as a wart.

papillomavirus: a type of *virus* that causes *papillomas.* See also *human papillomavirus.*

Pap test: a diagnostic test used to check *cells* from the cervix (the lower part of the uterus or womb) and the vagina. This test can find *precancerous* changes or *cancer* of the cervix or vagina. Also called Papanicolaou smear, Papanicolaou test, or Pap smear.

passive smoking: see *involuntary smoking.*

pelvic examination: an examination of a woman's uterus and other pelvic organs. It is used to help find cancers of the reproductive organs. The doctor will visually examine external structures and palpate (feel) the internal organs such as the ovaries and cervix.

peripheral vascular disease: a narrowing of the blood vessels that carry blood to the leg and arm muscles.

pesticides: a wide range of biologically active chemical compounds intended to kill pests: insects (insecticides), fungi (fungicides), rodents (rodenticides), and plants or weeds (herbicides).

physician's assistant (P.A.): someone who provides diagnostic, therapeutic, and preventive health care services under the supervision of a physician. They generally have to complete at least two years of college (although most have a bachelor's or master's degree).

polyp: a growth from a mucous membrane commonly found in the rectum, the colon, or other organs. Adenomatous polyps (a benign growth of glandular cells) sometimes turn into *cancer*. Many other types of polyps (inflammatory polyps, hyperplastic polyps) do not.

polypectomy: surgery to remove a polyp.

precancerous: a condition in which changes in *cells* have occurred that **may** (but does not always) lead to *cancer*. When detected, these early conditions are easily treated. Also called premalignant.

predisposition: susceptibility to a disease that can be triggered under certain conditions. For example, some women have a family history of breast cancer and are therefore more likely (but not necessarily destined) to develop breast cancer.

prevention: the reduction of cancer risk by eliminating or reducing contact with *carcinogenic* agents. A change in lifestyle, such as quitting smoking, for example, reduces the risk of lung and other cancers.

primary care physician: the doctor a person would normally see first when a problem arises. A primary care doctor could be a general practitioner, a family practice doctor, a gynecologist, a pediatrician, or an internal medicine doctor (an internist).

prostate: a gland found only in men. It is just below the bladder and in front of the *rectum*. The prostate makes a fluid that is part of semen. The tube that carries urine, the urethra, runs through the prostate.

prostate-specific antigen (PSA): a *protein* made by the *prostate* gland. Levels of PSA in the blood often go up in men with prostate cancer. The PSA blood test is used to help find prostate cancer and to monitor the results of treatment.

prostatitis: inflammation of the *prostate*. Prostatitis is not *cancer*.

protein: an essential *nutrient* found in foods such as meat, fish, eggs, and beans; required for human growth and tissue repair. Proteins are large molecules made up of a chain of smaller units called amino acids. They serve many vital functions within and outside of the cell.

psychiatrist: a medical doctor who specializes in mental health and behavioral disorders. They can also prescribe medications and provide counseling.

psychologist: a licensed mental health professional with a degree in psychology (Ph.D., Psy.D., Ed.D.) who offers workshops, counseling, and assessments of mental and emotional functioning.

psychoneuroimmunology: the scientific study of the mind and how it affects the body, specifically the associations between the brain, behavior, the immune system, and the onset and progression of disease.

radiation: the emission (sending out) of energy from any source, such as the sun, a heater, the human body, or radioactive materials.

electromagnetic radiation: a type of *nonionizing radiation* produced by moving electric charges. Sources of electromagnetic radiation include the sun, electronic devices, cellular phones, and power lines.

ionizing radiation: high-energy (or high-frequency) waves that are able to penetrate *cells* and can lead to a *mutation* in a cell's *DNA*, which could contribute to *cancer*.

irradiation: a process that involves exposing food to gamma rays or x-rays to kill bacteria, pests, or parasites without making the food radioactive or creating harmful chemical compounds. This term is also sometimes used to describe *radiation therapy*.

nonionizing radiation: low-energy (frequency) waves that do not have enough energy to penetrate cells to cause *mutations*. Forms of nonionizing radiation include microwaves, radio waves, and radar, as well as *electromagnetic radiation*.

ultraviolet radiation: also called UV rays, invisible high-energy rays coming from the sun that can damage *DNA*. Exposure to sunlight (UV radiation) causes almost all cases of *basal* and *squamous cell* skin cancer and is a major cause of skin *melanoma*.

radiation therapy: the use of high-energy *ionizing radiation* to destroy cancer *cells* in an effort to treat or control *cancer*.

radon: a naturally occurring radioactive gas produced by the breakdown of uranium in rock, soil, and water. When inhaled, it emits radioactive particles that can damage the *cells* in the lungs, which can increase a person's risk for lung cancer. It is colorless, odorless, and tasteless.

rads: the unit of measure for *radiation* exposure.

rectum: the section of the large intestine between the end of the colon and the anus.

registered dietitian: see *dietitian*.

registered nurse (R.N.): a nurse who has graduated from an approved nursing program and passed a national licensing examination to obtain a license. See also *nurse practitioner*.

retrospective study: a study that looks back in time to determine the cause of a present condition.

retrovirus: any of a group of viruses whose genetic material is in the form of ribonucleic acid (RNA) and produces the enzyme reverse transcriptase. This enzyme changes viral RNA into *DNA*, which is then incorporated into the host cell's DNA and may remain inactive for years or form new viruses. See also *HIV* and *HTLV-1*.

risk assessment: a process used to determine the potential hazards of a substance. It evaluates both the *cancer*-causing potential of a substance and the levels of the substance in the environment. Risks are assessed to protect people against unsafe exposures and to set appropriate environmental standards.

risk factor: anything that increases a person's chance of getting a disease such as *cancer*. For example, smoking is a risk factor for lung cancer. Some risk factors, such as smoking, can be controlled. Others, like a person's age, cannot be changed.

saturated fat: a type of *fat* found mostly in foods from animal sources; these fats in the diet are thought to raise *cholesterol* levels.

screening: the search for disease, such as cancer, in people without symptoms. For example, screening measures for prostate cancer include digital rectal examination and the PSA blood test. Screening may refer to coordinated programs in large populations.

secondhand smoke: also known as environmental tobacco smoke (ETS) or passive smoke, it is a mixture of two forms of smoke from burning tobacco products: sidestream smoke and mainstream smoke.

sexually transmitted disease (STD): a disease that can be spread or contracted through sexual intercourse or intimate contact. Intimate sexual contact may involve the genitals, mouth, or anus. Bacteria or *viruses* commonly cause STDs. Some common STDs include chlamydia, gonorrhea, syphilis, herpes, and AIDS.

sidestream smoke: the part of *secondhand smoke* that comes directly from a lighted cigarette, pipe, or cigar (as opposed to *mainstream smoke*).

smokeless tobacco: see *spit tobacco*.

social worker: a health care professional who has a degree in social work (B.S.W, M.S.W, or D.S.W) and is trained to help people deal with a range of emotional and practical issues.

spit tobacco: also called smokeless tobacco, a tobacco product available as snuff or chewing tobacco that increases the user's risk of developing *cancers* of the mouth and throat.

squamous cell: a flat scaly-looking *cell* that makes up much of the *epithelial* layers in the body.

squamous cell carcinoma: *cancer* that begins in *squamous cells,* such as those on the outer surface of the skin. These account for about 20 percent of all skin cancers. They commonly appear on sun-exposed areas of the body, such as the face, ear, neck, lip, and back of the hands. These cancers tend to be more aggressive than *basal cell carcinomas*. They are more likely to invade tissues beneath the skin and are slightly more likely to spread to *lymph nodes* and/or distant parts of the body.

stratum corneum: also called the horny layer, it is the outermost part of the *epidermis* that is composed of dead and living *keratinocytes*.

subcutis: the deepest layer of the skin containing vessels and nerves. This layer also conserves heat and has a shock-absorbing effect to protect the body from injury.

Sun Protection Factor (SPF): a number indicating the level of protection from UVB rays. For example, if you use a sunscreen with an SPF of 15, you will receive the equivalent of one minute of exposure for every fifteen minutes spent in the sun.

T cell: a type of *lymphocyte* that helps protect the body against *viruses*, fungi, and some bacteria. T cells recognize specific substances found in virus-infected *cells* and destroy these cells. T cells can also release substances that attract certain other types of white blood cells, which then digest the infected cells. T cells are also thought to destroy some types of *cancer* cells. Also called T lymphocyte.

target heart rate: a heart rate at approximately 50 to 75 percent of a person's maximum heart rate.

tissue: a collection of cells that performs a particular function.

toxic: poisonous.

transdermal nicotine system: also known as the nicotine patch, it is a method of nicotine replacement that provides a measured dose of nicotine through the skin. It is most effective when used at the beginning of a smoker's attempt to quit, in combination with other smoking cessation methods that address the psychological component of smoking. As the nicotine doses are lowered over a course of weeks, the person is weaned away from nicotine. Patches can be purchased without a prescription, and several types and different strengths are available. See also *nicotine replacement therapy*.

triglycerides: the form that *fats* take when circulating in the body; they make up the *lipid* portion of *lipoproteins*.

tumor: an abnormal lump or mass of tissue. Tumors can be *benign* or *malignant*.

ultraviolet radiation: a stream of invisible high-energy rays coming from the sun that can damage DNA, the genetic material of *cells*; also called UV rays, of which there are three types—UVA, UVB, and UVC.

UV Index: developed by the U.S. Environmental Protection Agency (EPA) and the National Weather Service, it is a prediction (ranging from 0 to 10+) of the probable intensity of *ultraviolet (UV) radiation* reaching the Earth's surface during the sun's highest peak (usually around noon); sometimes called the solar warning index.

vaginal cancer: *cancer* of the vagina. There are several types of vaginal cancer, most which begin in the *epithelial* lining of the vagina.

virus: a very small (smaller than bacteria) parasitic organism that can cause certain diseases. Viruses are too small to be seen with a regular microscope. Unlike bacteria, they cannot survive on their own—they can reproduce only in living *cells*.

vitamin: an organic *nutrient* (such as vitamins A, D, C, and so on) that can be found naturally in plant and animal sources and is essential for life. Vitamins produced synthetically are considered to be *dietary supplements*.

vulva: the external portion of the female reproductive system. The vulva includes two prominent skin folds known as the *labia majora* and two barely visible, hairless skin folds called the *labia minora*.

vulvar cancer: a malignancy that can occur on any part of the female external reproductive system but most often affects the inner edges of the *labia majora* or the *labia minora*.

waist-to-hip ratio: a formula for determining potential health risks based on measurements of abdominal fat using a ratio of waist size over hip size in inches. Lower ratios indicate better health, whereas higher ratios are associated with increased risk of disease.

Western blot: (sometimes called a Western or Western blot analysis) a sensitive laboratory test used to detect *antibodies* to the individual structural parts of the *virus* (unlike an enzyme-linked immunosorbent assay [ELISA], which detects the whole virus). A Western blot test is often used to confirm ELISA results.

x-ray: one form of radiation that can be used at low levels to produce an image of the body on film or at high levels to destroy cancer cells.

References

Chapter 1

American Cancer Society. 1999. *Talking with Your Doctor*. Atlanta, Georgia: ACS Publication No. 99-4638-HCP.

Eyre, Harmon J., Dianne Partie Lange, and Lois B. Morris. 2001. *Informed Decisions: The Complete Book of Cancer Diagnosis, Treatment, and Recovery*. 2d ed. Atlanta, Georgia: American Cancer Society.

Fries J. F. et al. 1993. "Reducing Health Care Costs by Reducing the Need and Demand for Medical Services: The Health Project Consortium." *New England Journal of Medicine* 329 (5):321-325 (July 29).

Harris Interactive Incorporated. 2001. "Chronic Illness and Caregiving: Survey of the General Public, Adults with Chronic Conditions and Caregivers." Survey conducted from March 17 to November 22, 2000.

Korsch, Barbara M., and Caroline Harding. 1998. *The Intelligent Patient's Guide to the Doctor-Patient Relationship: Learning How to Talk So Your Doctor Will Listen*. Reprint. New York: Oxford University Press.

Prochaska, James O., John C. Norcross, and Carlos C. Diclemente. 1995. *Changing for Good*. New York: Avon Books.

The Writing Group for the Activity Counseling Trial Research Group. 2001. "Effects of Physical Activity Counseling in Primary Care: The Activity Counseling Trial: A Randomized Controlled Trial." *Journal of the American Medical Association* 286 (6):677-687 (August 8).

Chapter 2

American Cancer Society 1996 Advisory Committee on Diet, Nutrition, and Cancer Prevention. 1996. "Guidelines on Diet, Nutrition, and Cancer Prevention: Reducing the Risk of Cancer with Healthy Food Choices and Physical Activity." *CA: A Cancer Journal for Clinicians* 46 (6):325-341 (November/December).

American Cancer Society. 2000. *The American Cancer Society's Guide to Complementary and Alternative Cancer Methods*. Atlanta, Georgia: American Cancer Society.

American Cancer Society. 2001. "Special Section: Obesity." *Cancer Facts and Figures 2001*, pp. 20-27. Atlanta, Georgia: ACS Publication.

American Cancer Society. 2002. "Nutrition and Physical Activity." *Cancer Facts and Figures 2002*, pp. 34-35. Atlanta, Georgia: ACS Publication.

American Cancer Society. 2002. "Nutrition and Physical Activity." *Cancer Prevention and Early Detection: Facts and Figures 2002*, pp. 10-21. Atlanta, Georgia: ACS Publication.

American Dietetic Association and Roberta Larson Duyff. 1997. *Monthly Nutrition Companion: 31 Days to a Healthier Lifestyle*. Minneapolis: Chronimed Publishing.

American Dietetic Association. 1996. *Cut the Fat!: More Than 500 Easy and Enjoyable Ways to Reduce Fat from Every Meal*. New York: HarperCollins, HarperPerennial.

American Dietetic Association. 1999. *Skim the Fat: A Practical and Up-to-Date Food Guide*. New York: John Wiley and Sons.

American Dietetic Association. 2000. "Nutrition and You: Trends 2000." Survey conducted by Wirthlin Worldwide in October 1999.

Brown, Jean et al. 2001. "Nutrition During and After Cancer Treatment: A Guide for Informed Choices by Cancer Survivors." *CA: A Cancer Journal for Clinicians* 51 (3):153-187 (May/June).

Byers, T. et al. 2002. "American Cancer Society Guidelines on Nutrition and Physical Activity for Cancer Prevention: Reducing the Risk of Cancer with Healthy Food Choices and Physical Activity." *CA: A Cancer Journal for Clinicians* 52 (2):92-119 (March/April).

Calle, Eugenia E. et al. 1999. "Body-Mass Index and Mortality in a Prospective Cohort of U.S. Adults." *New England Journal of Medicine.* 341 (15):1097-1105 (October 7).

Corle, Donald K. et al. 2001. "Self-Rated Quality of Life Measures: Effect of Change to a Low-Fat, High-Fiber, Fruit and Vegetable Enriched Diet." *Annals of Behavioral Medicine* 23 (3):198-207 (summer).

Dietary Guidelines Advisory Committee. 2000. "The Report of the Dietary Guidelines Advisory Committee on the Dietary Guidelines for Americans, 2000." United States Department of Agriculture. BMI Chart, p. 3.

Dietary Supplement Health and Education Act (DSHEA) of 1994. Public Law 103-417. 25 October 1994. Amendment to the *Federal Food, Drug, and Cosmetic Act.*

Doll, Richard and Richard Peto. 1981. "The Causes of Cancer: Quantitative Estimates of Avoidable Risks of Cancer in the United States Today." *Journal of the National Cancer Institute* 66 (6):1191-1308 (June).

International Food Information Council Foundation. 2001. "Functional Foods: Can They Reduce Your Risk of Cancer?" *Food Insight,* May/June. Published survey performed by the Food Marketing Institute.

Kant, Ashima K. et al. 2000. "A Prospective Study of Diet Quality and Mortality in Women." *Journal of the American Medical Association* 283 (16):2109-2115 (April 26).

Kune, Gabriel A., 1999. *Reducing the Odds: A Manual for the Prevention of Cancer.* St. Leonards, Australia: Allen and Unwin.

Mayfield, Eleonor. 1994. "A Consumer's Guide to Fats." *FDA Consumer.* Reprint and revisions made in November 1994, January 1996, and January 1999. Rockville, Maryland: FDA Publication No. 99-2286.

Michaud, Dominique S. et al. 2001. "Physical Activity, Obesity, Height, and the Risk of Pancreatic Cancer." *Journal of the American Medical Association* 286 (8):921-929 (August 22-29).

National Institutes of Health. 1998. "Clinical Guidelines on the Identification, Evaluation, and Treatment of Overweight and Obesity in Adults." Bethesda, Maryland: NIH Publication No. 98-4083.

Sbrocco, T. et al. 1999. "Behavior Choice Treatment Promotes Continuing Weight Loss: Preliminary Results of a Cognitive-Behavioral Decision-Based Treatment for Obesity." *Journal of Consulting and Clinical Psychology* 67 (2):260-266 (April).

Silverman, Debra T. 2001. "Risk Factors for Pancreatic Cancer: A Case-Control Study Based on Direct Interviews." *Teratogenesis, Carcinogenesis, and Mutagenesis* 21 (1):7-25.

United States Department of Agriculture and United States Department of Health and Human Services. 2000. "Nutrition and Your Health: Dietary Guidelines for Americans." 5th ed. Home and Garden Bulletin No. 232. Washington, D.C.: Government Printing Office.

Vachon, Celine M. et al. 2001. "Investigation of an Interaction of Alcohol Intake and Family History on Breast Cancer Risk in the Minnesota Breast Cancer Family Study." *Cancer* 92 (2):240-248 (July 15).

Whelan, Elizabeth M. 1994. *The Complete Guide to Preventing Cancer: How You Can Reduce Your Risks*. New York: Prometheus Books.

Whiting, Susan J. et al. 2000. "Relationship Between Carbonated and Other Low Nutrient Dense Beverages and Bone Mineral Content of Adolescents." *Nutrition Research* 21 (8):1107-1115 (August).

Chapter 3

American Cancer Society. 2001. "Adult Physical Activity." *Cancer Facts and Figures 2001*, p. 13. Atlanta, Georgia: ACS Publication.

American College of Sports Medicine Position Stand. 1998. "Exercise and Physical Activity for Older Adults." *Medicine and Science in Sports and Exercise* 30 (6): 992-1008.

American Heart Association. 1997. *Fitting in Fitness: Hundreds of Simple Ways to Put More Physical Activity into Your Life*. New York: Random House, Times Books.

American Heart Association and American Cancer Society. 1996. *Living Well, Staying Well*. New York: Random House, Times Books.

Anderson, R. E. et al. 1998. "Relationship of Physical Activity and Television Watching with Body Weight and Level of Fatness Among Children." *Journal of the American Medical Association* 279 (12):938-942 (March 25).

Annesi, James J., 2001. "Using Emotions to Empower Members for Long-Term Exercise Success." *Fitness Management*, August 2001.

Batty, David and Inger Thune. 2000. "Does Physical Activity Prevent Cancer? Evidence Suggests Protection Against Colon Cancer and Probably Breast Cancer." *British Medical Journal* 321 (7274):1424-1425 (December 9).

Byers, T. et al. 2002. "American Cancer Society Guidelines on Nutrition and Physical Activity for Cancer Prevention: Reducing the Risk of Cancer with Healthy Food Choices and Physical Activity." *CA: A Cancer Journal for Clinicians* 52 (2):92-119 (March/April).

Cronin, K. A. et al. 2001. "Evaluating the Impact of Population Changes in Diet, Physical Activity, and Weight Status on Population Risk for Colon Cancer (United States)." *Cancer Causes Control* 12 (4):305-316 (May).

Dorn, Joan et al. 2001. "Correlates of Compliance in a Randomized Exercise Trial in Myocardial Infarction Patients." *Medicine and Science in Sports and Exercise* 33 (7):1081-1089 (July).

Eickhoff-Shemek, JoAnn, and Kris Berg, *Physical Fitness: Guidelines for Success*. (College of Education, University of Nebraska-Omaha, photocopy).

Haskell, W. L. 1986. "The Influence of Exercise Training on Plasma Lipids and Lipoproteins in Health and Disease." *Acta Medica Scandinavica* 711: 24-37 (supplement).

Hulver, Matt. 2001. "Exercise Tips: Weight Control" *ACSM's Fit Society Page*, January/March. Quarterly publication of the American College of Sports Medicine.

Kampert, J. B. et al. 1996. "Physical Activity, Physical Fitness, and All-Cause and Cancer Mortality: A Prospective Study of Men and Women." *Annals of Epidemiology* 6 (5):452-457 (September).

Krucoff, Carol. 2000. "Moving Away from Cancer: Indications That Physical Fitness May Deter Various Types of Cancer." *Saturday Evening Post* 272 (6):16.

Lee, I. M., and R. S. Paffenbarger Jr. 1994. "Physical Activity and Its Relation to Cancer Risk: A Prospective Study of College Alumni." *Medicine and Science in Sports and Exercise* 26 (7):831-837 (July).

Lee, I. M., R. S. Paffenbarger Jr., and C. Hsieh. 1991. "Physical Activity and Risk of Developing Colorectal Cancer Among College Alumni." *Journal of the National Cancer Institute* 83 (18):1324-1329 (September 18).

Marcus, Bess H. et al. 1999. "The Efficacy of Exercise As an Aid for Smoking Cessation in Women: A Randomized Controlled Trial." *Archives of Internal Medicine* 159 (11):1229-1234 (June 14).

National Institutes of Health, National Heart, Lung, and Blood Institute. 1998. "Clinical Guidelines on the Identification, Evaluation, and Treatment of Overweight and Obesity in Adults." Bethesda, Maryland: NIH Publication No. 98–4083.

National Institutes of Health, National Institute of Diabetes and Digestive and Kidney Diseases (NIDDK), Weight-control Information Network (WIN). 1996. "Physical Activity and Weight Control." Bethesda, Maryland: NIH Publication No. 96-4031.

Nehlson-Cannarella, S. L. et al. 1991. "The Effects of Moderate Exercise Training on Immune Response." *Medicine and Science in Sports and Exercise* 23 (1):64-70 (January).

Nelson, Miriam E. and Sarah Wernick, 1999. *Strong Women Stay Slim*. New York: Bantam Dell Books.

Nelson, Miriam E. et al. 1994. "Effects of High-Intensity Strength Training on Multiple Risk Factors for Osteoporotic Fractures. A Randomized Controlled Trial." *Journal of the American Medical Association* 272 (24):1909-1914 (December 28).

Pate, R. R. et al. 1995. "Physical Activity and Public Health. A Recommendation from the Centers for Disease Control and Prevention and the American College of Sports Medicine." *Journal of the American Medical Association* 273 (5):402-407 (February 1).

Sherrill, Duane L., K. Kotchou, and S. F. Quan. 1998. "Association of Physical Activity and Human Sleep Disorders." *Archives of Internal Medicine* 158 (17):1894-1898 (September 28).

Shoff, S. M. et al. 2000. "Early-Life Physical Activity and Postmenopausal Breast Cancer: Effect of Body Size and Weight Change." *Cancer Epidemiology, Biomarkers, and Prevention* 9 (6):591-595 (June).

Stamford, Bryant, 1998. "Fitting in Fitness: Exercise Options for Busy People." *The Physician and Sportsmedicine*, Exercise Advisor, 26 (8); (August).

Strasburger, V. C. 1992. "Children, Adolescents, and Television." *Pediatric Reviews* 13 (4):144-151 (April).

Thune, Inger et al. 1997. "Physical Activity and Risk of Breast Cancer." *New England Journal of Medicine* 336 (18):1269-1275 (May 1).

Tracy, B. L. et al. 1999. "Muscle Quality II: Effects of Strength Training in 65- to 75-Yr-Old Men and Women." *Journal of Applied Physiology* 86 (1):195-201 (January).

United States Department of Health and Human Services, Centers for Disease Control and Prevention, National Center for Chronic Disease Prevention and Health Promotion. "1992 Behavioral Risk Factor Survey." Atlanta, Georgia: USDHHS Publication.

United States Department of Health and Human Services, Centers for Disease Control and Prevention, National Center for Chronic Disease Prevention and Health Promotion. 1996. "Physical Activity and Health: A Report of the Surgeon General." Atlanta, Georgia: USD-HHS Publication.

United States Department of Health and Human Services, Centers for Disease Control and Prevention, National Center for Chronic Disease Prevention and Health Promotion. 1998. "Adolescent and School Health: 1997 Youth Risk Behavior Surveillance System (YRBSS) Summary." *Morbidity and Mortality Weekly Report* 47 (No. SS-3).

United States Department of Health and Human Services, Centers for Disease Control and Prevention, National Center for Chronic Disease Prevention and Health Promotion. 2000. "Prevalence of Leisure-Time Physical Activity Among Overweight Adults – United States, 1998." *Morbidity and Mortality Weekly Report* 49 (15):326-330 (April 21).

Verloop, J. et al. 2000. "Physical Activity and Breast Cancer Risk in Women Aged 20-54 Years." *Journal of the National Cancer Institute* 92 (2):128-135 (January 19).

Wood, P. D., R. B. Terry, and W. L. Haskell. 1985. "Metabolism of Substrates: Diet, Lipoprotein Metabolism, and Exercise." *Federation Proceedings* 44 (2):358-363 (February).

Writing Group for the Activity Counseling Trial Research Group. 2001. "Effects of Physical Activity Counseling in Primary Care: The Activity Counseling Trial: A Randomized Controlled Trial." *Journal of the American Medical Association* 286 (6):677-687 (August 8).

Chapter 4

Altman, J. F. et al. 2000. "A Survey of Skin Cancer Screening in the Primary Care Setting: A Comparison with Other Cancer Screenings." *Archives of Family Medicine* 9 (10):1022-1027 (November/December).

American Cancer Society. 2002. "Sun Exposure." *Cancer Prevention and Early Detection: Facts and Figures 2002*, pp. 22-23. Atlanta, Georgia: ACS Publication.

Autier, P. et al. 1998. "Sunscreen Use, Wearing Clothes, and Number of Nevi in 6- to 7-Year-Old European Children. European Organization for Research and Treatment of Cancer Melanoma Cooperative Group." *Journal of the National Cancer Institute* 90 (24):1873-1880 (December 16).

Autier, P. et al. 1999. "Sunscreen Use and Duration of Sun Exposure: A Double Blind Randomized Trial." *Journal of the National Cancer Institute* 91 (15):1304-1309 (August 4).

Davis, Neville. 1978. "Modern Concepts of Melanoma and Its Management." *Annals of Plastic Surgery* 1 (6):628-629 (June).

Epstein D. S. et al. 1999. "Is Physician Detection Associated with Thinner Melanomas? *Journal of the American Medical Association* 281 (7):640-643 (February 17).

Friedman, Robert J. et al. 1991. "Malignant Melanoma in the 1990s: The Continued Importance of Early Detection and the Role of Physician Examination the Self-Examination of the Skin." *CA: A Cancer Journal for Clinicians* 41 (4):201-226 (July/August).

Gallagher, Rick P. et al. 2000. "Broad-Spectrum Sunscreen Use and the Development of New Nevi in White Children: A Randomized Controlled Trial." *Journal of the American Medical Association* 283 (22):2955-2960 (June 14).

Gilchrest, Barbara A. et al. 1999. "The Pathogenesis of Melanoma Induced by Ultraviolet Radiation." *New England Journal of Medicine* 340 (17):1341-1348 (April 29).

Perez, Martiza I. 2001. "Melanoma in Hispanics in the United States." *The Melanoma Letter* 19 (1):3-4 (January).

Reid, Craig D., 1996. "Chemical Photosensitivity: Another Reason to Be Careful in the Sun." *FDA Consumer* 30 (4). Rockville, Maryland: FDA Publication.

Rigel, Darrell S. and John A. Carucci. 2000. "Malignant Melanoma: Prevention, Early Detection, and Treatment in the 21st Century." *CA: A Cancer Journal for Clinicians* 50 (4):215-236 (July/August).

Skin Cancer Foundation. June 5, 2001. "Sun Alert: Dark-Skinned Races Get Skin Cancer, Too." Press release. New York.

Tucker, M. A. et al. 1997. "Clinically Recognized Dysplastic Nevi: A Central Risk Factor of Cutaneous Melanoma." *Journal of the American Medical Association* 277 (18):1439-1444 (May 14).

United States Department of Health and Human Services, Centers for Disease Control and Prevention. 1998. "Sun-Protection Behaviors Used by Adults for Their Children—United States, 1997." *Morbidity and Mortality Weekly Report* 47 (23):480-482 (June 19).

United States Department of Health and Human Services, Centers for Disease Control and Prevention, National Center for Chronic Disease Prevention and Health Promotion, Division of Cancer Prevention and Control. 1996. "National Skin Cancer Prevention Education Program." Atlanta, Georgia: USDHHS Publication.

United States Department of Health and Human Services, Centers for Disease Control and Prevention, National Center for Chronic Disease Prevention and Health Promotion, Division of Cancer Prevention and Control. 2001. "Skin Cancer: Preventing America's Most Common Cancer, 2001." Atlanta, Georgia: USDHHS Publication.

United States Department of Health and Human Services, Public Health Service, Food and Drug Administration. May 21, 1999. "Sunscreen Regulations Finalized." *FDA Talk Paper*. Rockville, Maryland: FDA Publication.

United States Department of Health and Human Services, Public Health Service, Food and Drug Administration. June 8, 2000. "Sunscreen Regulations Updated." *FDA Talk Paper*. Rockville, Maryland: FDA Publication.

United States Environmental Protection Agency, Office of Air and Radiation, Global Programs Division. 1998. "Stay Healthy in the Sun." Brochure, EPA430-K-98-004. Washington, D.C.: Government Printing Office.

United States Environmental Protection Agency, Office of Air and Radiation, Global Programs Division. September 1999. "UV Radiation." Fact Sheet, EPA430-F-99-024. Washington, D.C.: Government Printing Office.

United States Environmental Protection Agency, Office of Air and Radiation. June 1999. "The Sun, UV, and You: A Guide to SunWise Behavior." Brochure, EPA430-K-99-035. Washington, D.C.: Government Printing Office.

United States Environmental Protection Agency, Office of Air and Radiation. May 2001. "Sunscreen: The Burning Facts." Brochure, EPA430-F-01-015. Washington, D.C.: Government Printing Office.

Westerdahl, J. et al. 2000. "Risk of Cutaneous Malignant Melanoma in Relation to Use of Sunbeds: Further Evidence for UV-A Carcinogenicity." *British Journal of Cancer* 82 (9):1593-1599 (May).

Whitmore, S. Elizabeth et al. 2001. "Tanning Salon Exposure and Molecular Alterations." *Journal of the American Academy of Dermatology* 44 (5):775-780 (May).

Chapter 5

American Cancer Society. 2000. *The American Cancer Society's Guide to Complementary and Alternative Cancer Methods*. Atlanta, Georgia: American Cancer Society.

American Cancer Society. 2002. "Tobacco Use." *Cancer Facts and Figures 2002*, pp. 29-32. Atlanta, Georgia: ACS Publication.

American Cancer Society. 2002. "Tobacco Use." *Cancer Prevention and Early Detection: Facts and Figures 2002*, pp. 4-9. Atlanta, Georgia: ACS Publication.

Anderson, Kristin E. et al. 2001. "Metabolites of a Tobacco-Specific Lung Carcinogen in Non-smoking Women Exposed to Environmental Tobacco Smoke." *Journal of the National Cancer Institute* 93 (5):378-381 (March 7).

Boffetta, Paolo et al. 1999. "Cigar and Pipe Smoking and Lung Cancer Risk: A Multicenter Study from Europe." *Journal of the National Cancer Institute* 91 (8):697-701 (April 21).

Chao, Ann, et al. 2000. "Cigarette Smoking and Colorectal Cancer Mortality in the Cancer Prevention Study II." *Journal of the National Cancer Institute* 92 (23):1888-1896 (December 6).

Federal Trade Commission. 2000. "FTC Announces Settlements Requiring Disclosure of Cigar Health Risks: Landmark Agreements Require Strong Warnings on Both Packaging and Advertisements." FTC File Nos. 0023199-00023205. Washington, D.C.: Government Printing Office.

Fiore M. C., et al. 1995. "The Effectiveness of the Nicotine Patch for Smoking Cessation: A Meta-Analysis." *Journal of the American Medical Association* 273 (3):181 (January 18).

Goldstein, A. O., R. A. Sobel, and G. R. Newman. 1999. "Tobacco and Alcohol Use in G-Rated Children's Animated Films." *Journal of the American Medical Association* 281 (12):1131-1136 (March 24-31).

Halpern M. T. et al. 2001. "Impact of Smoking Status on Workplace Absenteeism and Productivity." *Tobacco Control* 10 (3):233-238 (September).

Joad, J. P. 2000. "Smoking and Pediatric Respiratory Health." *Clinical Chest Medicine* 21 (1):37-46, vii-viii (March).

Max, W. 2001. "The Financial Impact of Smoking on Health-Related Costs: A Review of the Literature." *American Journal of Health Promotion* 15 (5):321-331 (May/June).

McVary, K. T., S. Carrier, and H. Wessells; Subcommittee on Smoking and Erectile Dysfunction Socioeconomic Committee, Sexual Medicine Society of North America. 2001. "Smoking and Erectile Dysfunction: Evidence Based Analysis." *Journal of Urology* 166 (5):1624-1632 (November).

Murray, Robert P. et al. 1998. "Effects of Multiple Attempts to Quit Smoking and Relapses to Smoking on Pulmonary Function. Lung Health Study Research Group." *Journal of Clinical Epidemiology* 51 (12):1317-1326 (December).

National Institutes of Health, National Cancer Institute. 1995. *Clearing the Air: How to Quit Smoking... and Quit for Keeps*. Bethesda, Maryland: NIH Publication.

National Institutes of Health, National Cancer Institute. 1998. "Cigars: Health Effects and Trends." Smoking and Tobacco Control Monograph No. 9. Bethesda, Maryland: NIH Publication.

National Women's Health Resource Center. August 2001. "Adolescent Girls and Smoking." *National Women's Health Report* 23 (4). New Brunswick, New Jersey.

Nuorti, J. P. et al. 2000. "Cigarette Smoking and Invasive Pneumococcal Disease. Active Bacterial Core Surveillance Team." *New England Journal of Medicine* 342 (10):681-689 (March 9).

Pelkonen, Margit et al. 2001. "Smoking Cessation, Decline in Pulmonary Function and Total Mortality: A 30-Year Follow-Up Study Among the Finnish Cohorts of the Seven Countries Study." *Thorax* 56 (9):703-707 (September).

Shapiro, Jean A., Eric J. Jacobs, and Michael J. Thun. 2000. "Cigar Smoking in Men and Risk of Death from Tobacco-Related Cancers." *Journal of the National Cancer Institute* 92 (4):333-337 (February 16).

United States Department of Health and Human Services, Centers for Disease Control and Prevention. 1993. "Smoking—Attributable Mortality and Years of Potential Life Lost – United States, 1990." *Morbidity and Mortality Weekly Report* 42 (33):645-648 (August 27).

United States Department of Health and Human Services, Centers for Disease Control and Prevention. 2000. "Youth Tobacco Surveillance–United States 1998-1999." *Morbidity and Mortality Weekly Report* 49 (SS-10):1-93 (October 13).

United States Department of Health and Human Services, Centers for Disease Control and Prevention, National Center for Chronic Disease Prevention and Health Promotion, Office on Smoking and Health. 1990. "The Health Benefits of Smoking Cessation." DDHS Publication No. (CDC) 90-8416. Atlanta, Georgia: USDHHS Publication.

United States Department of Health and Human Services, Centers for Disease Control and Prevention, National Center for Chronic Disease Prevention and Health Promotion, Office on Smoking and Health. 1994. "Preventing Tobacco Use Among Young People: A Report of the Surgeon General." Atlanta, Georgia: USDHHS Publication.

United States Department of Health and Human Services, Centers for Disease Control and Prevention, National Center for Chronic Disease Prevention and Health Promotion, Office on Smoking and Health. 2000. "Tobacco Use Among Middle and High School Students— United States, 1999." *Morbidity and Mortality Weekly Report* 49 (3): 49-52 (January 28).

United States Department of Health and Human Services, Centers for Disease Control and Prevention, National Center for Chronic Disease Prevention and Health Promotion, Office on Smoking and Health. 2000. "Reducing Tobacco Use: A Report of the Surgeon General." Atlanta, Georgia: USDHHS Publication.

United States Department of Health and Human Services, Centers for Disease Control and Prevention, National Center for Chronic Disease Prevention and Health Promotion, Office on Smoking and Health. 2001. "Women and Smoking: A Report of the Surgeon General— 2001." Atlanta, Georgia: USDHHS Publication.

United States Department of Health and Human Services, Public Health Service, Agency for Healthcare Research and Quality. 2000. *Help for Smokers: Ideas to Help You Quit*. Based on the U.S. Public Health Service Tobacco Cessation Guideline, released June 2000. Rockville, Maryland: Government Printing Office.

United States Environmental Protection Agency, Office of Health and Environmental Assessment, Office of Research and Development. December 1992. "Respiratory Health Effects of Passive Smoking: Lung Cancer and Other Disorders." EPA/600/6-90/006F. Washington, D.C.: Government Printing Office.

United States Environmental Protection Agency, Office of Health and Environmental Assessment, Office of Research and Development. July 1993. "Secondhand Smoke: What You Can Do About Secondhand Smoke as Parents, Decision-Makers, and Building Occupants." EPA-402-F-93-004. Washington, D.C.: Government Printing Office.

World Health Organization. 1999. "Treatment for Tobacco Dependence: Addressing the World-wide Tobacco Epidemic through Effective Evidence-based Treatment, The Mayo Report."

Zhang, Zuo-Feng et al. 1999. "Marijuana Use and Increased Risk of Squamous Cell Carcinoma of the Head and Neck." *Cancer Epidemiology, Biomarkers, and Prevention* 8 (12):1071-1078 (December).

Chapter 6

American Social Health Association. 1998. "Sexually Transmitted Diseases in America: How Many Cases and at What Cost?" Menlo Park, California: Kaiser Family Foundation.

Antman K. and Y. Chang. 2000. "Kaposi's Sarcoma." *New England Journal of Medicine* 342:1027-1038 (April 6).

Anttila T. et al. 2001. "Serotypes of *Chlamydia trachomatis* and Risk for Development of Cervical Squamous Cell Carcinoma." *Journal of the American Medical Association* 285 (1):47-51 (January 3).

Bast, R. C. et al. (ed.) 2000. *Cancer Medicine*, 5th ed. Hamilton, Ontario (Canada): BC Decker Inc.

Bosch, F. X. et al. 1995. "Prevalence of Human Papillomavirus in Cervical Cancer: A Worldwide Perspective. International Biological Study on Cervical Cancer (IBSCC) Study Group." *Journal of the National Cancer Institute* 87 (11):779-780 (June 7).

Caselmann, W. H. and M. Alt. 1996. "Hepatitis C Virus Infection As a Major Risk Factor for Hepatocellular Carcinoma." *Journal of Hepatology* 24 (supplement 2):61-66.

Cassell, Gail H. 1998. "Infectious Causes of Chronic Inflammatory Diseases and Cancer." *Emerging Infectious Diseases* 4 (3):475-487 (July/September).

Cates, Willard et al. 1999. "Estimates of the Incidence and Prevalence of Sexually Transmitted Diseases in the United States." *Sexually Transmitted Diseases* 26 (supplement):S2-S7.

Cote, T. R. et al. 1997. "Non-Hodgkin's Lymphoma Among People with AIDS: Incidence, Presentation, and Public Health Burden." *International Journal of Cancer* 73 (5):645-650 (November 27).

DeVita, V. T. et al. (ed.) 1997. *Cancer: Principles and Practice of Oncology*. 5th ed. Philadelphia: Lippincott-Raven.

Di Bisceglie, A. M. et al. 1991. "The Role of Chronic Viral Hepatitis in Hepatocellular Carcinoma in the United States." *American Journal of Gastroenterology* 86 (3):335-338 (March).

Janicek, Mike F. and Hervy E. Averette. 2001. "Cervical Cancer: Prevention, Diagnosis, and Therapeutics." *CA: A Cancer Journal for Clinicians* 51 (2):92-114 (March/April).

Mitacek, E. J. et al. 1999. "Exposure to N-Nitroso Compounds in a Population of High Liver Cancer Regions in Thailand: Volatile Nitrosamine (VNA) Levels in Thai Food." *Food and Chemical Toxicology* 37 (4):297-305 (April).

Murphy, E. L. et al. 1989. "Modeling the Risk of Adult T-Cell Leukemia/ Lymphoma in Persons Infected with Human T-Lymphotropic Virus Type I." *International Journal of Cancer* 43 (2):250-253 (February 15).

Rubin, Stephen C. 2001. "Cervical Cancer: Successes and Failures." *CA: A Cancer Journal for Clinicians* 51 (2):89-91 (March/April).

Shah, K. V. 1997. "Human Papillomaviruses and Anogenital Cancers." *New England Journal of Medicine* 337 (19):1386-1388 (November 6).

United States Department of Health and Human Services, Centers for Disease Control and Prevention, National Center for HIV, STD, and TB Prevention, Division of Sexually Transmitted Diseases. September 2001. "Sexually Transmitted Disease Surveillance, 2000." Atlanta, Georgia: USDHHS Publication.

United States Department of Health and Human Services, Centers for Disease Control and Prevention, National Center for HIV, STD, and TB Prevention. 2000. "Tracking the Hidden Epidemics: Trends in STDs in the United States, 2000." Atlanta, Georgia: USDHHS Publication.

United States Department of Health and Human Services, Centers for Disease Control and Prevention. "1998 Guidelines for Treatment of Sexually Transmitted Diseases." *Morbidity and Mortality Weekly Report* 47 (No. RR-1).

Zhang, Z. F. et al. 1999. "*Helicobacter pylori* infection on the Risk of Stomach Cancer and Chronic Atrophic Gastritis." *Cancer Detection and Prevention* 23 (5):357-367.

Chapter 7

Andersen, Barbara L. et al. 1998. "Stress and Immune Responses After Surgical Treatment for Regional Breast Cancer." *Journal of the National Cancer Institute* 90 (1):30-36 (January 7).

Benson, Herbert. 2000. *The Relaxation Response*. Rev. ed. New York: Harper-Collins, Avon Books, WholeCare.

Carter, L. W. 1993. "Influences of Nutrition and Stress on People at Risk for Neutropenia: Nursing Implications." *Oncology Nursing Forum* 20 (8):1241-1250 (September).

Cohen, S., G. E. Miller, and B. S. Rabin. 2001. "Psychological Stress and Antibody Response to Immunization: A Critical Review of the Human Literature." *Psychosomatic Medicine* 63 (1):7-18 (January/February).

Contrada, Richard J. et al. 2000. "Ethnicity-Related Sources of Stress and Their Effects on Well-Being." *Current Directions in Psychological Science* 9 (4):136-139 (August).

Ettner, S. L. and J. G. Grzywacz. 2001. "Workers' Perceptions of How Jobs Affect Health: A Social Ecological Perspective." *Journal of Occupational Health and Psychology* 6 (2):101-113 (April).

Gump, B. B. and K. A. Matthews. 2000. "Are Vacations Good for Your Health? The 9-Year Mortality Experience After the Multiple Risk Factor Intervention Trial." *Psychosomatic Medicine* 62 (5):608-612 (September/October).

Harrell, Shelly P. 2000. "A Multidimensional Conceptualization of Racism-Related Stress: Implications for the Well-Being of People of Color." *American Journal of Orthopsychiatry* 70 (1):42-57 (January).

Heiney, Sue P. et al. 2001. *Cancer in the Family: Helping Children Cope with a Parent's Illness*. Atlanta, Georgia: American Cancer Society.

Hobson, Charles J. et al. 1998. "Stressful Life Events: A Revision and Update of the Social Readjustment Rating Scale." *International Journal of Stress Management* 5 (1):1-23 (January).

Landrine, Hope and Elizabeth A. Klonoff. 1996. "The Schedule of Racist Events: A Measure of Racial Discrimination and a Study of Its Negative Physical and Mental Health Consequences." *Journal of Black Psychology* 22 (2):144-168 (May).

Roberts, Felicia D. et al. 1996. "Self-Reported Stress and Risk of Breast Cancer." *Cancer* 77 (6):1089-1093 (March 15).

Rogers, N. L. et al. 2001. "Neuroimmunologic Aspects of Sleep and Sleep Loss." *Seminars in Clinical Neuropsychiatry* 6 (4):295-307 (October).

Smith, A. P. 1998. "Breakfast and Mental Health." *International Journal of Food Sciences and Nutrition* 49 (5):397-402 (September).

Spiegel D. and S. E. Sephton. 2001. "Psychoneuroimmune and Endocrine Pathways in Cancer: Effects of Stress and Support." *Seminars in Clinical Neuropsychiatry* 6 (4):252-265 (October).

Stevens, Judy A. et al. 1999. "Surveillance for Injuries and Violence Among Older Adults." *Morbidity and Mortality Weekly Report* 48 (SS08):27-50.

Swanson, Naomi G. 2000. "Working Women and Stress." *Journal of the American Medical Women's Association* 55 (2):76-79 (Spring).

Thompson, Vetta L. 1996. "Perceived Experiences of Racism as Stressful Life Events." *Community Mental Health Journal* 32 (3):223-233 (June).

United States Department of Health and Human Services, Centers for Disease Control and Prevention. 1995. "Suicide Among Children, Adolescents, and Young Adults – United States, 1980-1992." *Morbidity and Mortality Weekly Report* 44 (15):289-291 (April 21).

United States Department of Health and Human Services, Centers for Disease Control and Prevention, National Center for Injury Prevention and Control. 2002. "Injury Fact Book 2001-2002." Atlanta, Georgia: USDHHS Publication.

Wood, C. 1993. "Mood Change and Perceptions of Vitality: A Comparison of the Effects of Relaxation, Visualization and Yoga." *Journal of the Royal Society of Medicine* 86 (5):254-258 (May).

Chapter 8

Altekruse, S. F., S. J. Henley, and M. J. Thun. 1999. "Deaths from Hematopoietic and Other Cancers in Relation to Permanent Hair Dye Use in a Large Prospective Cohort Study." *Cancer Causes and Control* 10 (6):617-625 (December).

American Cancer Society. 1999. *Understanding Chemotherapy: A Guide for Patients and Families*. Rev. April 2000. No. 9458-HCP. Atlanta, Georgia: ACS Publication.

American Cancer Society. 2002. "Environmental Cancer Risks." *Cancer Facts and Figures 2002*, p. 35-36. Atlanta, Georgia: ACS Publication.

Axelson, O. 1995. "Cancer Risk from Exposure to Radon in Homes." *Environmental Health Perspective* 103 (supplement 2):37-43 (March).

Boice, J. D. and J. H. Lubin. 1997. "Occupational and Environmental Radiation and Cancer." *Cancer Causes and Control* 8 (3):309-322 (May).

Bradbard, Laura. 1993. "On the Teen Scene: Cosmetics and Reality." *FDA Consumer*. Reprint May 1994. Rockville, Maryland: FDA Publication No. 94-5015.

Cogliano, J. 1998. "Assessing the Cancer Risk from Environmental PCBs." *Environmental Health Perspective* 106:317-323.

Gago-Dominguez, M. et al. 2001. "Use of Permanent Hair Dyes and Bladder Cancer Risk." *International Journal of Cancer* 91 (4):575-579 (February 15).

Gertig, D. M. et al. 2000. "Prospective Study of Talc Use and Ovarian Cancer." *Journal of the National Cancer Institute* 92:249-252 (February 2).

Hall, Eric J. 1984. *Radiation and Life*. 2nd ed. New York: McGraw-Hill Companies, Elsevier Science.

Harvard Report on Cancer Prevention; Volume 2: Prevention of Human Cancer. 1997. "Work-Related Cancers." *Cancer Causes and Control* 8 (supplement 1):S35-S38 (November).

Henkel, John. November/December 1999. "Sugar Substitutes: Americans Opt for Sweetness and Lite." *FDA Consumer* 33 (6). Rockville, Maryland: FDA Publication.

Henkel, John. May/June 1998. "Irradiation: A Safe Measure for Safer Food." *FDA Consumer* 32 (3). Revised June 1998. Rockville, Maryland: FDA Publication No. 98-2320.

Hornung, R. W. 2001. "Health Effects in Underground Uranium Miners." *Occupational Medicine* 16:331-344 (April/June).

Inskip, P. D. et al. 2001. "Cellular-Telephone Use and Brain Tumors." *New England Journal of Medicine* 344 (2):79-86 (January 11).

International Agency for Research on Cancer (IARC). 1988. "Man-Made Mineral Fibres and Radon. IARC Monographs on the Evaluation of Carcinogenic Risks to Humans." 43:173.

International Agency for Research on Cancer (IARC). Updated 1998. "Talc Not Containing Asbestiform Fibres (Group 3), and Talc Containing Asbestiform Fibres (Group 1)." 42 (Supplement 7):349.

Kimbrough, R. D., M. L. Doemland, and M. E. LeVois. 1999. "Mortality in Male and Female Capacitor Workers Exposed to Polychlorinated Biphenyls." *Journal of Occupational and Environmental Medicine* 41 (3):161-171 (March).

Laden, F. et al. 2001. "1,1-Dichloro-2,2-bis(p-chlorophenyl)ethylene and Polychlorinated Biphenyls and Breast Cancer: Combined Analysis of Five U.S. Studies." *Journal of the National Cancer Institute* 93 (10):768-776 (May 16).

Marcinowski, F., R. M. Lucas, and W. M. Yeager. 1994. "National and Regional Distribution of Airborne Radon Concentrations in U.S. Homes." *Health Physiology* 66 (6):699-706 (June).

National Research Council (NRC), Subcommittee to Update the 1999 Arsenic in Drinking Water Report, Committee on Toxicology, Board on Environmental Studies and Toxicology. 2001. *Arsenic in Drinking Water: 2001 Update*. Washington, D.C.: National Academy Press.

National Research Council (NRC), Committee on the Biological Effects of Ionizing Radiation. 1998. *Health Effects on Exposure to Low Levels of Radon: BEIR VI*. Washington, D.C.: National Academy Press.

National Research Council (NRC), Committee on Risk Assessment of Exposure to Radon in Drinking Water. 1999. *Risk Assessment of Radon in Drinking Water*. Washington, D.C.: National Academy Press.

Olsen, S. F., M. Martuzzi, and P. Elliott. 1996. "Cluster Analysis and Disease Mapping – Why, When, and How? A Step by Step Guide." *British Medical Journal* 313 (7061):863-866 (October 5).

Robb-Nicholson, C. 2001. "By the Way, Doctor. I recently received an e-mail warning about a risk for breast cancer associated with using antiperspirants. Are you familiar with this theory? Is it valid?" *Harvard Women's Health Watch* 8 (7):7 (March).

Thomas, T. L. and P. A. Stewart. 1987. "Mortality from Lung Cancer and Respiratory Disease Among Pottery Workers Exposed to Silica and Talc." *American Journal of Epidemiology* 125 (1):35-43 (January).

United States Department of Health and Human Services, Public Health Services – Agency for Toxic Substances and Disease Registry (ATSDR). 1997. *Toxicological Profile for Benzene*. Atlanta, Georgia: USDHHS Publication.

United States Department of Health and Human Services, National Institutes of Health, National Institute of Environmental Health Sciences. 1999. *NIEHS Report on Health Effects from Exposure to Power-Line Frequency Electric and Magnetic Fields*. Research Park Triangle, North Carolina: NIH Publication No. 99-4493.

United States Department of Health and Human Services, National Institutes of Health, National Institute of Environmental Health Sciences, Public Health Services – National Toxicology Program. *Report on Carcinogens – 9th Edition*. Revised January 2001. Research Triangle Park, North Carolina: USDHHS Publication.

United States Environmental Protection Agency, Office of Air and Radiation, Office of Radiation and Indoor Air. August 1992. "Consumer's Guide to Radon Reduction: How to Reduce Radon Levels in Your Home." Booklet, EPA 402-K-92-003. Washington, D.C.: National Center for Environmental Publications (NSCEP).

United States Environmental Protection Agency, Office of Water. Spring/Summer 2001. *Water Quality Criteria and Standards Newsletter*. EPA 823-N-01-004. Washington, D.C.: National Center for Environmental Publications (NSCEP).

United States Food and Drug Administration, Center for Food Safety and Applied Nutrition, Office of Cosmetics. July 2001. *Color Additives Fact Sheet* based on Henkel, John. December 1993. "From Shampoo to Cereal: Seeing to the Safety of Color Additives." *FDA Consumer 27* (10). Rockville, Maryland: FDA Publication.

Wergeland, E., A. Andersen, and A. Baerheim. 1990. "Morbidity and Mortality in Talc-Exposed Workers." *American Journal of Industrial Medicine* 17 (4):505-513.

Yin, S. N. et al. 1989. "A Retrospective Cohort Study of Leukemia and Other Cancers in Benzene Workers." *Environmental Health Perspective* 82:207-213 (July).

Chapter 9

American Cancer Society. 2001. *Breast Cancer Facts and Figures 2000-2001*. Atlanta, Georgia: ACS Publication.

American Cancer Society. 2002. *Cancer Facts and Figures 2002*. Atlanta, Georgia: ACS Publication.

American Cancer Society. 2002. *Cancer Prevention and Early Detection: Facts and Figures 2002*, pp. 24-30. Atlanta, Georgia: ACS Publication.

American Cancer Society. 2002. "Special Section: Colorectal Cancer and Early Detection." *Cancer Facts and Figures 2002*, pp. 20-27. Atlanta, Georgia: ACS Publication.

Eyre, Harmon J., Dianne Partie Lange, and Lois B. Morris. 2001. *Informed Decisions: The Complete Book of Cancer Diagnosis, Treatment, and Recovery*. 2d ed. Atlanta, Georgia: American Cancer Society.

Gotzsche, P. C. and O. Olsen. 2000. "Is Screening for Breast Cancer with Mammography Justifiable?" Lancet 355 (9198):129-134 (January 8).

Smith, Robert A. et al. 2002. "American Cancer Society Guidelines for the Early Detection of Cancer." *CA: A Cancer Journal for Clinicians* 52 (1):8-22 (January/February).

Solomon, D., M. Schiffman, and R. Tarone; ALTS Study Group. 2001. "Comparison of Three Management Strategies for Patients with Atypical Squamous Cells of Undetermined Significance: Baseline Results from a Randomized Trial." *Journal of National Cancer Institute* 93 (4):293-299 (February 21).

Tarr, Peter. July 2001. "Joe and Ali Torre: Teaming Up to Fight Prostate Cancer." *Intouch — Cancer Prevention and Treatment: The Good Health Guide* 3 (4):22-26, 31. Melville, New York: PRR, Inc.

Vogel, Victor G. 2000. "Breast Cancer Prevention: A Review of Current Evidence." *CA: A Cancer Journal for Clinicians* 50 (3):156-170 (May/June).

Winchester, D. J. 1996. "Male Breast Cancer." *Seminars in Surgical Oncology* 12 (5):364-369 (September/October).

Index

and food irradiation, 285–286
Helicobacter pylori, 228
Basal cell carcinoma, 152, 166
Basal cell nevus syndrome, 152
Behavior change. *see* Lifestyle changes
Benign *versus* malignant tumors, 9
Benson, Herbert, 254
Benzene, 303
Bicycling, 123
Bidis, 175–176
Bioengineered foods, 57
Birth control pills and smoking, 180
Bladder cancer
    and hair dyes, 274
    risk factors for, 76–77
    and saccharin, 287–288
    and smoking, 173, 178
Body mass index (BMI), 80–81
Body piercing, 234
Body shape and weight distribution, 79
Bone density, 96–98, 114
Brain cancer, 277–280
Breakfast, 49
Breast cancer
    and alcohol, 65
    American Cancer Society guidelines for
      early detection of, 312–313
    and breast self-exam, 3, 311–313, 317–319
    cell behavior, 9
    and clinical breast exams, 316–317
    and exercise, 91, 96
    and mammography, 3, 277, 297–298,
      314–317, 341–342, 390
    in men, 319
    and pesticides, 282
    prevention, 354
    and radiation therapy, 297–298
    resources, 390–392
    risk factors for, 76–77, 314, 354
    screening, 311, 314–319, 355
    treatment with tamoxifen, 299
Breathing exercises, 253
British Journal of Cancer, 149
Bupropion, 197
Burkitt's lymphoma, 225

avoiding boredom in, 107–108
and back pain, 97
beginner's rules, 125
benefits of, 96–98, 112
and bone density, 96–97
and cancer risk, 5, 54, 91, 96
children and, 101–103, 119–120
companionship and, 110, 130
consulting physicians before, 115–116, 118–119
convenience of, 130
cost of, 106–107
dangers of, 116
defining, 89–90, 121
duration, intensity, and frequency, 121
excuses for not participating in, 105–111
and fatigue, 109
fit test, 92–95
and fitness assessment, 92–95, 117
and the FITT test, 127–128
goals, 131
guidelines, 119–120, 125
and heart rate zone, 126–127
and the immune system, 97
injuries, 109, 116
journaling, 120
making time for, 102–106, 128–129
and metabolism, 114–115
and middle age weight gain, 113
and motivation, 129–132
and muscle mass, 112
myths of, 111–115
and pain, 113
predictors for success in, 104–105
and prevention of disease, 96
reasons why people stop or continue, 111
resources, 377–380
scheduling, 124, 130
and seven myths about exercise, 111–115
in short sessions, 120
specific types of, 123
starting, 115–117, 122–125
statistics, 99–101
and staying motivated, 129–132
strength training, 114–115

and stress, 97, 255
suggested activities, 122–123
sweating during, 110
taking breaks from, 131–132
talking during, 126
television viewing replacing, 101–102, 105–106
variety, 130–131
warming up before, 124
and weight control, 97, 108, 112–114
women and, 99, 114–115
Physician assistants (PAs), 29–30
Physician Data Query (PDQ), 32
Physicians
academic, 36
advice for patients, 26–27
assessment of health, 25–26
board certified, 33
communicating with, 37–43
dermatologist, 165–166
exercise consultations with, 115–116, 118–119
experience and expertise among, 33–35
and improving the doctor-patient relationship, 43
interviewing, 34
involved in research, 35
practice environment and hospital affiliations, 35
primary care, 28–29
and problems with communication, 42
questions to ask, 34, 38–42
reputations, 36
resources for information about, 32–33
selecting, 31–37
specialized, 29
style of practice and personality, 36–39
teaching affiliations, 36
and trust, 37
types of, 27–29
worksheets for visits to, 345–367
Phytochemicals, 59
Pipe smoking, 178–179
Polychlorinated biphenyls (PCBs), 294
Polyunsaturated fats, 63, 65